DISCLAIMER

The author of this work has no medical qualifications of any nature and has no expertise in the diagnosis or treatment of diabetes or any other medical condition. Advice and treatment in respect of such conditions can only be provided by an appropriately qualified medical professional.

Inappropriate physical activity can have a highly detrimental effect on your health and consequently readers are advised in the strongest possible terms to seek comprehensive advice from an appropriately qualified medical professional before engaging in physical activity of any nature. This is particularly important where you have a serious underlying medical condition such as diabetes.

Any change in your diet can lead to serious health complications and this is particularly so where you have a serious underlying medical condition such as diabetes. Anyone considering changing their diet, whether in line with suggestions contained in this work or otherwise, should ensure that they do not do so until they have taken comprehensive advice from an appropriately qualified medical professional.

The author of this work accepts no responsibility for any injuries, illnesses or accidents caused by or arising out of dietary or exercise choices taken by readers who have not sought appropriate medical advice prior to making those choices.

ACKNOWLEDGEMENTS

I firstly want to thank the thousands of clients I have coached over the last six years – whether I have worked with you on a one-to-one basis or online. Thank you for believing and trusting in my skills as a coach. You can rest assured your success has been responsible for my success and I truly hope I have served you well. This includes everyone from my first client Michelle to Tom, who I coached the other day.

I also want to thank the thousands of individuals who have followed my work online. Whether you read my articles, listen to my podcasts or put up with my day-to-day ramblings on social media – thank you for taking the time out of your day to read, share and test my philosophies on nutrition and training. This also includes all those that have travelled from afar to hear me speak at major exhibitions and private seminars.

I want to give a massive thank you to my one and only Claire Graham. Thank you for putting up with my stubborn and highly focused mindset throughout the course of my career.

Another major thanks goes to my family for pushing me to further my education when I was younger. Without their motivation and support I most surely wouldn't be where I am today. I know we have our differences and that at first you didn't agree with what I decided to do with my life after I finished higher education. I hope you're proud of what I have achieved so far and will continue to support me doing what I love best. Thank you for everything!

I also want to thank my best friend Michael Rea who has believed in me from day one. Mike is one of those guys I could ring at any time of the day or night. He has been there at the darkest and happiest times of my life and provided a shoulder to cry on, someone to bounce ideas off and a motivator who has pushed me on to bigger and better things. Thank you, mate.

Gavin Sloan (my right-hand man) who's expertise and level of commitment has been invaluable. A lot of this book wouldn't have been possible without you! Thank you!

David Lewis, who designed the beautiful front cover of the book. Thank you!

Rich Urwin, who has designed the inside of the book along with the member's website. Thank you for sharing your ultra-creative talents!

I want to say a special thank you to Duane Mellor, PhD APD and Dr Islam Afzal who were extremely helpful with proof reading the book and giving their valuable feedback.

Duane Mellor, PhD APD is the Associate Professor & Discipline Lead for Nutrition and Dietetics for the School of Public Health and Nutrition at the University of Canberra, Australia. Duane is also the joint deputy chair of the Evidence and Research Based Practice committee of the European Federation of Associations of Dieticians (EFAD). Duane has published exciting research on the effects of chocolate on diabetes and other dietary bioactives.

Dr Islam Afzal graduated from the University of Birmingham Medical School in 2005. Since then he has gone on to specialise in vascular disorders and complications including cancer, pregnancy and diabetes. Dr Afzal has featured a number of times in national media as a specialist in glucose homeostasis. A published researcher and a bodybuilding competitor himself, Dr Afzal is currently based at Aston Medical School, Aston University, UK and is currently leading research into the effects of supplemental intervention on sarcopenia in patients with type 2 diabetes and frailty in the ageing population.

Also!

Thanks to everyone who doubted and wanted to see me fail from the start. I'm sorry my work ethic and level of success scared you. Jealousy is an awful disease – get well soon and enjoy the book.

The last thank you I want to give may sound rather strange.

Diabetes – thank you.

Without being diagnosed with type 1 diabetes at the tender age of 16 (12 years ago) I most definitely would not have discovered or ventured into the amazing world of health and fitness.

The Obstacle Is The Way...

CHAPTER 1: INTRODUCTION

WE ALL HAVE OUR FEARS

Modern people faces many fears, such as running around on 5% phone battery, having too much body fat and too many emails. But people with diabetes have even more things to worry about, including loss of sight, multiple organ failure, limb amputation and shorter life expectancy, to name just a few.

For most people, having good health and a better body seem like a nice idea. But for each and every person with diabetes on the planet, they're a MUST HAVE. However, ask yourself this: how many fellow people with diabetes have you seen in good health and great shape? My guess is not many.

The reason for this is that many people with diabetes feel powerless and don't have a clue where to start when it comes to building a healthy, strong, good-looking physique. Like many other people with diabetes, this fear and confusion have played on my mind from time to time. So I decided to do something about it and write this book.

The fact you're reading it indicates you're mindful of your health. You might be an experienced fitness fanatic looking for an edge on your diet and training; you might be a complete beginner, looking for the most effective way to improve your health and get in shape; or you might be a personal trainer who works with people with diabetes.

If you are, The Diabetic Muscle and Fitness Guide has plenty to offer, whether it's knowledge bombs that entirely change the way you think about building a stronger, leaner and healthier body, a crash course in diet, exercise and mindset or some actionable tools and tactics you might not have considered.

Before diving in, I would like you to honestly answer a few questions:

- Are you unhappy with how you look and feel right now?

- Are you willing to dedicate yourself fully to the diet and training programmes outlined in this book?

- Are you willing to accept the process won't be easy?

- Are you willing to share your new-found knowledge and experiences to help other people in the same or worse boat than you?

If you answered 'no' to any of these questions, please put this book down and read something else. It's not for you. But, if you answered 'yes' you're about to discover the exact ins and outs of how I overcame diabetes and built a body I respect and am very proud of. This book is effectively a dossier of all my experiences (the highs and lows), knowledge (including what I've learned from others) and secrets to date.

Please note, it is not a clinical guide. I am not a doctor and you should always consult your GP. But besides being a personal trainer with diabetes, I have trawled through many texts about the disease and the evidence I present here is backed by scientific studies.

I've spend a great deal of time researching this book and am certain it will provide clarity and direction for those of you wanting to build a leaner, stronger and better-looking body.

WHY I'M WRITING THIS BOOK

Not many people know I'm diabetic. I've always kept it to myself bar the odd occasion when I've been asked to share my experiences on a fitness podcast or when another diabetic has approached me for advice.

I never wanted sympathy or unnecessary attention because I suffer from an autoimmune disease. It was my way of coping. After all, why would I want to be reminded I had a disease and was more likely to die younger than most people? But now I've decided to take the plunge and put my condition to good use.

I've lost count of the number of requests I've had over the years to write about fat loss and muscle building strategies for people with diabetes. So I am writing this in the hope that my knowledge and experience of living with diabetes, dealing with it and basically giving it the two fingers will help you, your loved ones or clients overcome it.

Things To Consider;

1. I'm an extremely curious person and an obsessive self-experimenter.

2. I've had the pleasure of networking with some of the best minds in the health and fitness industry.

3. I've coached thousands of clients to become healthier and stronger.

4. I want to know what I can learn from this, so I might apply it to others and myself.

WHAT THIS BOOK IS

People think too far ahead when they want to build a better-looking body. The constant pressure to look perfect means many overlook the actual process needed to get there. They get confused, look for quick fixes and end up not knowing what they really ought to be doing.

This book is a complete summary of everything I know about rapid body redesign in the diabetic body. I've spent years striving for mastery of this subject. All the diet, training and mindset strategies are based on real life experience, countless hours of trial and error and evidence-based study.

I have considered current diabetic research, highlighting key findings, scrutinized particular research methods (bad science does exist) and made valid suggestions for future research. None of the studies I've used to back up my claims have been cherry-picked.

Prescribing the best diet and training approach is never a matter of a 'yes' or 'no' answer. There is always a degree of certainty or doubt. For areas that lack research, we can only hypothesize based on what we know, using the closest available research and – where appropriate – trial and error.

Another hugely beneficial aspect of this text is the fact it's written by a person with diabetes for people with diabetics. I can directly relate to the underlying frustration and ever-changing challenges of diabetes. Not many fitness professionals can say that!

Credible advice on diabetes isn't easy to find. The information and advice you'll read here will allow you to make more efficient and effective use of your time, money and effort. I know only too well how easy it is to waste these precious resources on poor information.

The effort and detail I go into here should leave you with plenty of time, spare change and energy to direct on other areas of your life. Life is for living!

WHAT THIS BOOK IS NOT

Let me reiterate: I'm not a doctor. I don't have a PhD. I am a lifelong person with diabetes committed to learning all about his condition.

This book is not intended to be a comprehensive text on diabetes nor does it claim to treat, cure or diagnose the condition. It is a personal overview of essential key principles for rapidly redesigning the body and enhancing performance in diabetics.

All opinions are my own and are in no way intended to replace the medical advice of a health care professional, medical doctor, GP, registered dietician or nurse.

This book is also not:

- A boring clinical text overloaded with scientific terms and devoid of real life experience and practical tips.

- A magic bullet. If you want incredible results overnight you may as well ask for your money back. Training to become lean and as strong as physically possible requires serious work, day after day.

- A runner's or endurance athlete's guide, although I do discuss how different types of exercise affect diabetes management.

HOW TO USE THIS BOOK

This book isn't written for everyone. It is exclusively for people living with Type 1 (T1D) and Type 2 (T2D) diabetes who are serious about building a better body and want to understand both the 'how' and the 'why' behind everything they do.

It contains everything you need to know from a theoretical and practical perspective on how to build muscle and shred fat whilst living with diabetes.

The information is written in an easy-to-digest format, but will occasionally delve into deeper scientific language so you'll empower yourself with the knowledge, structure and methods of assessment needed to ensure you're constantly progressing.

You may be aware this book was co-launched in association with diabeticmuscleandfitness.com, an online community of likeminded training enthusiasts who share one uber-important goal – to kick diabetes' ass and build the best-looking body possible.

The site contains a number of important online resources, which you will read about here. I'm constantly updating it with articles, videos and much more.

Members get access to my 'Diabetic Muscle Dossier', which is a monthly newsletter loaded with nutrition, training, diabetes research, mindset and whatever else I can squeeze in there. I also do a monthly webinar discussing various topics and answering members' questions. As the community grows, so will opportunities for seminars and training camps, which is something I am super pumped about!

FITNESS PROFESSIONALS

Today's fitness professionals work with more people than ever living with diabetes (especially T2D). This presents a major challenge, particularly with the market for personal trainers and coaches growing. It's imperative you stand out by knowing your stuff. This book will educate you on diabetes and increase your awareness of how a person living with diabetes responds to the exercises and nutrition you prescribe.

BOOK BREAKDOWN

I suggest you start on chapter 1 and read the following chapters in order. You may be tempted to skip straight to the plan but don't: the 'why' must come before the 'what'.

CHAPTER 1 (you're reading it now) gives a general overview of what this book is and what it is not.

CHAPTER 2 tells the story of how I transformed from a fat, depressed, unhealthy person with T1D into a much healthier, stronger and leaner version of myself. I also outline how my obsession for learning about diabetes, the human body, nutrition and exercise helped me become a leading personal trainer and fitness educator.

CHAPTER 3 covers all things diabetes. This includes everything from understanding the underlying physiology (what's actually wrong with me) to the detrimental effects of not looking after your condition.

CHAPTER 4 focuses on mindset. I cover many of the depressing, annoying and emotional issues people with diabetes face and outline the coping strategies I've used to successfully change my perception and overcome the fear and self-doubt associated with diabetes.

CHAPTER 5 takes a closer look at T1D and T2D medications. I discuss the most recent innovations in diabetic health care.

CHAPTER 6 focuses on nutrition and how to develop a smart, sustainable diet that fuels maximum muscle gain and shreds fat. I'll also discuss how supplements can be used to build a better you.

CHAPTER 7 teaches everything you need to know about building an effective training programme. I cover a ton of often-overlooked training principles for long-term success in the weights room. You'll never enter the gym without a clear plan of action again.

CHAPTER 8 is a step-by-step guide on how to evaluate and adjust your programme for daily and long-term success. There is zero room for guesswork.

CHAPTER 9 focuses on lifestyle management by highlighting everything you can do outside the gym to promote mind and body development.

CHAPTER 10 provides an overview and some closing thoughts, including 50 tips I wish I knew when I was first diagnosed. I also talk about my exclusive Diabetic Muscle and Fitness online community and how I plan to stay at the forefront of the diabetic strength and fitness scene.

MY STORY

I've dedicated the last ten years of my life to understanding the world of iron, and the science and lifestyle that accompanies it. Now, after many requests, I've finally decided to sit down and put pen to paper.

LET'S ROLL BACK A FEW YEARS…

It all goes back to Tuesday morning on the 16 June 2009 when I was on my usual bus ride to school. I did the same journey five times a week for more than five years. You hopped on, had some banter with the boys, ate sweets, slapped the back of people's heads when they fell asleep and waved out the window at passing cars.

When you're in a routine it soon becomes obvious when something is out of place. On that particular day I distinctly remember my eyesight wasn't as sharp as normal. Reading passing car number plates was difficult. My first thought was: 'I need glasses'. For a 16 year old who was guilty of shouting 'specky four eyes' at other kids, wearing glasses this didn't go down well.

As the day progressed I felt increasingly tired. By break time, I was half asleep. I also seemed to be going to the toilet more than usual. Something was wrong. I told my mum, who booked an appointment with my GP and I was diagnosed with Type 1 Diabetes (T1D).

I was told T1D was a hereditary condition that inevitably would have developed. But I am sure my teenage lifestyle didn't help. As the saying goes, 'genetics load the gun, lifestyle pulls the trigger.' My lifestyle would have pulled several triggers: I was overweight, inactive, stressed and unhealthy.

I didn't know what to expect. I knew one kid in my year with diabetes who was allowed to eat Fruit Pastilles whenever he felt funny. This seemed pretty cool - what better medication than sweets! My opinion soon changed when I was taken to the diabetic education ward at Belfast City Hospital. Waiting to see the nurse, I noticed various posters on the walls giving graphic warnings of what could happen if you didn't manage diabetes: loss of sight, limb amputation, organ failure… you name it. Worst of all: shorter life expectancy. Lets just say 'the fear' hit me pretty badly at that particular moment.

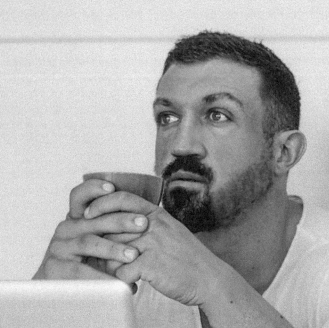

"NO WAY, YOU HAVE TO INJECT YOURSELF EVERYDAY. I COULDN'T."

I WOULD REPLY: "WELL, IF I DON'T, I DIE. PRETTY BIG MOTIVATOR!"

The nurse on duty, Margaret Devlin, managed to calm me down and talk me through how my new blood sugar meter and insulin pens were going to replace my somewhat useless pancreas.

And so I became a walking pincushion.

I had to prick myself multiple times each day to check the level of glucose in my blood. Think the odd pinprick hurts? At first I had to prick myself up to 25 times a day to make sure I was within the target range of 4.5-7.4 mmol/L (or 80 - 134 mg/dl). My fingers were pincushions.

Friends would say: "No way, you have to inject yourself everyday. I couldn't." I would reply: "Well, if I don't, I die. Pretty big motivator!"

With T1D, blood sugar levels can rise and rise until they reach toxic levels. This is caused by the pancreas' failure to produce the essential hormone insulin, which transports metabolic traffic (including glucose, protein and fatty acids) from blood to tissue. Consequently metabolites build up, cells starve and there is a negative effect on the normal, healthy workings of the body.

Think of how you feel after an enormous Christmas dinner: this is similar to how high blood sugar feels. I can get sleepy and pissed off pretty quickly if I don't monitor things.

Food and stress can cause blood sugar levels to rise. Injecting exogenous (artificial) insulin and increasing lean body mass through exercise can prevent it.

There is another danger on the flip side. Blood sugar levels can plummet into a hypoglycemia (low) state, which also has negative implications for health and energy. Going without food for too long and/or taking too much insulin are the main causes. Hypoglycemia can be quickly resolved by consuming carbohydrates but hunger levels can soar uncontrollably, which encourages you to eat far too many calories, which is partly why so many people with T1D are overweight.

When I was diagnosed I was bombarded with all sorts of information, flyers and pamphlets. It would have been better used as papier-mâché. None of it motivated me. It seemed vague, out-dated and soul destroying. The last thing I wanted was have a nurse cut my toenails and to wear one of those silly diabetic dog collar bracelets.

I soon realised that if I wanted to control my diabetes, I needed to understand how my body works so I set about educating myself.

POST DIAGNOSIS

I quickly morphed from an obese, highly inactive, inflamed and depressed person with diabetes into a much healthier, leaner and stronger person with diabetes with an undying passion to learn more and to question everything in a quest to achieve optimal health, body composition and performance.

I can't remember a single day since my diagnosis when I haven't had my head stuck in a physiology or strength training book, or a research paper, or been questioning an expert on all things relating to diabetes, nutrition, exercise and mindset. In those 11 years I have made radical changes to my health, physique and performance.

Picture this – 16 years old, 17 stone, 5 ft 11, extremely overweight and with a fasting blood sugar level of 16 mmol/L (288 mg/dl)

Fast forward to the present day – I'm currently 18 st 7 lbs, just below 11% body fat and have a fasting blood sugar level of 4.7 mmol/L (80 mg/dl). I can lift double or more than my body weight on the three key lifts: squat, bench and deadlift. And I can run 100m in 19.8 seconds.

This most certainly didn't happen overnight. It took years of hard work and commitment. But I'm much better off now. Don't get me wrong: the first few years of the journey were rough. I cringe at some things I did, such as excessive training and highly restrictive eating, I also had an empty wallet due to trying every supplement under the sun. But I learned from my mistakes and refined my approach to get to where I am today.

My deep fascination with human physiology, nutrition and exercise, and desire to better myself, are the reason I am where I am today. You could say I turned adversity into advantage. Now I want to pass on my knowledge.

THEY TOLD ME I WAS MAD

I've lost count of the number of times I've been told I was wasting my time and that I should accept the norms of being diabetic, such as feeling like shit, worrying about everything I ate and having a shorter life expectancy. But being average didn't go down well with me. I made an undying commitment to learn more, eat smarter and train harder. I became obsessed with my quest to beat diabetes and it paid of - I'm far from your average person with diabetes nowadays.

MY FIRST DAY AT THE GYM

I never liked sports. I was one of those kids that always tried to skip PE. I forged many a sick note (sorry, Mr Peake) so I could sit on my ass and mess around instead. So plucking up courage to go to the gym was difficult – really difficult. But nothing motivated me more than fear and having my health on the line.

The prospect of going blind or having a limb amputated seemed worse than death itself and that forced me to get creative and work very hard. Trust me, fear is a blessing in disguise.

First I needed a gym. It was a toss-up between the local leisure centre or a bodybuilding gym. I knew plenty of people who went to the leisure centre. But circuit training and yoga didn't really appeal to me, especially as the majority of members were over 40 years old and female. I wanted a great body and knew the bodybuilding gym was my best bet.

My first trip there was an experience. I distinctly remember three things: the pumping sound of electronic dance music; the aroma of iron, steel and sweat and an atmosphere conducive to an undying motivation for self-improvement.

As time went by, I went from training two days a week to four then eventually five. I made new friends and secured a great training partner. It was a friendship forged by an identical goal – to become better versions of our original selves.

I soon realised I loved the gym and everything that came with it. I dedicated a huge chunk of my life to eating, sleeping and training. Unlike other teenagers I had no interest in going out, getting drunk and meeting girls. My sole focus was to better my health and body. I felt proud, in control and unique for being able to exercise self-control at such a difficult time in my life.

At first I was fairly clueless about what I was doing. I just followed odd pieces of advice from somebody senior. Still I enjoyed the process but as I progressed and invested more time, money and effort I realised I needed to be more effective and efficient.

The only way to do this was to chase knowledge and mastery of my new found love. In those early years I spent every bit of pocket money on textbooks, magazines, videos and workout programmes. You should see the backlog of learning materials in my attic.

Gradually my knowledge developed and so did my results. I began to earn the respect of my peers and wanted to display the fruits of my hard work. Bodybuilding was the perfect format for me: it involved setting a date and showcasing my results while competing against other likeminded individuals.

Each and every one of you reading this book is effectively a bodybuilder. Think about it – you want to lose fat and sculpt a well-shaped, muscular physique. That's bodybuilding! The only thing you're not doing is stepping on stage, unless you're one of the growing numbers of people that do.

GAME ON!

My steepest learning curve came during my years as a junior bodybuilder. I learned so much from the process of building a solid base of size and strength offseason then shredding fat while retaining all that muscle I'd worked so hard for.

The first show or two were tough. I overdid things, lost muscle and nearly burned myself out. But I learned and ended up travelling the world, securing a few sponsors and winning or placing highly in a number of national and international contests.

During this stage of my life I also pursued a degree in nutrition from Queen's University Belfast, which took five years and included one year's work placement as a health improvement officer in areas of economic disadvantage. I acquired a wealth of information on everything from human physiology, biochemistry, clinical nutrition, interpreting and conducting research to a deep understanding of food manufacturing processes and legislation.

I was engrossed in learning as much as I could about human physiology, nutrition and exercise. I admit I became obsessed, selfish and neglected other important areas of my life, including family and friends, which later came back to bite me on the butt. But my life had direction, clarity and structure and my commitment to learning was the springboard for where I am today.

If I hadn't acquired this sense of direction I don't know what I would be doing today. Possibly sitting on the couch, reading this book.

And So I Began Helping Others...

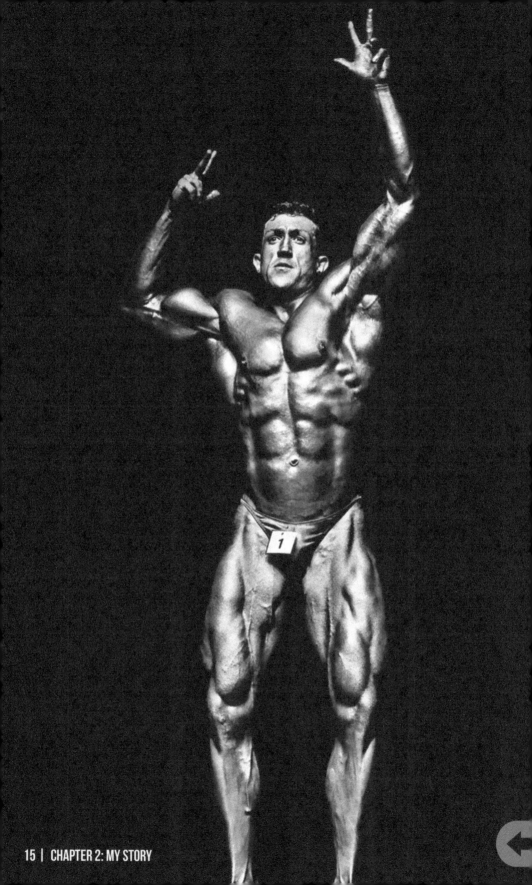

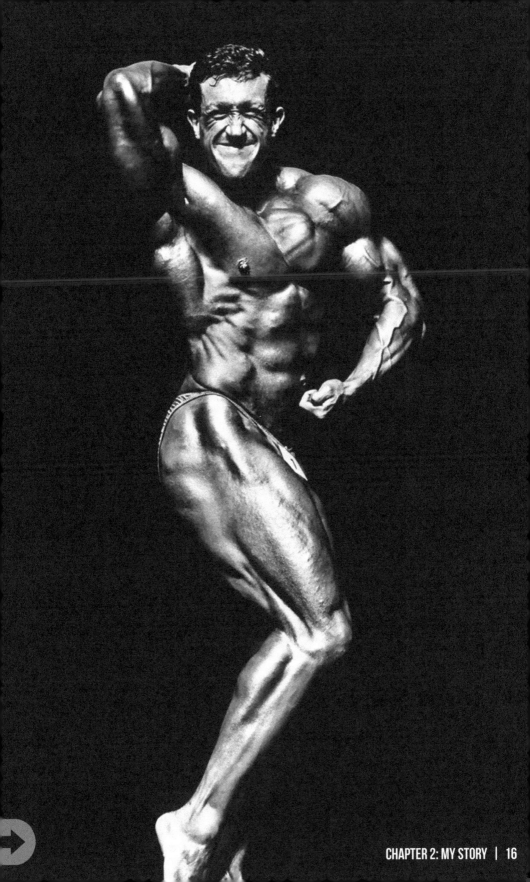

I loved talking about diet and training, writing programmes and generally helping people. I quickly got a name as the go-to guy for all things nutrition and training. Soon I was working around the clock on it as well as doing my health promotion job. Eventually I left my job and started my own personal training and nutrition consultancy. I haven't looked back since.

Demand for my services grew and grew. Soon I had a two-to-three month waiting list. It's still as long today.

I've lost count of the number of men and women I've helped over the years. I've worked with professional athletes from a wide range of sports to the everyday fitness bunny. It's safe to say I've played a considerable role in helping many people become healthier, leaner and stronger versions of their original selves.

HARD WORK BEGAN TO PAY OFF!

Soon my efforts and results got noticed beyond my client base. I was asked to write for some local newspapers, lifestyle magazines and online forums. Now I write for some of the world's top fitness publications including Train International, FLEX, Muscle&Fitness and Iron Life.

I speak at some of the world's biggest health and fitness expos and educate around 2,000 fitness professionals each year through private seminars. You could say, my hard work is paying off.

I'M NOT A SAINT

Over the years I came to terms with diabetes and learned to accept the bumpy ride. The good always outweighed the bad but I'm no saint. I've forgotten the odd hospital check up, overeaten at times, delayed treating hypos, forgotten to test my blood sugar level, drunk too much alcohol and even told people I wasn't diabetic, just to save hassle and small chat. I'm human. I'm not perfect and this disease is part of who I am.

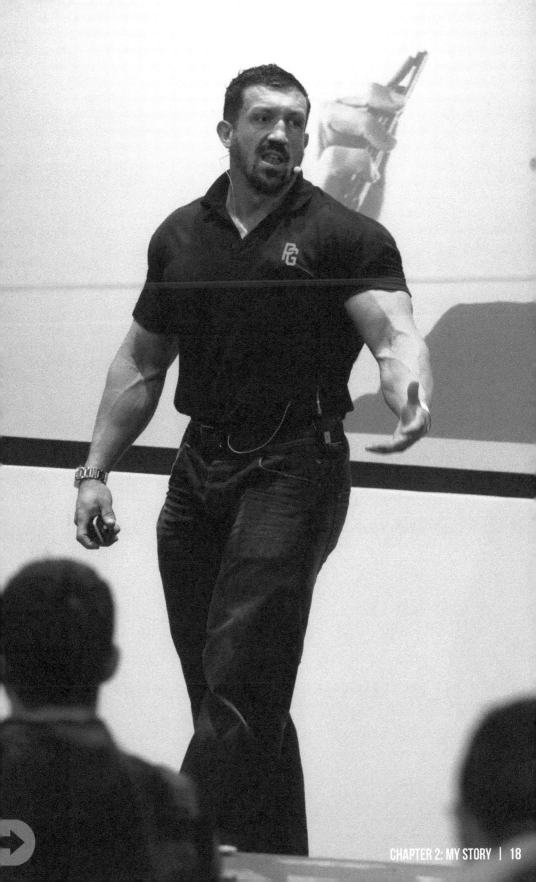

BECOME AN OUTLIER...

If your reading this book, respect! You've shown commitment to beating diabetes and improving your health.

If you're T1D (Type 1 Diabetes), like me, the best thing you can do is accept what you have and do your best to control it. If you're T2D (Type 2 Diabetes), it's time to change your ways. Imagine how it will feel living with a health problem you could have prevented? That would be a hard pill to swallow, right?

Break your life with diabetes down into two parts: before reading this book and after reading this book. Commit to investing time, money and effort into your goal. Nothing will happen without dedicated focus and behaviour change.

This book isn't loaded with fluff. It contains knowledge acquired from extensive study, years of hands-on experience and lots of trial and error. Follow its advice and you will make the most efficient and effective use of your time in the gym and kitchen. I honestly can't wait to see your results.

Why settle for normal? Why settle for unhealthy? Why settle for a shorter life? Especially when you can do something about it.

Let's Get Started!

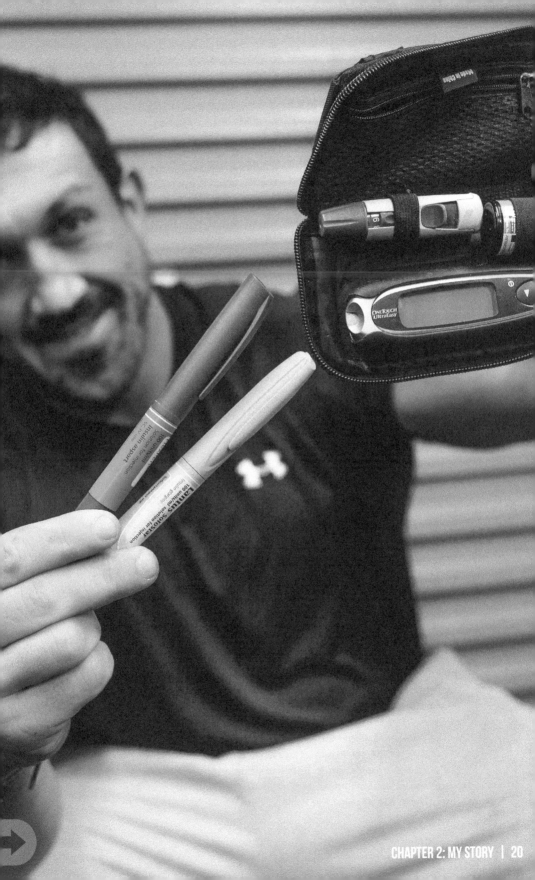

CHAPTER 3: THE DIABETIC MONSTER

LEARNING OUTCOMES

After reading this chapter, you should be able to

- Define what diabetes is and its different forms

- Acknowledge the function and abnormalities of all the essential hormones and organs involved with diabetes.

- Realise the complications associated with diabetes.

- Become familiar with how to diagnose diabetes using various clinical tests.

- Appreciate the importance of regular self-assessment and blood glucose testing.

- Dispel popular myths about diabetes.

DEFINING DIABETES

About 1,900 years ago, one of the most celebrated Greek physicians, Aretaeus of Cappadocia, described diabetes as 'a melting down of the flesh and limbs into the urine'. His observations were remarkably accurate even by the standards of today.

POORLY MANAGED DIABETES LEADS TO SERIOUS COMPLICATIONS AND EARLY DEATH.

This section attempts to explain what diabetes is, the effects it can have on the human body and strategies for successful management. Please understand that the pathology of diabetes is incredibly vast and complex. In fact, many details are well beyond the scope of this text and beyond what the everyday fitness enthusiast with diabetes or personal trainer needs to know.

I have presented what I feel are the fundamentals in a simplified, practical and easy to understand way. If you wish to further expand your knowledge, the online member's community www.diabeticmuscleandfitness.com is loaded with valuable information. I've also outlined key educational resources in the appendix at the end of this text.

WHAT IS DIABETES MELLITUS?

Diabetes mellitus is a group of metabolic diseases characterised by raised levels of glucose in the blood. It occurs when the body cannot produce enough insulin or cannot use the insulin it produces effectively. Insulin, which is a hormone manufactured in the pancreas in beta-cells, assists with the transport of glucose from the bloodstream into the body's cells for use as energy.

There are three main types of diabetes mellitus:

- **Type 1 Diabetes** results from the pancreas failing to produce enough insulin.

- **Type 2 Diabetes** is a condition of defective insulin signalling.

- **Gestational Diabetes** is a condition where women without previously diagnosed diabetes exhibit high blood glucose (blood sugar) levels during pregnancy, especially in the third trimester.

This text will focus exclusively on the two most popular forms of diabetes: T1D and T2D.

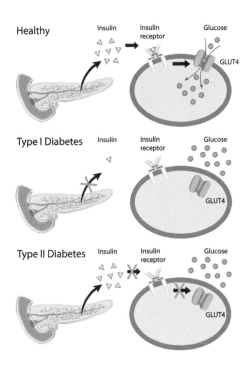

MAJOR COMPLICATIONS OF DIABETES

When insulin isn't produced or acts ineffectively, glucose remains circulating in the blood, leading to a condition known as hyperglycemia. Long-term hyperglycemia can result in the dysfunction and failure of various organs and systems, including the eyes, kidneys, nerves, heart and blood vessels.

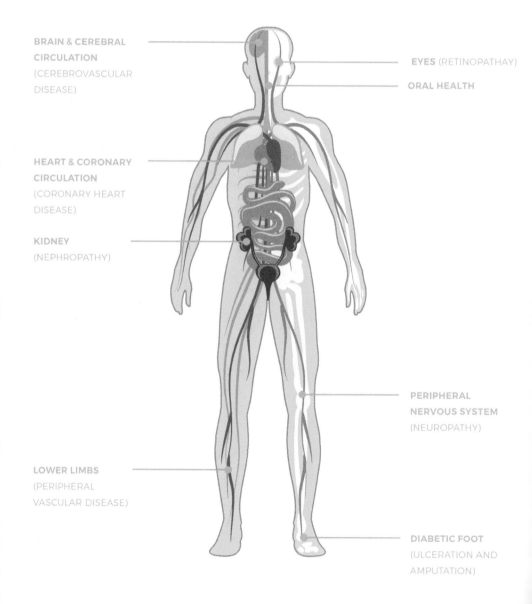

BRAIN & CEREBRAL CIRCULATION (CEREBROVASCULAR DISEASE)

EYES (RETINOPATHAY)

ORAL HEALTH

HEART & CORONARY CIRCULATION (CORONARY HEART DISEASE)

KIDNEY (NEPHROPATHY)

PERIPHERAL NERVOUS SYSTEM (NEUROPATHY)

LOWER LIMBS (PERIPHERAL VASCULAR DISEASE)

DIABETIC FOOT (ULCERATION AND AMPUTATION)

DIABETES INSIPIDUS: A RARER FORM OF DIABETES

Diabetes insipidus is a highly rare form of diabetes said to affect about one in 25,000 people. Excessive thirst and urination are among the complications, with some people reported to pass up to 20 litres of urine in a day [1].

It is not related to diabetes mellitus, but it does share some of the same signs and symptoms.

Typically in diabetes insipidus, problems occur with the production of the hormone vasopressin (AVP), also called antidiuretic hormone (ADH), which plays a vital role in regulating fluid in the body. The lack of AVP produced means the kidneys cannot make enough concentrated urine, resulting in massive water loss through urine.

EFFECTIVE TREATMENTS FOR DIABETES MELLITUS

Treatment for diabetes aims to keep blood glucose levels as close to normal as possible to reduce the risk of developing complications. Treatment will vary depending on the type of diabetes. Lifestyle modification in conjunction with medications like insulin is often needed.

> EFFECTIVE MANAGEMENT OF DIABETES IS A TEAM EFFORT BETWEEN THE PERSON WITH DIABETES AND RESPECTED AND SUITABLY EXPERIENCED HEALTH PROFESSIONALS.

KEY PLAYERS - THE PANCREAS AND LIVER

Before we go into greater detail on the different types of diabetes it is important to gain a fundamental understanding of how the liver and pancreas work. These two organs play a vital role in regulating blood glucose.

Skeletal muscle tissue also plays a vital role, which I'll discuss in the exercise section of this text.

THE PANCREAS

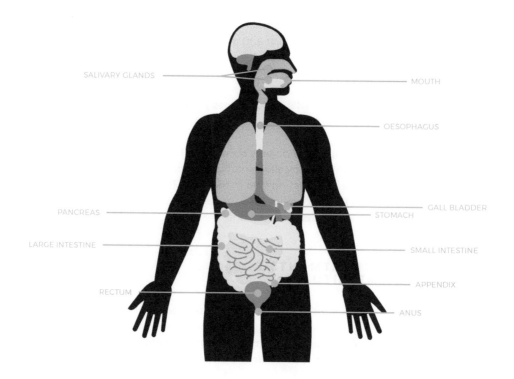

SALIVARY GLANDS
MOUTH
OESOPHAGUS
GALL BLADDER
PANCREAS
STOMACH
LARGE INTESTINE
SMALL INTESTINE
APPENDIX
RECTUM
ANUS

The pancreas is a long and slender organ shaped a little like a Christmas tree. It sits behind the stomach, in a bend of the duodenum (large intestine).

It is both an endocrine and exocrine gland.

Exocrine refers to a gland that releases its contents through a tube or duct from inside to outside the body.

The exocrine function helps with digestion by producing important enzymes that break down food, which allows the body to absorb the nutrients.

The endocrine function primarily involves the secretion of the two primary hormones relevant to diabetes management, insulin and glucagon.

The endocrine-producing cells of the pancreas are known as pancreatic islets or islets of Langerhans. There are approximately three million pancreatic islets cell clusters present in the pancreas (2).

Within these cells, there are four types of cells involved in the production of hormones that assist in the regulation of blood glucose levels.

Each type of cell secretes a different kind of hormone (3):

- α alpha cells secrete glucagon (increase glucose in blood)
- β beta cells secrete insulin (decrease glucose in blood)
- δ delta cells secrete somatostatin (regulates/stops α and β cells)
- PP cells, or γ (gamma) cells, (secrete pancreatic polypeptide)

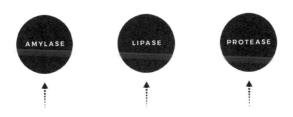

ENZYMES (DIGESTIVE SYSTEM)

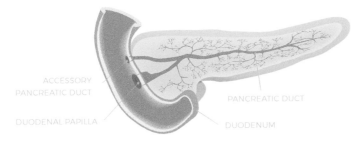

HORMONES (ENDOCRINE SYSTEM)

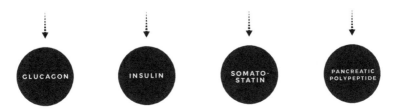

PANCREATIC HORMONES: GENERAL OVERVIEW

Insulin is considered the trademark hormone of diabetes. It is a peptide-based anabolic hormone produced by beta cells in the islets of Langerhans in the pancreas.

INSULIN INCREASES THE STORAGE OF GLUCOSE, FATTY ACIDS AND AMINO ACIDS IN CELLS AND TISSUES AND IS CONSIDERED AN ANABOLIC HORMONE.

The major actions of insulin include:

1. Facilitates the transport of glucose through certain membranes (e.g. adipose and muscle cells).

2. Stimulates the conversion of glucose to glycogen (liver and muscle cells).

3. Slows the production of glucose (gluconeogenesis) in liver and muscle cells.

4. Regulates the storage of fat (lipogenesis) in liver and adipose cells.

5. Regulation of muscle mass by suppressing muscle protein breakdown as opposed to increasing protein synthesis.

6. Facilitates the metabolism of minerals.

In people who do not have diabetes:

- Insulin secretion is pulsatile in response to high blood sugar.

- Counter-regulatory hormones can inhibit insulin secretion when blood glucose levels are low.

- Besides carbohydrate, insulin secretion can be stimulated by amino acids, fat and intestinal hormones and other factors such as stress and illness.

INSULIN IS A KEY PLAYER IN THE STORAGE AND USE OF FUELS WITHIN THE BODY.

Disorders in insulin production and signalling, which indicate uncontrolled diabetes have widespread and devastating effects on the body's organs and tissues. Glucagon is a peptide hormone produced by alpha cells in the pancreatic islets in the pancreas.

The pancreas releases glucagon when blood sugar levels fall too low, for instance during fasting or exercise. It opposes the action of insulin by raising the concentration of glucose in the blood by signalling the liver to release its carbohydrate stores into the blood. It also promotes the breakdown of fat in fat cells. Therefore, glucagon is a catabolic hormone.

In diabetes, where insulin is lacking or produced in limited amounts, the effects of glucagon are unopposed, which can lead to hyperglycemia if left unmanaged.

When glucose levels rise, the pancreas releases insulin to help get glucose out of the bloodstream and into cells, and when glucose levels drop too low, the pancreas releases glucagon to help increase glucose to a healthy level.

SOMATOSTATIN

Somatostatin essentially means stagnation of the body. The primary purpose of somatostatin is to inhibit the production of endocrine hormones, prevent the unnatural reproduction of cells (e.g. tumours) and serve as a neurotransmitter in the central nervous system. Neurotransmitters are brain chemicals that relay messages throughout the body, between nerve cells.

Somatostatin can inhibit the following:

- **Pituitary Gland**
  Growth hormone (GH)
  Thyroid stimulating hormone (TSH).

- **Pancreas**
  Secretion of pancreatic hormones, including insulin and glucagon.

- **Gastrointestinal Tract**
  Gastric secretion of key hormones and digestive enzymes

PANCREATIC POLYPEPTIDE (PP)

PP is a gut hormone with several functions that contribute to the maintenance of energy balance. It helps regulate pancreatic secretion activities (both endocrine and exocrine) and promotes satiety by reducing food intake, the rate of gastric emptying and gallbladder contraction [4].

It sounds like an appealing option for use as a weight loss agent and indeed it was used for this purpose until pharmaceutical tests showed it was unsuccessful long-term [5].

Other hormones produced in other organs, affecting carbohydrate metabolism include; epinephrine, thyroid hormones, glucocorticoids, and growth hormone.

THE LIVER

The liver is the largest solid organ in the body, weighing on average 1.8 kg in men and 1.3 kg in women. It holds approximately 13% (about one pint or 0.57 litres) of your total blood supply at any given time and has over 500 functions [6].

Some key functions include:

- Getting rid of waste products
- Fighting infection
- Storage of energy
- Production of glucose and fat
- Processing of amino acids
- Digestive roles, including the production of bile
- Storing iron, vitamins and other essential chemicals

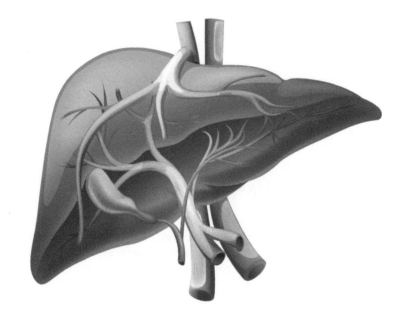

It is important to understand the liver's role in diabetes and energy metabolism.

Let's first review its function from the perspective of someone without diabetes then highlight the changes that occur within the body of a person living with diabetes.

THE LIVER AND ENERGY METABOLISM

Dietary carbohydrates are not essential. However, the body needs glucose. The brain typically requires approximately 130 g of glucose every day. Not all glucose has to come from the diet because the liver has the ability to synthesise it. The liver can also produce fatty acids from excess carbohydrate.

THE LIVER SERVES AS A WAREHOUSE FOR GLUCOSE STORAGE AND PRODUCTION. IT CAN ALSO PRODUCE FATTY ACIDS UNDER CERTAIN CONDITIONS.

As blood glucose and insulin levels increase, the liver increases its absorption of glucose. Glucose is packaged and joined into bundles of stored energy known as glycogen. The amount of glycogen stored depends on circulating insulin, and glucose levels.

This process is known as glycogenesis.

When blood glucose levels drop, insulin production falls. The shortage of insulin signals the liver to release its assets by sending glucose back into the blood to keep the body nourished.

This kind of scenario typically occurs during long periods between meals and during sleep and exercise.

This process is known as glycogenolysis.

When energy is low, such as during a calorie-restricted diet, fast or as a result of poorly controlled diabetes, where nutrients can enter their respected cells the liver has the ability to produce glucose from scratch.

This process is known as gluconeogenesis and involves the creation of glucose from non-carbohydrate sources, notably amino acids and glycerol in the liver.

FASTING BLOOD GLUCOSE LEVELS DEPEND ENTIRELY ON THE FASTING RATE OF GLUCOSE PRODUCED IN THE LIVER.

Another biochemical process that takes place in the liver during periods of fasting or carbohydrate restriction is ketogenesis.

When carbohydrate intake is restricted, it lowers blood sugar and insulin levels.

As insulin levels fall and energy is needed, fatty acids leave their respected fat cells and enter the bloodstream. From here they are taken up by specific cells and metabolised via a process called beta-oxidation into a molecule called acetyl-coA.

Acetyl-coA in the liver is converted to certain molecules, which are: acetoacetate, beta-hydroxybutyrate and acetone. These molecules are collectively known as ketone bodies.

Once created, the liver pushes the ketone bodies into the blood stream where they are utilised by skeletal and heart muscle cells as fuel. Also, the brain begins to use ketones as an alternate fuel source when blood levels are high enough to cross the blood-brain barrier. When this happens a person is said to be in nutritional ketosis.

Ketogenic Diets

Ketogenic diets are growing in popularity, and their ability to suppress insulin has been shown to be effective in the treatment and management of obesity and T2D [7], as well as a host of other diseases [8,9,10]. But the severe restriction of carbohydrate (often below 30 g) may increase the potential for hypoglycemia of people with T1D, rendering a ketogenic diet potentially problematic [11].

NUTRITIONAL KETOSIS IS NOT KETOACIDOSIS

Ketoacidosis is a severely out of control ketoic state in which blood levels of ketone bones rise above 10-25 mmol/L. The problem occurs when the acidic effects of ketones can no longer be buffered and controlled in the blood. It typically only occurs if insulin levels fall too low.

This type of metabolic derangement is typical of an uncontrolled diabetic who does not take enough insulin. Due to the lack of insulin, nutrients cannot get into cells. This results in an elevated flow of fatty acids out of fat cells, which are then converted to ketone bodies and dumped into the blood stream.

A combination of high blood sugar and high levels of ketone bodies results in a very acidic blood pH, which has implications for health.

OTHER ENERGY PRODUCING ROLES OF THE LIVER

Lipogenesis is the term used to describe the biochemical process of creating fat (fatty acid and triglycerides) within the body from glucose or other substrates.

This process takes place predominantly in the liver. Adipose tissue, which is the fat under the skin, plays a lesser role – even under conditions of substantial carbohydrate overfeeding.

Hepatic De Novo Lipogenesis occurs in the liver during times of calorific excess and overfeeding, which is a typical scenario associated with obesity.

The liver converts excess glucose to fatty acids using various enzymes. These fatty acids can be stored in the liver or transported via specific carriers called lipoproteins to muscle and fat tissue for future fuel use and/or storage. The ratio that is stored or used is highly dependent on energy intake vs. energy expenditure.

STORAGE OF LIVER FAT CAN ONLY OCCUR WHEN DAILY CALORIE INTAKE EXCEEDS EXPENDITURE.

IMPLICATIONS FOR DIABETES

In a healthy liver, insulin halts the production of glucose and instead promotes glycogen storage or generates fatty acids during times of energy excess.

The liver of a person with T1D has no internal break system. Insulin deficiency allows glucose production in the liver to go uncontrolled, leading to hyperglycemia and ketoacidosis if unmanaged.

WHY DOES THIS HAPPEN?

When insulin is deficient glucose cannot enter its respected cell for use as energy.

The liver produces even more glucose in an attempt to provide energy for the starved cells. The fact insulin is not available means none of this newly-formed glucose can enter the cells. It builds up and starves the cells even further

If untreated, the situation will only get worse. Consequently, administration of insulin medication is needed to facilitate the entry of glucose into cells.

In those suffering from T2D, the liver's ability to produce glucose is less of a concern due to the fact insulin is still present. However, the creation and storage of fat within the liver remains a possibility. It occurs due to overeating and positive energy balance, which is a common trait in those living with T2D.

FATTY LIVER DISEASE

A fatty liver is a dysfunctional and insulin-resistant liver. Commonly termed non-alcoholic fatty liver disease, it is one of the earliest stages in the etiology of T2D and metabolic syndrome [12].

However, in people living with T1D this isn't always the case. The fact that insulin is injected into the subcutaneous tissue means there is a relatively low insulin concentration in the portal vein, which is the main vein responsible for carrying blood to the liver from the spleen, stomach, pancreas, and intestines [13].

In fact, people living with T2D who start subcutaneous insulin therapy have been shown to experience a decrease in portal vein insulin concentrations and deliver by suppressing pancreatic insulin secretion and, consequently a decrease in liver fat [13]. However, further research is needed in this area.

INSULIN INCREASES GLUCOSE UPTAKE IN THE LIVER BY FACILITATING THE CREATION OF GLYCOGEN AND DECREASES GLUCOSE OUTPUT.

PROLONGED ELEVATIONS IN INSULIN THAT RESULT FROM AN ENERGY SURPLUS INCREASE THE BODY'S ABILITY TO PRODUCE FAT VIA THE PROCESS OF LIPOGENISIS.

GENERAL OVERVIEW:
REGULATION OF BLOOD GLUCOSE

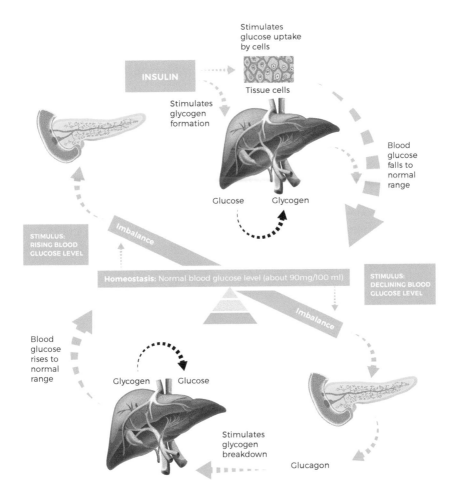

OTHER DIABETIC HORMONES WORTH KNOWING ABOUT

There are other important **hormones** worth knowing about when it comes to diabetes. These include

GLP-1 (Glucagon-like-peptide-1) and **GIP** (glucose-dependent insulinotropic polypeptide) are a group of hormones released from inside the gut, which stimulate insulin secretion while at the same time decrease the production of glucagon. GLP -1 also slows down the rate at which the stomach empties, and also signals the brain to make us feel full or satisfied.

These hormones explain why someone who consumes glucose via the mouth has a greater insulin response than someone who injects it. These hormones signal to the pancreas that glucose is coming and insulin needs to be secreted before glucose even reaches the blood stream.

Amylin is produced alongside insulin and has a similar effect to GLP-1. It reduces glucagon levels and also reduces the liver's ability to produce glucose and decreases appetite.

In those living with T1D with absent or malfunctioning beta cells the hormones insulin, amylin and GLP-1 cannot work properly. This could explain why people with diabetes fail to suppress glucagon during meals and afterwards become hyperglycemic. GLP-1 and amylin are available as medications, which I talk about later in this book.

Glucose counter-regulatory hormones or 'stress' hormones work to maintain blood glucose levels. They often come into play during stressful situations, including infections, serious illness or significant emotional stress. They oppose the actions of insulin. Key examples include:

Cortisol, which is often termed 'the stress hormone' is a life-sustaining steroid hormone produced in the adrenal glands.

It is essential for the maintenance of homeostasis (balance) within the body during times of stress.

It plays a key role in helping stabilise blood glucose levels by stimulating the:
• Breakdown of stored glucose in the liver
• Production of glucose from fatty acids
• Break down of protein (proteolysis), often from skeletal muscle

Cortisol also inhibits the creation of new proteins via the process of protein synthesis.

It also serves various other roles within the body, including:
• Mental clarity
• Immune responses
• Anti-inflammatory actions
• Blood pressure
• Heart and blood vessel tone and contraction
• Central nervous system activation

Cortisol levels tend to be at their highest first thing in the morning after a prolonged period of sleep. This response is known as the 'cortisol awakening response' and provides us with a 'get up go'.

As the day goes on cortisol levels, naturally begin to decline, and end up lowest later in the evening. This response is known as the 'diurnal rhythm' and is important for winding down in preparation for sleep.

Physical and emotional stress can increase cortisol production. Certain stimulant-based drugs and compounds, such as caffeine, yohimbine and similar ergogenic aids can have a similar effect.

Cortisol is vital for human health but should only peak when needed. Levels should return to normal after a stressful event.

Today's high-stress culture hammers cortisol production more than any time in history.

We drink too much coffee, watch horror movies and play video games before bed, scroll through social media and get anxious at the thought of getting stuck in traffic before work in the morning. All of the behaviours make it difficult to wind down and achieve deep restful sleep.

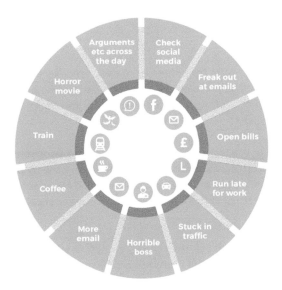

Epinephrine (adrenaline) released from the adrenals and nerve endings works as a counter insulin hormone by stimulating the liver to release glucose via the breakdown of glycogen, or glycogenolysis. It also promotes the breakdown of fat cells that make their way to the liver for transformation into glucose and ketones.

Growth Hormone is released from the pituitary gland in the brain. It is important in human development but also acts as a stress hormone that raises the concentration of glucose and free fatty acids in the blood. It, too, opposes the action of insulin.

TYPE 1 DIABETES

T1D (formerly known as insulin-dependent diabetes or juvenile diabetes) is an autoimmune disease.

Autoimmune Disease: When the body's immune system attacks normal working cells and tissues.

T1D develops because the body attacks its insulin-producing beta cells in the pancreas. When the number of beta cells diminishes to a certain level, the body is unable to produce enough insulin to control blood glucose.

Blood glucose rises, hyperglycemia develops, and diabetes is the result.

There may be some beta cell reformation (by cell division or by new cell formation) that replaces the destroyed cells. However, over the years the net destruction is greater than the replacement. Additionally, there is some evidence that the alpha cells that produce glucagon can also be destroyed in the pancreas of people with T1D.

PEOPLE WITH TYPE 1 DIABETES STRUGGLE TO REGULATE BLOOD GLUCOSE LEVELS.

When a person living with T1D continues to eat, especially foods containing carbohydrates, blood sugar levels rise uncontrollably in the blood and urine. Consequently, the cells of the body are deprived of their primary fuel source - glucose (energy).

To compensate for the lack of glucose inside cells, the body resorts to creating energy from amino acids and fat. Ketones are the by-product of this process and are produced in the liver. When the body uses ketones for fuel, it is said to be in a state of ketosis, which indicates a state of carbohydrate deprivation.

How is this possible if glucose, the primary carbohydrate in human metabolism is abundant in the blood stream? Even though glucose is elevated, it cannot get into cells due to a lack of insulin. Consequently, the cells are starved of their primary fuel source and must resort to other measures for fuel.

Low levels of ketosis are perfectly healthy. However, chronically high levels in combination with high blood sugar (due to insulin deficiency) can result in a potentially life-threatening medical state known as diabetic ketoacidosis, or DKA, whereby the blood becomes very acidic and dangerous.

Other profound changes in energy metabolism of someone with T1D include [14,15]:

- Poor nutrient and mineral absorption, which may lead to nutritional deficiencies
- Dehydration
- Reduction in bone density
- Increased metabolic rate – yes this may be good for fat burning but the context in which this occurs is detrimental to long-term health.
- Increased catabolism of muscle protein
- Increased breakdown of fat (in an unhealthy context)
- Altered mitochondrial function
- Abnormal levels of oxidative stress
- Abnormal levels of glycation
- Chronic inflammation

Key Symptoms Include [14,16]:

- Abnormal thirst and a dry mouth
- Frequent urination
- Lack of energy, extreme tiredness
- Constant hunger
- Unexplained weight loss
- Recurrent infections and slow wound healing
- Blurred vision
- Laboured or 'Kussmaul breathing' (associated with severe metabolic acidosis)

MANAGEMENT

People with T1D can lead a perfectly normal life if they respect and manage their condition.

This involves a well-structured self-management plan focused on the following:

- Insulin therapy – T1D diabetics need insulin every day in order to control the levels of glucose in their blood.
- Blood glucose monitoring
- Healthy diet
- Regular physical exercise (especially if overweight)

In many economically developing countries, especially in low-income families, access to diabetes self-management education, insulin and other medical tools is limited. This leads to severe disability and early death in children with diabetes.

Self-management of T1D is a challenge, presenting a number of issues.

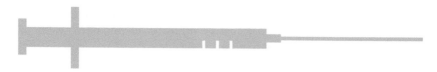

PEOPLE WITH TYPE 1 DIABETES WILL DIE WITHOUT INSULIN

Hypoglycemia is defined as a blood sugar level of 3.5 mmol/L (65mg/dl) It is advisable to be treated once levels fall below 4 mmol/L (72mg/dl)

A number of factors can increase the likelihood of hypoglycemia. They include:

• Injecting too much insulin
• Delaying or missing meals or snacks
• Doing unplanned or too much physical activity
• Drinking large quantities of alcohol

Common symptoms usually include sudden weakness, cold sweats and dizziness.

Hyperglycemia is the biochemical hallmark of diabetes and is a prerequisite for diagnosis. A blood sugar level higher than 11.1 mmol/L (200 mg/dL) is considered hyperglycemic and can be caused by various factors, including anaerobic exercise and stress. Common causes are:

• Mistimed or forgotten medication
• Eating too much food between medication
• Stress
• Infection
• Eating too much food to treat a hypo
• Certain medications

THERE CAN BE A HIGH DEGREE OF DIFFERENCES BETWEEN INDIVIDUALS WHEN IT COMES TO RECOGNISING THE SYMPTOMS OF HYPO AND HYPERGLYCEMIA.

DIABETIC KETOACIDOSIS (DKA)

Consistently high blood glucose levels can lead to a condition called diabetic ketoacidosis (DKA). It occurs due to a severe lack of insulin, which prevents the body using glucose for energy. Consequently the body starts to break down other tissues as alternative energy sources. Ketones are the by-product of this process.

Ketones contain energy, much of which gets wasted when they're excreted via urine. This causes a negative effect on energy balance. Certain ketones like beta hydroxybutrate are acidic by nature and can also be termed keto acids. High ketone levels and an inability to manage acid-base balance disrupt electrolyte balance and, if left uncontrolled, can result in severe complications. If blood glucose levels are consistently above 12 mmol/L (216 mg/dl) you should check for ketones.

Long-term complications can impact on a wide variety of body parts, including:
- Eye problems (retinopathy)
- Cardiovascular disease
- Kidney problems (nephropathy)
- Problems with the nerves and feet (neuropathy)

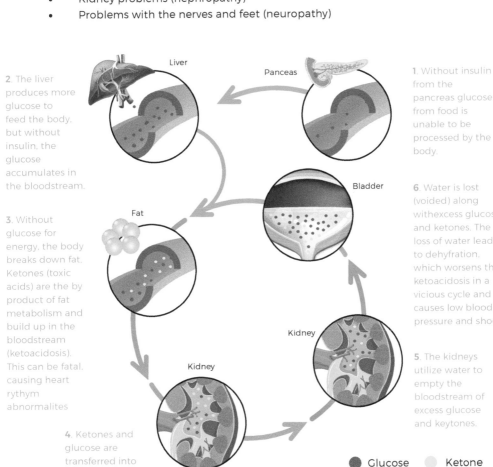

2. The liver produces more glucose to feed the body, but without insulin, the glucose accumulates in the bloodstream.

3. Without glucose for energy, the body breaks down fat. Ketones (toxic acids) are the by product of fat metabolism and build up in the bloodstream (ketoacidosis). This can be fatal, causing heart rythym abnormalites

4. Ketones and glucose are transferred into the urine.

Liver

Panceas

Fat

Bladder

Kidney

Kidney

1. Without insulin from the pancreas glucose from food is unable to be processed by the body.

6. Water is lost (voided) along withexcess glucose and ketones. The loss of water leads to dehyfration, which worsens the ketoacidosis in a vicious cycle and causes low blood pressure and shock.

5. The kidneys utilize water to empty the bloodstream of excess glucose and keytones.

● Glucose   ○ Ketone

CAUSES

The causes of T1D are still unclear [14,16]. The working theory for most autoimmune diseases is that the following three things create a perfect storm [17]:

1. Genetics
2. Trigger factors (e.g. diet, environment, early events in the womb and infection)
3. Intestinal permeability

However, much work remains to be done in understanding the role of environmental trigger factors and the gut in the development of T1D.

WHO'S AT RISK?

T1D is less common and accounts for only 5-10 % of people with diabetes.

However, the number is increasing. The disease can affect people at any age but usually occurs in children or young adults [14,16].

What are the implications for performance, muscle building and fat loss?

- Muscle loss due to increased protein turnover and reduced rates of protein synthesis.

- Dehydration and disruptions in electrolyte balance hinder mental clarity and physical performance.

- Reduced aerobic capacity.

- Fluctuations in blood sugar levels can affect mood, energy and desire to train.

- Frequent trips to the toilet can prove annoying and impair performance, especially in timed events.

- The hassle of administering insulin in public. Some individuals may avoid it due to embarrassment.

You can reduce the risk of complications by making an undying commitment to respect your diabetes and health. This involves controlling blood sugar levels through close monitoring and tactful administration of necessary medications, eating a quality diet, keeping active, being mindful of stress and getting enough rest.

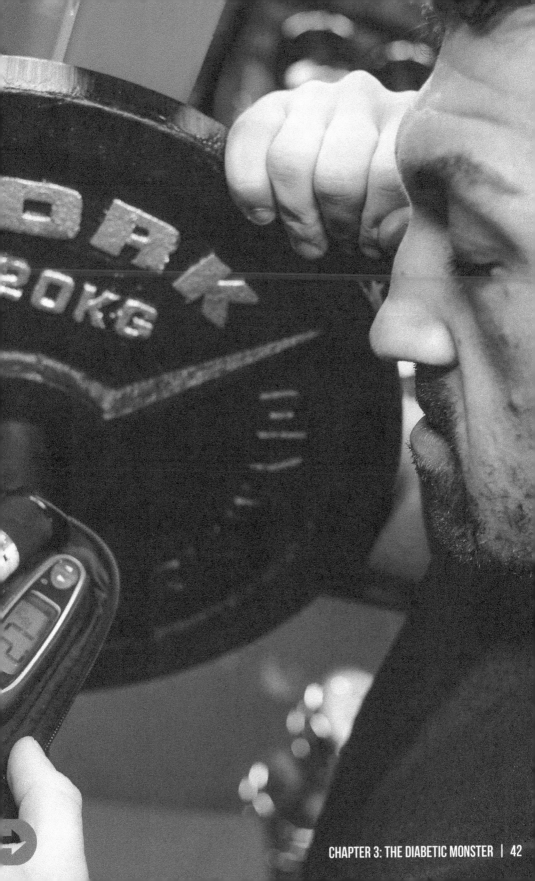

TYPE 2 DIABETES AND PRE-DIABETES

T2D is the most common form of diabetes today and typically indicates two key problems:

1. **Insulin resistance Muscle**, liver and fat cells do not use insulin properly.

2. **Reduced insulin production Glucose** builds up in the blood, overflows into the urine and is excreted out of the body, never fulfilling its role as the body's main source of fuel.

Pre-diabetes is a metabolic condition closely linked to obesity. Blood glucose levels are higher than normal but not yet high enough to be classified as T2D. If undiagnosed or untreated, people with pre-diabetes can develop T2D.

T2D often can go unnoticed and undiagnosed for years until a health complication manifests itself.

HOW TO TELL THE DIFFERENCE BETWEEN TYPE 1 AND TYPE 2 DIABETES

A variety of lab tests can determine which type of diabetes someone has [18].

Two important tests include:

*   **C-Peptide**: This blood test can reveal how much insulin the pancreas is making.

C-peptide does not affect blood glucose levels in the body but is produced during the synthesis of insulin. It is produced by the beta cells in the pancreas and makes up 50% of the precursor molecule to insulin, proinsulin. The peptide splits away from insulin once manufactured.

Significantly low levels of C-peptide are indicative of T1D. Normal or abnormally high levels of C-peptide are indicative of T2D.

A C-peptide test can also help identify cases of low blood sugar (hypoglycemia) due to excessive use of insulin therapy or a noncancerous tumour in the pancreas (insulinoma). Synthetic insulin causes C-peptide to be released. Therefore a person who suffers from low blood glucose as a result of too much insulin will have a low level of C-peptide but a high degree of insulin.

A C-peptide test is advisable when blood glucose reaches a hyperglycemic state of 200 mg/dL (11.1 mmol/L).

- Antibody Blood Test:

The autoimmune aspect of T1D is brought on by the actions of specific antibodies that attack the insulin-producing cells of the pancreas.

Antibody blood tests measure the body's production of particular types of antibodies, which destroy cells and promote T1D.

Known antibodies include:

- Islet cell cytoplasmic antibodies (ICA)
- Glutamic acid decarboxylase (GAD)
- Insulinoma-associated protein 2 (IA-2)
- Insulin autoantibodies (IAA)

Antibody tests are particularly useful for:

- Identifying the type of diabetes when an original diagnosis is doubtful, for instance a person with T2D who is not overweight or obese.
- Establishing whether gestational diabetes is T1D.
- Measuring the progression of T1D or indicating a risk of T1D diabetes or LADA.

OTHER BIOMARKERS AND CLINICAL SIGNS, SUCH AS KETONES, URIC ACID AND BLOOD LIPIDS CAN BE CROSS-REFERENCED WITH INITIAL TESTS TO BACK UP DIAGNOSIS AND HIGHLIGHT DIABETES COMPLICATIONS.

RISK FACTORS

Although the exact reasons for developing T2D are still unknown, there are some important risk factors.

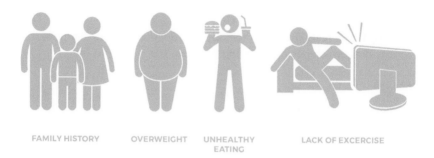

FAMILY HISTORY   OVERWEIGHT   UNHEALTHY EATING   LACK OF EXCERCISE

It usually occurs in adults, but increasingly is being seen in adolescents and even children.

The American Diabetes Association recommends testing to detect pre-diabetes and T2D in adults who are overweight or obese and have one or more of the following risk factors.

- Physically inactive.
- Have a family member with diabetes.
- Have a family background that is African American, Alaska native, American Indian, Asian American, Hispanic/Latino or Pacific Islander.
- Given birth to a baby weighing more than 9 lbs.
- Been diagnosed with gestational diabetes when the diabetes was first found during pregnancy.
- Having high blood pressure (>140/90 mmHg) or being treated for high blood pressure.
- HDL cholesterol below 35 mg/dL, or a triglyceride level above 250 mg/dL.
- Diagnosed with polycystic ovary syndrome (PCOS).
- Impaired fasting glucose (IFG).
- Impaired glucose tolerance (IGT) on previous testing.
- Having other conditions associated with insulin resistance, such as severe obesity or a condition called acanthosis nigricans, characterized by a dark, velvety rash around the neck or armpits.
- History of cardiovascular disease.

If results appear normal, retests should be taken at least every three years. However, doctors may recommend more frequent testing depending on initial results and risk status. In those without these risk factors, testing should begin at age 45.

OBESITY AND TYPE 2 DIABETES

Rates of T2D in conjunction with obesity are increasing worldwide.

There are many contributory factors, which are often deemed the sole cause of obesity. They include:

- Too many carbs (especially refined carbohydrates).
- Too much fat.
- Decreasing participation rates in formal exercise.
- Unhealthy food additives, environmental toxins and genetically modified organisms.
- Lowering of willpower of new generations.
- Too many processed foods.
- Not enough healthy meals.
- A culture of obesity.
- Fast food.

However, in my opinion the main culprits are:

1. **An increase in workplace mechanisation and other lifestyle technologies.**

Machines have replaced a huge proportion of the global workforce. More people are playing sports on computers than in real life. We sit more, move less and preserve more energy.

It is normal to be active throughout life so it's no surprise that a lack of physical activity permits the body to accrue various kinds of problems, including obesity, T2D and heart disease.

2. Cheaper Food

Food is much cheaper than it used to be. Just look at some of the deals in your nearest supermarket. This is especially true for high calorie junk food like ice cream, pizza and biscuits.

People often buy on impulse.

You know what it's like. You go into a shop and come out with way more than you needed. What the heck, it was on offer at the time, so why lose out?

This means there is more food lying around your house, and a greater chance of overeating.

3. Improved Access to Food

Nowadays we have vending machines in waiting areas, supermarkets in every town, petrol stations serving food 24/7 on our highways and streets lined with coffee shops, takeaways and restaurants all serving delicious food.

Food is everywhere, especially in economically developed countries, where obesity is at an all time high.

4. More Convenience

If you went food shopping 50 years ago, you had to buy your ingredients, sometimes from different shops then carry them home (driving was only for the rich) and cook them from scratch.

Sounds like a lot of effort doesn't it?

Fast forward to today.

We can walk into a shop and buy a ready-made meal of the shelf. No cooking, no fuss, just rip the package off and eat. Convenience food has allowed us to consume more energy than ever before while at the same time expend less energy preparing it.

Our ancestors would have spent days hunting and chasing their food. Nowadays, we simply click speed dial.

Pizza

NEW

5.   Improved Taste

Food manufactures are constantly putting their products through extensive organoleptic testing. This ensures the food tastes, smells, feels and looks just right for public consumption.

Ingredients are tweaked and refined to achieve the best product possible.

It doesn't take a rocket scientist to work out that the end goal is to increase product consumption. Which allows for more eating and greater calorie consumption.

Food also lasts longer nowadays, meaning less wastage and more calories to eat.

It's important to keep all of these factors in mind when thinking of solutions or approaches to combating obesity and T2D.

> TYPE 2 DIABETES BECOMES PROGRESSIVELY MORE DIFFICULT TO MANAGE IF IT ISN'T LOOKED AFTER. THE BODY BECOMES MORE RESISTANT TO INSULIN AND THE PANCREAS LOSES THE ABILITY TO PRODUCE SUFFICIENT AMOUNTS OF INSULIN.

CHECK YOUR ENVIRONMENT

It has also been suggested that T2D has the potential to spread within environments [19].

For example, take a typical overweight couple who:

A.   Lack an understanding of health.
B.   Lack the skills to cook a meal from scratch.
C.   Are highly inactive.
D.   Go to bed too late and lack sleep.
E.   Have a social network of similarly overweight friends and relatives.

Is it fair to say these behaviours are more likely to be reinforced between two people who live in the same home?

What if they bring kids up? Will they be influenced by their parents' attitude to health, eating and physical activity?

What happens if one individual goes on a health kick, loses weight and feels better about themselves?

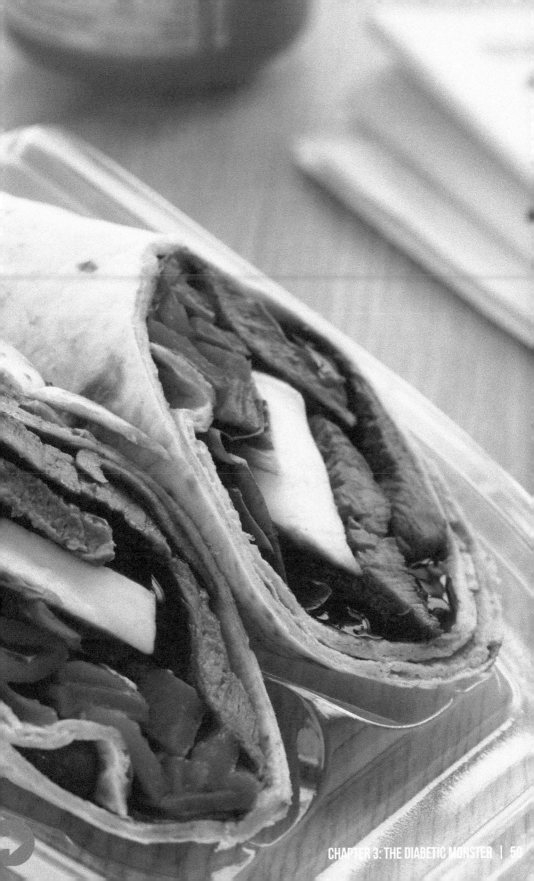

Is it likely to motivate the other to do the same?

Food Poverty: The ability to afford, access, and/or cook the right amount and quality of food for proper health.

Correlation does not always imply causation. There are always exceptions.

However, I personally feel individuals are a product of their environment and that behaviours catch on and habits get shared.

If you hang around five people who don't care about their health, eat too much, play too many video games and hate going to the gym – do you have a fair chance of becoming the sixth?

You bet.

SELF-AWARENESS OF HEALTH AND LIFESTYLE ARE ESSENTIAL FOR GOOD HEALTH.

OUR MODERN DAY CULTURE PUTS US AT INCREASED RISK OF EATING MORE AND MOVING LESS.

HEALTH COMPLICATIONS

While T2D and T1D differ in nature, they share similar symptoms and complications if left unmanaged.

Obesity, which is a hallmark of most people with T2D, is a particular issue.

High levels of body fat are unhealthy. The list of health problems associated with it is ever growing.

Obesity is directly linked to increased risk of T2D, cardiovascular disease, depression, sleep apnoea, osteoarthritis and cancer.
It is thought the increased risk of disease and illness associated with obesity is due to a number of factors:

1. **Sex hormone** imbalance Excessive fatty tissue alters the balance between the key sex hormones testosterone, oestrogen and progesterone. This can pose problems relating to fertility, cancer, muscle recovery and body composition;

2. **Insulin resistance Obesity** often results in higher insulin production. As tissues become resistant to the hormone they require more of it to control blood glucose levels. But high levels of insulin in the blood are associated with an increased risk of breast and colon cancer (the two most common forms of cancer);

3. **Chronic low-grade total body inflammation** obese individuals tend to exhibit low-grade, long-term inflammation. Inflammation isn't all bad: it's a useful protective mechanism but chronic long-term inflammation isn't healthy. Inflammation breeds inflammation and is said to be the root cause of many diseases and illnesses. Obese people often have high levels of tumour necrosis factor (TNF), interleukin-6 (IL-6) and C-reactive protein (CRP), which are all link to increased risk of disease;

•   Where you store body fat is more important than the total amount of body fat. Storing fat in your arms and legs, resembling a pear-shaped body is relatively safe.

•   Storing the majority of fat in the abdominal area, which surrounds your organs and is known as visceral fat is increasingly dangerous for cardiovascular disease, diabetes and other health complications.

MANAGEMENT

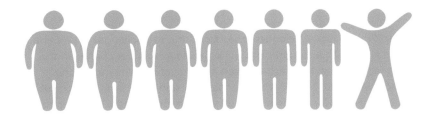

DIET AND LIFESTYLE

Although we cannot change our genetic risk of developing T2D, many epidemiologic studies and randomised clinical trials show that it is largely preventable through diet and lifestyle modifications.

One of the greatest triumphs in diabetes research came from the massive Diabetes Prevention Program (DPP) in 2002.

The programme, which involved 1,079 participants, set out to test which treatments were most effective. Participants were divided into three groups, which experienced either:

- Intensive lifestyle changes – exercise (30 minutes, 5 days a week), a healthy diet, and weight loss (loss of 7% of initial weight)
- Administration of the diabetic drug metformin
- A placebo (disguised as metformin)

The lifestyle group was 58% less likely to develop diabetes compared to the placebo group. The metformin group was 31% less likely to develop diabetes compared to the placebo group. This suggests lifestyle changes (weight loss, healthy diet and activity) are the most effective intervention known to date.

My only concern is many of these studies are conducted in controlled environments, under medical supervision and impose somewhat sudden nutrition and exercise variables over specific time frames, including very low calorie diets.

What about long-term adherence to these approaches after trials have finished?

Are the individuals educated to pursue progress once the trial period finishes?

It doesn't take a rocket scientist to work out that such changes in diet and lifestyle along with accountability will promote a healthier change in the people who adhere. Newcastle University conducted some interesting research, which put 30 T2D diabetic volunteers on a diet of 600-700 kcals per day for eight weeks. The end result was very promising with participants losing on average 14 kg. Thirteen subjects who'd had the condition for up to 10 years were able to reverse it and remain diabetes free six months after the study. Participants were eating about one third less after the study than before it. I would love to know if these individuals were able to keep their T2D in remission for the rest of their lives.

This research encouraged the charity Diabetes UK to fund a larger trial, involving 280 patients to examine how successfully people can reverse T2D through weight loss simply under the care of their family doctor and nurse over a two-year follow-up period. This measurement of adherence is something many research projects don't do.

Imagine what a lifetime of healthy living could do?

Translating the findings into real world action requires fundamental change in public policies, especially within the food and health sectors [20].

Promotion of healthy diet and lifestyle should be a global public policy priority.

EXERCISE

There is a myriad of evidence to support the role all types of physical exercise play in improving metabolic control in T2D [21] and gestational diabetes [22].

Weights resistance exercise, the main form of exercise promoted in this book, has been proven more beneficial than aerobic [23] exercise or diet [24] alone at improving body composition and decreasing the likelihood of complications [25].

BARBELLS VS. CARDIO?

Resistance training increases muscle mass more significantly than any other form of exercise. This has a number of key benefits to anyone living with T2D.

Having more muscle speeds up the metabolic rate, which means your body burns more energy when it's resting.

Muscle mass serves as the body's major port of entry for glucose use and storage. Resistance training facilitates the uptake of glucose in muscle tissue and reduces the need for insulin [26, 27, 28].

Resistance training has also been shown to increase the liver's sensitivity to insulin, which means improvements in metabolic control and uptake of glucose [29].

MEDICATION

If blood sugar levels cannot be controlled by diet, weight loss and exercise, medication is required.

T2D medication works in various ways. Some drugs reduce insulin resistance, others increase the amount of insulin in the blood and some even slow the rate food leaves the gut. Medication can be taken orally or by injection.

I talk more about medications in chapter 5.

Many people with T2D also suffer from other obesity-related complications like elevated levels of fat in the blood (high triglycerides and cholesterol) and high blood pressure and therefore may require additional medication.

IMPLICATIONS FOR MUSCLE BUILDING AND PERFORMANCE

Individuals who fail to control their T2D compromise their ability to build muscle and perform at their best.

There are a host of implications, including:

- Derangements in key hormones that are involved in the muscle building process, notably insulin and testosterone.
- Chronic levels of inflammation, which may hinder recovery, jeopardise immunity and increase risk of illness.
- Poor cardiovascular fitness as a result of chronic low levels of physical activity can hinder exercise performance.
- Mobility problems caused by excess body fat that restricts exercise performance.
- Depression and anxiety.

INDIVIDUALS WHO HAVE ZERO EXERCISE EXPERIENCE MUST DEMONSTRATE INCREDIBLE FOCUS AND PATIENCE TO THE PROCESS, RATHER THAN FOCUS ON THE OUTCOME ALONE.

OTHER FORMS OF INSULIN RESISTANT DIABETES

In addition to Type 1 and Type 2 Diabetes, there is a huge range of other forms of insulin resistance and diabetes. Many of them are well beyond the scope of this resource, so I've solely focused on the more commonly seen and defined types of diabetes.

Unfortunately, many of these conditions are misdiagnosed leading to delays in treatment.

Similar to all forms of Diabetes, self and professional monitoring are necessary. Treatment can differ, ranging from diet and lifestyle right through to injectable and oral diabetic medication or only just a dietary/lifestyle change.

If left uncontrolled health complications are inevitable.

TYPE 1.5 OR LATENT AUTOIMMUNE DIABETES IN ADULTS (LADA)

Latent autoimmune diabetes in adults (LADA) is a slowly progressing form of autoimmune diabetes. The progression of autoimmune β-cell failure is slow, meaning insulin production slowly declines over time and eventually results in a straight deficiency [39].

With the retention of internal insulin production, glucose levels are easier to control for more years. Lowering the risk factors typically found in Type 2 Diabetes associated with blood lipids, blood pressure, or cardiac and vascular problems.

Correct diagnosis of LADA is important because insulin treatment will be required much sooner in Type 1.5 than Type 2 diabetes as the condition progresses.

GESTATIONAL DIABETES

Gestational diabetes mellitus (GDM) is any degree of glucose intolerance with onset or first recognition during pregnancy [40]. It usually occurs during the second or third trimester of pregnancy.

A 'perfect storm' of hormonal and inflammatory responses, typical of pregnancy are responsible for causing insulin resistance in liver, muscle, and adipose tissue as the body aims to drive nutrients to the developing baby leads to Gestational Diabetes.

Women with gestational diabetes don't have diabetes before their pregnancy and the condition usually passes after birth. However, it's important to consider genetic predisposition, poor diet and lifestyle may influence diabetes in later life. Also in rare cases, it can be a case of diabetes developing for the first time in pregnancy.

If Gestational diabetes is left uncontrolled, excessive sugar circulating in the blood will enter the baby's bloodstream via the placenta. Consequently, jeopardising the health of both mother and child.

The symptoms of hyperglycemia during pregnancy can be difficult to distinguish from normal pregnancy symptoms, but may include increased thirst and more frequent urination. Also, targets for diabetes in pregnancy are tighter than those generally recommended for people with diabetes, so what is considered high glucose levels in pregnancy are lower than those that would result in symptoms.

Testing for Gestational diabetes is usually assessed by using a glucose tolerance test at 24-28 weeks into pregnancy. Diet and exercise are often enough to control the condition, but if proven ineffective, supplementary insulin or oral diabetes medication may be prescribed.

> DUE TO FETAL AND MATERNAL RISKS, TIGHT MATERNAL GLUCOSE CONTROL IS REQUIRED FROM CONCEPTION TO DELIVERY IN ALL PREGNANT WOMEN WITH T1D.

NEONATAL DIABETES

Neonatal diabetes is an extremely rare genetic form of diabetes that is diagnosed in infants less than 6 months of age. It results from specific mutations in the gene, which affects insulin production. Consequently, resulting in hyperglycemia.

The condition can often result in development delay and epilepsy (41). There are two types; Transient and Permanent Neonatal Diabetes Mellitus.

Transient Neonatal diabetes is known to disappear within a year of birth, but can come back in later life.

WOLFRAM SYNDROME

Wolfram Syndrome is a rare genetic disorder, causing diabetes, eye trouble, deafness and various other possible diseases.

ALSTRÖM SYNDROME

Alström Syndrome is a rare genetically inherited syndrome, which has some standard features including Type 2 Diabetes.

OTHER CONDITIONS
POLYCYSTIC OVARY SYNDROME (PCOS)

PCOS is Polycystic Ovary Syndrome, also known as Stein-Leventhal Syndrome, is one of the most common hormonal endocrine disorders in premenopausal women characterised by significant metabolic as well as reproductive morbidities (42,43). It is considered one of the leading causes of reduced fertility (44).

PCOS is caused by an imbalance between hormones in your brain and ovaries. In particular levels of Luteinizing Hormone (from the pituitary gland) and insulin (from the pancreas) run too high, resulting in extra testosterone production by the ovary and varying degrees of insulin resistance (45,46). This hormonal imbalance can cause irregular periods, unwanted hair growth, and acne. The condition is known as "the diabetes of bearded women."

The most common form of treatment for PCOS is the birth control pill and/or Metformin to help correct the hormone imbalances (45,46).

As already mentioned there are many other unusual types of diabetes ranging from haemochromatosis to Leprechaunism. To learn more, I've included some excellent resources at the end of this chapter for further research.

DIABETES DIAGNOSTICS: KEY MEASURES

You've probably heard it said before: what gets measured gets managed. Therefore to measure is to know...

People living with diabetes must undergo regular assessments to assess the effectiveness of their treatment and detect any signs of complications.

Yet millions of people go undiagnosed until its too late, and complications take over.

DON'T TRY TO PREDICT THE FUTURE. ASSESSMENTS AND REGULAR SCREENING OR CHECK-UPS SAVE LIVES AND SERIOUS HASSLE.

This section will discuss the main biomarkers every person living with diabetes must respect. It will also highlight the importance of regular health check-ups as part of the long-term management strategy for people living with T1D.

The World Health Organisation and the International Diabetes Foundation established methods and criteria for diagnosing T1D and T2D. They include (34):

- HbA1C greater than 6.5% (48mmol/mol)

- A random blood sample taken from a vein showing a blood glucose concentration of >200 mg/dl or ≥ 11.1 mmol/L.

- A fasting blood sample showing a glucose concentration of >126 mg/dl or ≥ 7.0 mmol/L (whole blood ≥ 6.1 mmol/L).

- A blood sample taken 2 hours after an oral glucose tolerance test (OGTT) showing a blood glucose concentration of >200 mg/dl or ≥ 11.1 mmol/L.

- Additionally T1D is suspected if ketones are detected in the urine or blood. Additional tests, including checks on other markers like c-peptide levels and antibodies, may be necessary to determine this.

WHAT'S AN ORAL GLUCOSE TOLERANCE TEST?

An OGTT is a medical test in which a set amount of glucose (usually 75 g) is consumed within a 5-minute window and blood samples are taken every 30 minutes for 2 hours to determine how quickly it is cleared from the blood.

DAILY BLOOD GLUCOSE MONITORING

Tracking blood sugar levels is an essential aspect of diabetes management, especially for those with T1D. Blood glucose levels fluctuate, literally on a minute-by-minute basis.

When first diagnosed with T1D, I became obsessed with tracking my blood glucose levels. I tracked the dips, peaks and everything else in between. I wanted to gather essential feedback on how my sugars reacted to different foods, exercise, stress and anything else life threw at me.

Over time I became familiar with how my body reacted to different foods, exercise and lifestyle circumstances. I was passionate to learn about human physiology, especially insulin and its counter-regulatory hormones like cortisol and adrenaline.

I've now reached a stage where I pretty much know my blood glucose levels based on how I feel. Occasionally I get it wrong, especially during periods of fatigue, high levels of stress or when I'm under the influence of alcohol. In these circumstances, it's always best to assess, no matter how experienced you are.

My current monitoring revolves around the following key times:
- First thing in the morning.
- Before bed.
- Pre-exercise.
- 20 mins post-exercise (when stress hormones start to fall).
- Instinctively when I feel off.
- Before driving and during breaks in long journeys.
- When I'm under the influence of alcohol.

Establish a routine with your healthcare professional on how often and when to test your blood glucose levels.

10 SUPER USEFUL TIPS FOR SUCCESSFUL BLOOD SUGAR MONITORING

1. Wash hands for both hygiene and accuracy reasons.
2. Be careful to let only the blood, not your skin, touch the strip. Residue from food or medication may affect test results, which can lead to unnecessary administration of medication and unwanted hypos.
3. Close the bottle of test strips to avoid contamination with dirt or moisture.
4. Use a clean lancet for every test. Re-using the same lancet increases the risk of infection.
5. Rotate sample sites to avoid build-up of scar tissue.
6. Squeeze sample finger gently until tips of finger appear red, this encourages blood flow and makes it easier to get a sample.
7. Test in public if you need to – your health matters more than a few people staring.
8. If you suspect your meter is wrong, test again, preferably using another meter.
9. Make sure your test strips are within their expiry date.
10. Carefully dispose of needles, pens, test strips and lancets. Nobody likes to see these lying around, and it gives people with diabetes a bad name.

UK VS. INTERNATIONAL MEASURES OF BLOOD GLUCOSE

UK and most of Europe measure in mmol/L.
USA and most other non-European countries measure in mg/dL.

WHAT'S THE DIFFERENCE?

Both units are used to measure blood glucose levels, which is the concentration of glucose in the blood, But they do so in slightly different ways.

mmol/L outlines the number of molecules of substance within a specified volume, in this case 1 litre.

mg/dL measures the concentration of glucose in the blood by the ratio of weight to volume, in this case milligrams per decilitre.

HOW TO CONVERT UNITS

Formula to calculate mmol/L from mg/dL: mmol/L = mg/dL / 18
Formula to calculate mg/dL from mmol/L: mg/dL = 18 × mmol/l

Testing Long Term Blood Glucose Control: Hemoglobin A1c (HbA1c)
Hemoglobin A1c (HbA1c) testing is a successful clinical test to determine
long-term blood glucose control.

The term HbA1c refers to glycated hemoglobin, which develops when
hemoglobin, a protein in red blood cells that carries oxygen throughout the
body, joins with glucose in the blood and becomes 'glycated'.

Haemoglobin molecules tend to live for 8-12 weeks and a HbA1c value gives
a good indication of how high or low your blood glucose levels have been
over that period.

For people with diabetes, this is important because the higher the HbA1c,
the greater the risk of developing diabetes-related complications (35).

HbA1c provides a superior measure of blood glucose control compared to
fasting and 2 hour Oral Glucose Tolerance Tests, which only gauge a
snapshot of blood glucose levels at a particular time of day.

HbA1c can be measured anytime, irrespective of fasting or feeding.

However, both diagnostic tools are essential for effective diabetes
management (35).

**SHORT TERMS TESTS, ALTHOUGH USEFUL AT A PARTICULAR
MOMENT, CAN BE MISLEADING IN DESCRIBING THE CHRONIC AND
COMPLEX CLINICAL CONDITIONS OF DIABETES.**

HBA1C TARGETS

According to the charity Diabetes UK, the HbA1c target is below 48
mmol/mol as evidence shows this reduces the risk of developing
complications, such as nerve damage, eye disease, kidney disease and heart
disease.

Guidelines by the National Institute for Health and Care Excellence (NICE)
in the UK suggest adults with T1D should aim for a target HbA1c level of 48
mmol/mol (6.5%) or lower to minimise the risk of long-term vascular
complications.

MEASUREMENT

In the UK, NICE guidelines suggest measuring HbA1c levels every 3–6 months in adults with T1D and more frequently in individuals whose blood glucose control is expected to change rapidly – for example, people starting new forms of medication or suffering illness (36).

HbA1c can be expressed as a percentage (DCCT unit) or as a value in mmoL/mol (IFCC unit). Since 2009, mmoL/mol has been the default unit to use in the UK.

DON'T CONFUSE AN HBA1C MEASUREMENT IN MMOL/MOL, WITH BLOOD GLUCOSE LEVELS, WHICH ARE OFTEN MEASURED IN MMOL/L.

A lot of people get confused about the units used to measure HbA1c. See the table below for reference.

Fig: HbA1c & Glucose Blood Levels

HbA1c (%)	HbA1c (%) (mmol/mol)	Ave. Blood Glucose (mmol/L)	Ave. Blood Glucose (mg/dL)
13	119	18 mmol/L	324 mg/dL
12	108	17 mmol/L	306 mg/dL
11	97	15 mmol/L	270 mg/dL
10	86	13 mmol/L	234 mg/dL
9	75	12 mmol/L	216 mg/dL
8	64	10 mmol/L	180 mg/dL
7	53	8 mmol/L	144 mg/dL
6	42	7 mmol/L	126 mg/dL
5	31	5 mmol/L	90 mg/dL

WORTH KNOWING

- Finger-prick HbA1c should not be used unless the methodology and the healthcare staff and facility using it can demonstrate their procedures match the standardised quality assurance of the International Federation of Clinical Chemistry and Laboratory Medicine (IFCC). Finger prick tests must be confirmed by laboratory venous HbA1c in all patients.

- In many parts of the world HbA1c is not available and its cost is so high that it is meaningless to even discuss whether it should be given priority over simple and inexpensive glucose measurements.

This effectively divides the world into two categories: the most developed societies, which diagnose diabetes using HbA1c, and less developed societies, which diagnose based on plasma glucose.

This kind of division must be avoided at all costs. It adds to the inequities in health and healthcare. The NICE guidelines for diagnosing gestational diabetes are slightly different (38):

- A fasting plasma glucose level of 5.6 mmol/L or above.
- A 2-hour plasma glucose level of 7.8 mmol/L or above.

TAKE HOME

Since many cases of diabetes are undiagnosed. It is important to increase public awareness of the main signs and symptoms associated with diabetes. Catching the condition early can safeguard against heart disease, and many other health problems including death.

People living with diabetes must consistently measure their blood glucose levels in order to assess the effectiveness of their blood glucose control.

A GLOBAL ISSUE

Diabetes is a life-long, incurable and costly non-communicable disease that poses a major health challenge to society in the 21st century.
It can be generally classed into four categories:

- Type 1 diabetes (T1D)
- Type 2 diabetes (T2D)
- Gestational diabetes (GDM)
- Diabetes resulting from other specific origins e.g. genetic defects, neonatal diabetes, drugs, pancreatic diseases, infections and surgery.

A NON-COMMUNICABLE DISEASE (NCD) IS A MEDICAL CONDITION OR DISEASE THAT IS NON-INFECTIOUS OR NON-TRANSMISSIBLE. NCDS CAN REFER TO CHRONIC DISEASES, WHICH LAST A LONG PERIOD OF TIME AND PROGRESS SLOWLY. HOWEVER, SOME CONSIDER T2D TO BE SOCIABLY TRANSMISSIBLE, AS SHARING A SEDENTARY LIFESTYLE AND POOR DIET CAN INCREASE RISK OF DEVELOPING THE CONDITION.

THE MAJORITY OF T2D CASES CAN BE PREVENTED.

All forms of diabetes are responsible for millions of deaths each year, debilitating complications and profound human misery. It is considered such a major public health challenge that the United Nations issued a resolution in 2006 declaring it to be a major global health threat, which gives it the same status as HIV/AIDS.

ARE WE FIGHTING A LOSING BATTLE AGAINST DIABETES?

Recent statistics from the respected International Diabetes Federation, an umbrella body for national diabetes associations, confirm an unavoidable truth: despite considerable global investment in medical interventions, research and health promotion, the ongoing battle to protect people from all forms of diabetes and its associated life-threatening health complications is well and truly being lost. Currently, more people are living with diabetes than are citizens of the United States.

DIABETES

Type 1 diabetes is a less common form of diabetes. But the majority of diabetes found in children and adolescent is T1D.

Type 2 diabetes is the most popular form of diabetes, accounting for 85%-95% of all cases (16). The majority of these are preventable.

Gestational diabetes is increasingly prevalent, like T2D. Women diagnosed with gestational diabetes (GDM) are at least seven times more likely to develop T2D than women without GDM (30).

PREVALENCE

According to recent statistics from the International Diabetes Federation, 415m people worldwide suffer from diabetes. An estimated one in two adults with diabetes is undiagnosed (16).

DIABETES: FACTS AND FIGURES

WORLDWIDE

2015   415 MILLION PEOPLE WITH DIABETE
2040   642 MILLION PEOPLE WITH DIABETES

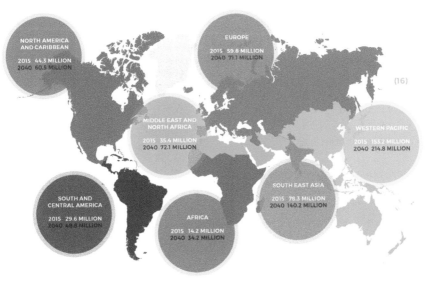

NORTH AMERICA
AND CARIBBEAN

2015 44.3 MILLION
2040 60.5 MILLION

EUROPE

2015 59.8 MILLION
2040 71.1 MILLION

(16)

MIDDLE EAST AND
NORTH AFRICA

2015 35.4 MILLION
2040 72.1 MILLION

WESTERN PACIFIC

2015 153.2 MILLION
2040 214.8 MILLION

SOUTH AND
CENTRAL AMERICA

2015 29.6 MILLION
2040 48.8 MILLION

AFRICA

2015 14.2 MILLION
2040 34.2 MILLION

SOUTH EAST ASIA

2015 78.3 MILLION
2040 140.2 MILLION

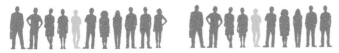
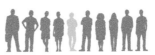

2015 ONE IN 11 ADULTS HAS DIABETES

2040 ONE IN 10 ADULTS WILL HAVE DIABETES

ONE IN TWO ADULTS
WITH DIABETES IS
UNDIAGNOSED

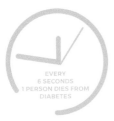

EVERY
6 SECONDS
1 PERSON DIES FROM
DIABETES

5.0 MILLION DEATHS IN 2015

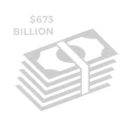

$673
BILLION

12% OF GLOBAL HEALTH EXPENDITURE
IS SPENT ON DIABETES

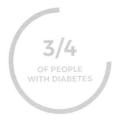

3/4

OF PEOPLE
WITH DIABETES

LIVE IN LOW AND MIDDLE
INCOME COUNTRIES

ABOUT 80% OF PEOPLE SUFFERING FROM DIABETES LIVE IN LOW AND MIDDLE-INCOME COUNTRIES. (16)

THE GREATEST NUMBER OF PEOPLE LIVING WITH DIABETES IS BETWEEN 40 AND 59 YEARS OF AGE. (16)

FUTURE PREDICTIONS

It is suggested that if trends continue, by 2040, 642 million people, or one adult in 10, will have diabetes.

COST

The costs associated with diabetes are colossal and include:

- Increased use of health services Diagnosis/treatment
- Medication
- Medical research
- Disability services

Average diabetes-related healthcare spending per country varies enormously. For example, people diagnosed with diabetes in the United States incur an average medical expenditure of about $13,700 per year (31), compared to $87 per person with diabetes in Tajikistan (32).

GLOBAL HEALTH EXPENDITURE DUE TO DIABETES
(20-79 YEARS)

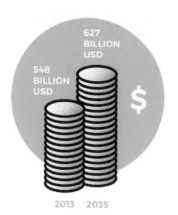

627 BILLION USD

548 BILLION USD

2013   2035

DIABETES CAUSED **5.1 MILLION DEATHS** IN 2013. EVERY SIX SECONDS A PERSON DIES FROM DIABETES

URGENT NEED FOR FOCUS

As diabetes continues to grow on a daily basis, it places increasingly more social and economic stress on societies.

Coordinated advocacy between governments and key diabetes-related federations are needed.

The following global priorities need to be addressed:

- Prevention of T2D.
- More cost-effective treatments for all forms of diabetes.
- Improved health outcomes for people with diabetes, including universal access to essential medicines and technologies.

If these issues aren't addressed, more people will suffer and spending will need to rise to levels that health services are unable to afford.

THE MAJORITY OF PEOPLE WITH DIABETES LIVE IN THE ECONOMICALLY LESS-DEVELOPED REGIONS OF THE WORLD. (16) MANY OF THESE PEOPLE FACE HEALTH INEQUITY, DISCRIMINATION AND STIGMA.

MORE THAN 3.2M PEOPLE IN THE UK WERE DIAGNOSED WITH DIABETES IN 2013. THIS IS OVER 163,000 MORE THAN THE PREVIOUS YEAR.

EUROPE HAS THE HIGHEST NUMBER OF CHILDREN WITH T1D. THE REASON FOR THIS IS NOT ENTIRELY CLEAR. (16)

DIABETIC MYTHS

Having lived with diabetes for more than 10 years, I've seen all the stigmas attached to it, and heard plenty of confusion about what it is. It hasn't only come from healthy folk, but also from people with diabetes and, in some cases, healthcare professionals.

Here's a list of popular diabetic myths.

Myth #1: Type 1 and Type 2 diabetes are the same.

Fact: Although T1D and T2D are both classified by higher than normal blood glucose levels, the cause, pathology and progression of the conditions are different.

Some would even say they are completely different diseases due to the different defective mechanisms and that they simply happen to share the same consequence of high glucose levels.

Myth #2: Diabetes Isn't Serious.

Fact: If you think sizing up a wheelchair, going blind or having a prosthetic limb sounds like a laugh you're on your own. Or how does falling into a coma and dying from it sound? It's simple – there is no such thing as mild diabetes.

Myth #3: Diabetics must avoid sugar.

Fact: Sugar is in every food that contains carbohydrate. Some sugars affect blood glucose quicker than others. Glucose, the simplest form of carbohydrate, will cause a rapid increase in blood glucose, whereas the fructose from fruit will not.

There is no such thing as a good or bad food, just good or bad diets or patterns of eating. A diet dominated by fast-acting carbohydrates at the expense of essential protein and healthy fats will hinder health, body composition and performance.

If you consume sugary-based food within your diet, consider this:
- Medication must cover the quantity of food consumed.
- Overall calorie intake must be respected. Carbohydrates don't fill us up and are often overeaten.
- Essential nutrient requirements for both protein and essential fatty acids (omega 3 and 6).

Myth #4: Diabetics should buy and eat special 'diabetic food.

Fact: It's revolting, expensive and encourages regular toilet breaks.

Are you having a laugh, food manufacturers? Do one!

Myth #5: Treat Hypos With Chocolate.

Not only did this myth increase the time it took me to get out of a hypo, it also encouraged me to gorge down many unnecessary calories and contributed to unwanted fat gain. The best way to treat hypos I've found is a glucose-based liquid sports drink or sweets. Both are quick to work, convenient and easy to transport. Be mindful of over-treating hypos and causing hyperglycemia

Myth #6: Diabetes will hold you back in life.

ONLY IF YOU LET IT.

Take pride in getting to grips with your condition. Understand it and do your best. You have a choice in the matter.

The better your control, the better your mind and body will work.

Don't get me wrong: you might struggle to enroll as the next James Bond. A hypo wouldn't go down too well under fire. Nor is it easy to obtain a heavy goods vehicle licence.

But things are changing. Police forces are no longer barring people with diabetes, and some local authorities do allow people with diabetes to hold licenses as taxi drivers provided their medical records show proof of good control and healthy eyesight.

Myth #7: You can catch diabetes

DIABETES IS A NON-COMMUNICABLE DISEASE (NCD), A MEDICAL CONDITION OR DISEASE THAT IS NON-INFECTIOUS OR NON-TRANSMISSIBLE.

There is a genetic component involved in developing T1D and T2D. The risk of diabetes is increased if you have parents or siblings with the condition.

Other forms of diabetes can also be directly inherited, including maturity-onset diabetes in the young (MODY) and diabetes that results from mitochondrial DNA mutation.

The environment is another factor, especially in the development of T2D, the preventable form of diabetes. If you live in a household with poor dietary habits, low levels of physical activity, smoking and stress you are at greater risk of mirroring these high-risk behaviours, consequently increasing your chances of developing T2D.

Myth #8: Diabetics are more likely to get ill

IF YOU DON'T LOOK AFTER YOUR CONDITION YOU WILL INEVITABLY PLACE MORE STRESS ON YOUR BODY'S SYSTEMS LIKEWISE, IF YOU'RE SICK YOU INCREASE THE POTENTIAL FOR BLOOD SUGAR ISSUES, WHICH CAN AGGRAVATE THE ILLNESS EVEN FURTHER. THIS IS THE REASON WHY VACCINATIONS, INCLUDING THE FLU JAB ARE RECOMMENDED FOR PEOPLE WITH DIABETES.

Myth #9: Diabetes is easy to manage

DIABETES IS A FULL-TIME EXPERIMENT THAT REQUIRES 24/7 ATTENTION.

Blood glucose levels don't always behave as they should. Always be prepared to change your game plan with food, activity and medication.

Myth #10: Type 1 is the 'bad kind' of diabetes

BOTH FORMS OF DIABETES BRING VERY LITTLE BENEFIT TO THE HUMAN BODY. BOTH ARE HARMFUL IF UNCONTROLLED.

There are plenty more myths and confusion especially when it comes to diet and exercise. I will go into much more detail later in the book.

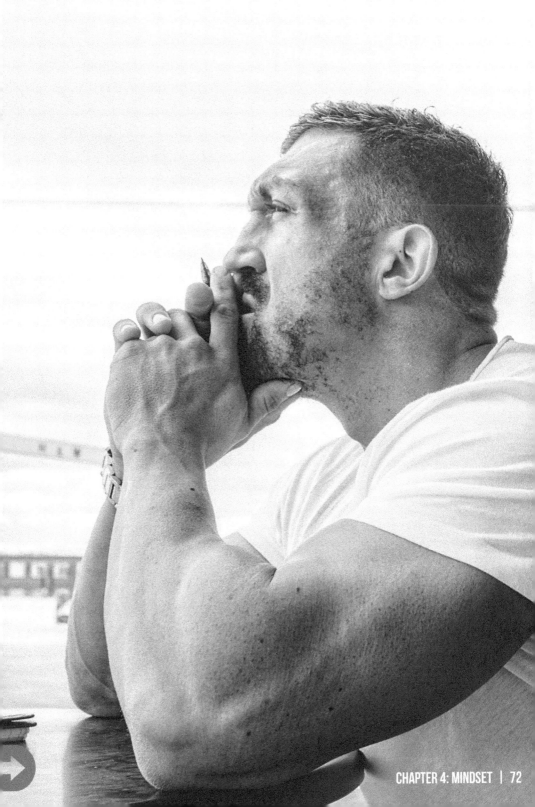

CHAPTER 4: MINDSET

In this chapter I want to outline the importance of mindful living for overcoming diabetes.

I also want to highlight the importance of lifestyle, particularly sleep and stress management for improving health, diabetic control and progress in the gym.

First, and most importantly.

Relax – It's one of the best secrets to elite health and performance.

MINDSET

In the year 170, during a brutal war in Germania, the great Roman Emperor Marcus Aurelius sat down to write these words:

'Our actions may be impeded. But there can be no impeding our intentions or dispositions because we can accommodate and adapt.

The mind adapts and converts to its own purposes the obstacle to our acting.

The impediment to action advances action. What stands in the way becomes the way... '

In layman's terms, Aurelius was saying that problems are always to be expected and instead of dwelling on them we should turn those obstacles upside down and use them to empower us and guide the way.

I work with thousands of clients every year. A small proportion has diabetes but the majority are everyday people without the condition who want to look, feel and perform better.

Each and every one of them (people with and without diabetes) has a different mindset.

Some are incredibly negative; some are incredibly inspiring; and some are just downright confused.

"The mind is a beautiful servant, but a terrible master."

WHICH IS IT FOR YOU?

Diabetic or not, everyone is subject to life's struggles; no one gets it easy, so stop thinking you're special.

We all have flaws, limiting beliefs, insecurities, disappointments, mistakes and past experiences to contend with.

How you deal with each of these is entirely up to you.

BUILDING A HEALTHY MINDSET: KEY ELEMENTS

Let me outline what I feel are the most important aspects of getting your mind(set). It applies to everything from overcoming diabetes to making healthy life choices.

Your Life – Your Choice

How you look and feel right now is a direct result of the choices you've made in life.

This includes everything from what you eat to the people you hang around with, and even controlling your diabetes.

Happy?

Maybe you are, maybe you aren't

If not, realise you have complete control of your attitudes and actions!

This is where mindset comes in.

A confused or troubled mind won't work!

Perception (is everything)

For me diabetes is a way of life, an obstacle with specific rules and guidelines that need to be respected.

When it comes to my personal diabetic management I take two clear perspectives.

1.   Try my very best to control the condition. I achieve this through regular assessments and by following key eating, lifestyle and therapeutic measures.

2. Accepting things will never be perfect. I'll not get it right every time. When things do mess up, snap out of it, learn from it and move on!

Acceptance (Break The Trance)

First things first.

You're diabetic.

You have two choices,

Come to terms with the condition, embrace it, understand it and do everything you can to control it.

Or... Deny the truth, get on with your life and hope for the best.

The problem is many people with diabetes simply don't care or know enough to change. But their very existence is under threat. It doesn't matter how much you're worth, how popular or good looking you are – without your health you're good to nobody, including yourself!

Break The Trance! Do something about it – you have control!

5 FACTORS YOU MUST ACCEPT

1. Medication, nutrition, exercise, rest and mindfulness are essential for helping you overcome diabetes.

2. Perfect control doesn't happen overnight. It takes time to become proficient. Don't stress when you lose control. Note down each and every problem and ask yourself why it's happening.

3. Accept some aspects of the condition are beyond your control. They can include unexplained rises or drops in blood sugar or fluctuations in mood. Accept the situation and do your best to fix it.

4. You will screw up (on many occasions), whether you forget to bring insulin to a dinner party, over eat when you suffer a hypo or forget to take a dose of medication. Don't freak out. You forgot, You're human, ride it out and learn from your mishap - you'll not do it again in a hurry.

5. People will joke about your condition. Laugh it of, and never take it to heart. Stress is self-harm – perception is everything! See it for what it is... white noise.

Before you start your diet and training, ask yourself this:

If my body didn't look any better than how it is now, could I be happy?

If the answer is 'yes', great, get stuck in and enjoy the journey to a healthier body!

If you answered 'no', it might be wise to first of all address your underlying emotional state.

Is health or visual appearance your end goal? For most, appearance comes before health. This often originates from deep-routed insecurity and a need for significance. I've been there myself: I was overweight and felt out of place for a great deal of my life.
Feeling 'out of place' drove me down many rabbit holes in life, one to the next – it got me nowhere.

Take it from me: no diet or training regime will fix underlying unhappiness in your life, unless it's primarily focused on health.

Get your shit together, address your emotional demons and know that you already are all that you seek. And, that most of the opinions you have of yourself are made up and stem from your perception of how other people see you.

Like that really matters?

Don't waste another minute...

THE POWER OF NOW

Ever travelled into the future? Or back in time?

I've done both!

Every time I travel I conjure up a particular emotion. That emotion depends entirely on where I travel to within my mind.

Sometimes I smile, sometimes I cry, sometimes I clench my fist and plot the most creative revenge stories ever. At other times I think 'what if?' or 'why did that happen?'

Rarely do I visit the past now except when there are practical reasons for doing so, such as learning from previous experiences (i.e don't do that again) and/or planning future appointments/business.

Again, dipping in and out of the future except occasionally for practical purposes isn't beneficial to living, especially when you dwell on negative experiences.

Worrying about what certain people will think when you begin striving for a goal, or getting angry over someone that has wronged you, are examples of this.

Living like this will kill you – slowly!

Such limiting beliefs are merely fragments of your imagination based on past experiences.

They don't exist!

There's a lot of truth to the meaning FEAR – False Evidence Appearing Real... Focus on what you're doing right now – not last year or last week, but now – this very second. That is living!

SELF CONTROL

"The man who acquires the ability to take full possession of his mind may take possession of anything else to which he is just entitled" – Andrew Carnegie

I set myself a rule when I was 16.

That rule was: "Never say F**k it!"

Don't get me wrong: I've broken this rule on many occasions, usually because of impulse or boredom. Bar the odd exception, the end result has never been good.

This rule could relate to anything: diet, business, drinking, lifestyle habits or taking up something new. Each circumstance is unique and may or may not justify a F**k it attitude.

This rule was particularly important in three key areas of my health: lifestyle, diet and exercise. I resolved never to take the attitude of saying: 'F**k it I'll not train, F**k it I'm not diabetic I'll eat what I want, F**k it I'll give into that situation and create never-ending stress for myself over short-term satisfaction'.

I knew the F**k it attitude to life would catch me out in the long term.

5 KEY STEPS TO ACHIEVING SELF-CONTROL

These steps could apply to any walk of life: health, physique, performance, business, finance or relationships. Apply as you wish.

1.   Picture what you want. Study every detail.

2.   Ask yourself the following

Q.   What key behaviours result in the end product?
Q.   What do I need to do more of to achieve my end goal?
Q.   What do I need to do less of?
Q.   Can I do any better? If so, how?

3.   The answers to these questions now serve as your official standards, values and benchmarks to every action you make.

4.   When challenged with trouble or a F**k it moment, ask yourself: is this choice/potential action in line with my values? Does it match the behaviour needed to get towards my end goal?

5.   Act.

If the answer is yes – do it!
If the answer is no – move on!

Failing from taking action or failing to take action – which is it for you?

SELF TALK

How many times have you thought?
- I can't
- I don't deserve it!
- It's impossible!
- No way!
- Not a chance!
- I'll fail miserably

Guess what? You're right: you can't, don't and won't do what you WANT/NEED to do!

On the other hand if you think you're awesome, you most certainly are! If you think you can do it, you can and will...

The mind is an incredibly powerful tool. Be careful with your thoughts and how you speak to yourself. If you belittle yourself with can't and won't all you are doing is simply reinforcing ideas and reasons why you CAN'T!

Word choice determines thought choice; thought choice determines actions. You fix the words; you fix the thoughts.

I'm a firm believer life is down to the quality of questions you ask.

Why am I struggling?

Why do I want to change?

What would happen if I don't change my habits?

What do I need to do next?

You'll surprise yourself with some pretty powerful life changing answers that would otherwise be disregarded if you didn't question yourself. Question everything! Find meaning!

HAVE PURPOSE

Have a reason to wake up in the morning.

This will give you direction and keep you moving forward. The more purpose you inject into your life, the brighter your internal sparkle will burn, the longer you will live and the more productive you will be while you're alive. What's your purpose?

For me it's the following:

1. To build a healthy, happy strong body and mind.
2. To help others.
3. To be valuable.

BE HONEST

Be honest when it comes to your personal life and diabetic management. Lying to yourself may create short-term comfort but over the long-term, pain is the only outcome.

If you're wrong – own up and fix it.

The stress and aftermath aren't worth it – trust me.

You get weaker every time you lie.

BLOODY HARD WORK

You need to put the work in. No gadget, app or book (including this one) is going to help you unless you put the work in.

I can't stress this enough.

A great looking physique doesn't come easy. You get out what you put in. The same goes for mastering control of your diabetes.

SIMPLICITY

K.I.S.S – Adopt the Keep It Simple, Stupid principle.

If It's Important, Do It Daily!

In order to build a healthy body and mind you'll need the following (daily):

- Great food,
- Regular movement,
- Laughter,
- Great company
- Relaxation
- Quiet time to think, read & write.

REALISTIC VS. POSITIVE THINKING

Thinking positively will set you up for a fall.

You must be realistic in your goal setting.

This is especially true when it comes to chasing physical perfection.

Let me elaborate...

When you see an incredibly shaped physique on your social media newsfeed, the front of a magazine or the beach, how do you feel?

Motivated? Inspired? Invincible?

Or does it leave you feeling uncomfortable and a million miles away from building the physique you truly want?

From the minute we wake up to the minute we go to bed we are constantly exposed to images, videos and social media posts that portray the idea of physical perfection and the idyllic fitness lifestyle.

Many people, myself included, are guilty of seeing a photo or video online and instantly thinking 'that's what I want to look like.'

Don't get me wrong, it's important to be regularly inspired and to have an ideal target of what you are working so hard to achieve.

There are plenty of individuals within the fitness industry that can prove extremely motivating, especially when you look at their personal stories or how they've overcome certain challenges to build the body and live the life to which you aspire.

However, there is a fine line between setting a positive and realistic goal, and aiming for a physique or performance ideal that doesn't really exist.

For instance, you don't know how long that person you admire has been training, whether they are genetically gifted, or have used chemical assistance. What's more, you don't know how recent that photo is, or whether it's been digitally altered, or had a filter applied, or the time and effort that's gone into getting that one shot. Lighting makes a huge difference to how a physique looks in front of a camera.

Have you ever been happy with your first selfie pic? Or does it take another 10 takes to get the right one?

FITNESS MEDIA - THE REALITY

A professional fitness model may do one shoot in a day, using different locations and outfits, then drip feed images on their social media accounts over the next few weeks and months, which creates the impression of them being physical perfection all year round.

The truth is that it's very hard to maintain peak physical condition 24/7, 365 days a year, especially when you take into account the metabolic abnormalities that occur during a prolonged hypo-caloric state, as well as the everyday stress life throws at us.

Yet if you take these pictures at face value they can soon become not sources of inspiration but constant reminders of your self-perceived failure to make giant improvements week-in, week-out, or of the time it's taken you to get closer to your dream body.

I've lost count of the number of times my clients have complained about feeling demotivated, depressed and wanting to give up because they've gone on social media and it's left them feeling dissatisfied with their progress, even after they've had a great session.

This can be very destructive in your journey to building a better body. It's therefore extremely important to be able to look at inspiring images and let them motivate you to be the best you can be without piling on internal pressure that you must reach that pinnacle of perfection or else you are a failure.

Thinking positively in this sense means when you see an image of a physique that you aspire to emulate you can look at it and say that while you respect and admire what you see, it is not a realistic goal for you right now and you shouldn't place all your focus on looking like that anytime soon. Rome wasn't built in a day, and neither was an impressive physique.

And remember that some people add muscle easily and never seem to put on fat. They are genetically gifted and find it relatively easy to build and maintain a great body. Just think back to when you were at school. There was always that one kid who was ripped to shreds no matter what they ate (bastard), another who was the best at every sport (not me), and one who was super strong without ever having trained a day in their life (usually the farmer kid).

It's down to their genes, which determine how easy or hard we find it to build muscle and burn fat.

Whatever your starting point, with the right training and nutrition plan and the right mentality, drive and determination - and the right coaching if required - you can make a remarkable change to your physique.

Don't benchmark without knowing all the facts. Sometimes there's a lot more to meets the eye.

BE FUSSY

This may sound a little far fetched but you should be fussy about who you surround yourself with, the environment you socialise in and the material you expose your mind to.

Doing this, can be very fruitful.

Try your best to surround yourself with high achievers, motivators and inspirational people. They'll serve you so much better than the energy vampires we all know.

Identify the unhealthy people, circumstances and material in your life by asking yourself: is this adding value or taking value from me?

If they're taking value – your best to cut ties and move on.

DON'T PAY ATTENTION TO SOCIAL MEDIA

Strangely, the human brain can't distinguish between real life and social media.

How many times have you caught yourself benchmarking yourself against someone else's social media profile? I used to do this all the time when I first exposed myself to Facebook, Twitter and Instagram. It used to really get to me.

It doesn't matter if it's personal or business related. I'm sure you've subject yourself to the following questions:

"Why do they get so much attention and I don't?"

"Why has so-and-so liked that photo?"

" I'm not doing well enough based on what I see."

" Look who they know!"

Firstly, understand social media is a communication tool. People and business interact by generating attention with each other.

Some of the tactics used to generate attention are 100% legitimate. This includes individuals, businesses and agencies that put up credible content or sell a product that genuinely adds value or solves the needs of the person observing.

Then there is the self-glorifying attention seeker who blows everything out of proportion to seek the approval of others. The only uploads you see are never-ending snapshots of their 'perfect life'. The reality is the darker normal side of their life remains hidden.

This gives the false perception that certain individuals' lives are a constant stream of happiness, accomplishments and power. The problem lies when you benchmark and feel pathetic in comparison.

Let me put it straight – take it with a pinch of salt.

I could easily sit down beside Arnold Schwarzenegger, ask him for a selfie and then upload it to social media and tell the world I'm 'spending time with my good pal Arnold'.

I wish...

On a business note, you can easily buy a few thousand fake Facebook likes for £10 and come across as super popular...
I know a few people who fake it until they make it (or, should I say, didn't ever actually make it).

Social media has been lying to you since you set up your account.

Rise above and don't fall prey to the bullshit!

PERFECT CONTROL, PERFECT BALANCE... WHATEVER

There is no such thing as perfect for you or I. I used to hate myself for not being perfect with my personal life, business, diabetic management, strength, physique - the list is endless.

The reality is, we all struggle. We all fall off the wagon from time to time.

Seeking perfection will drive you mad. Seek perfection and you seek procrastination and ultimately failure. Nothing messes up your life more than trying to be perfect.

You will have days when your sugars are all over the place, messy hair, low earnings, troublesome customers, friends who let you down and everything else in between. The reality is, it doesn't matter.

Stop thinking of life as an absolute straight road from A to B. Start thinking of life as a journey from A-Z, with all kinds of stops, roundabouts and obstacles along the way.

Life is a sliding scale. One day you might reach L then have to turn around again and work everything over again from B. You're human - it happens so anticipate it, be kind to yourself and realise you aren't perfect and never will be.

Understanding you're not perfect is the day you set yourself free from the ball and chain you've been carrying all along.

SET STANDARDS

Start showing a level of strength people don't associate you with, by learning to say 'no'. People will begin to respect you more. Trust me on that.

What are you willing to put up with in life? If you're willing to put up with constant BS in the form of negativity, unprofessionalism, poor standards and timewasters they will dominate your life.

What are you going to do about it?

If you're not strong enough to stick to your values, people are going to take advantage of you.

I used to put up with a lot of BS. The result? My tough decisions controlled me. Health, success, happiness, decision making - the list was endless.

UNTIL I cut all unnecessary BS from my life.

What are your values and standards? Do you have any? If not, why not?

What are you going to eliminate from your life right now?

Where is all your time and energy being wasted?

Can you visualize your life without these things?

That's the life you're after - go get it!

Take control - ditch the negative, relish the positive!

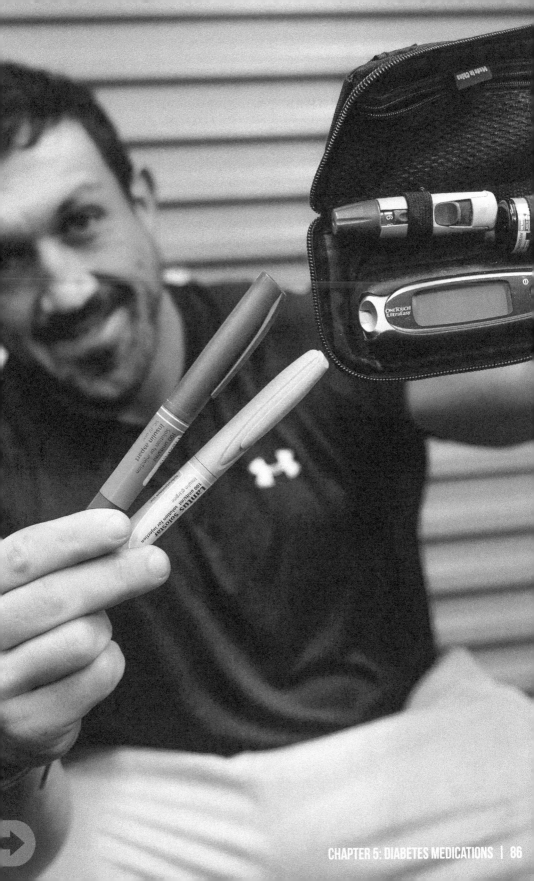

CHAPTER 5: DIABETES MEDICATIONS

LEARNING OUTCOMES

After reading this chapter, you should be able to understand and respect:

- The need for medication in the treatment of diabetes.
- All the different types of diabetes medication. Including their actions, side effects and administration.
- Everything there is to know about injectable insulin.
- The pros and cons of using multiple daily injections (MDI) over a continuous subcutaneous insulin infusion pump (CSII).
- Key strategies and equipment for measuring blood glucose.
- Future research and therapies in diabetes management.

A CLOSER LOOK AT THE MEDICINES USED IN THE MANAGEMENT OF DIABETES

There are many different types of medications used to treat people with diabetes. People with T1D will always require insulin for the rest of their lives. It will need to be either injected by a pen device (occasionally a syringe) or a pump (continuous subcutaneous insulin infusion).

People living with T2D can be less reliant on drugs, and in some cases require no medication. This is only possible if they modify their lifestyles and embrace diet and exercise. But unfortunately most people with T2D struggle to control their condition through lifestyle modification alone and usually require medication.

BEFORE TAKING MEDICATION

An appropriate level of knowledge is needed to use diabetes medications successfully. After all, anyone with diabetes can take medication just because their doctor tells them to.

In order to fully reap the benefits of medication, the person living with diabetes must be motivated to:

- Learn about the basic underlying physiology behind diabetes. Especially how and why blood glucose behaves the way it does in relation to diet, activity and lifestyle.
- Handle regular injections and attachment of infusion sets.
- Conduct regular blood tests (including finger prick tests and/or application of CGM devices)
- Record data and self-adjust insulin, diet and lifestyle in response to findings.
- Work in conjunction with a collaboration of health care specialist especially an endocrinologist, dietitian and exercise physiologist (exercise specialist).

FUTURE RESEARCH

There is a lot of work looking to develop new treatments and even vaccines to prevent the development of diabetes. Research is vital to develop new, more effective and safer treatments for diabetes. Drugs licensed for the treatment of diabetes must undergo various clinical testing for effectiveness and safety as well as any long-term adverse health implications.

EVERY DRUG HAS SIDE EFFECTS

Every medication for diabetes has the potential for side effects, some worse than others, and everyone can be affected differently. If you use any form of diabetes medication, talk with your doctor and diabetes care team about their possible impact on body weight, appetite and energy.

I discuss many of the common side effects in the drug profile section later on in this chapter.

ALWAYS SEEK MEDICAL ADVICE DURING ANY FORM OF DRUG TREATMENT. NEVER CHANGE YOUR DOSE OR DISCONTINUE ANY MEDICINAL TREATMENT WITHOUT TALKING TO YOUR DOCTOR FIRST.

I firmly believe anyone living with diabetes should try their absolute best to use diet and lifestyle to minimise their requirements for medication and the risks of side effects.

MEASUREMENT BEFORE TREATMENT

Before I go into detail about different kinds of diabetes medications, I want to discuss the personal blood glucose monitoring tools available. These are absolutely crucial for managing diabetes.

> PEOPLE WITH DIABETES MUST MONITOR THEIR BLOOD GLUCOSE BEHAVIOR DURING ANY DRUG TREATMENT.

BLOOD GLUCOSE METERS

There is a broad range of blood glucose meters available. Since I was diagnosed with diabetes, there have been remarkable advancements in the technology of meters. They are now relatively small, painless and can even be hooked up to your smartphone for highly organised tracking. It depends on the type of diabetes you have and your local health care system whether meters are available free of charge or at a cost. You may be able to get test strips on prescription from your doctor, or you may have to buy them, which can be expensive.

Either way, they'll save you, your life and your leg. Literally!

Your health care team should be able to advise on choosing a meter. I personally use an Accu-Chek Mobile because it's compact and saves the hassle of carrying and changing individual test strips. Some devices do provide the option of plugging in insulin doses and set dietary intake. However, this just takes too long. However, this is entirely personal.

Some devices also let you test for ketones. This feature is pretty cool and advisable for those who are struggling to gain good control.

WHEN TO TEST?

People living with T1D or those using any form of injectable insulin therapy need to test more frequently than those just using oral only medications.

KEY TIMES TO TEST INCLUDE:

- Upon awakening.
- Instinctive testing (if something doesn't feel right, test).
- Before meals.
- Before driving (depending on your treatment).
- 1-1.5 hours post-meals.
- Pre-exercise.
- Intra-exercise (if needed).
- Post-exercise.
- Two hours post-exercise.
- If you are consuming alcohol.
- Pre-bedtime.

SAMPLE SITES

- Avoid the extreme tips of the fingers. It is also better not to use your thumb or first finger as they can easily smear blood everywhere if you are not careful.
- The side of the fingers can be tested. However, I personally find 1 cm below the nail on the top of the finger most comfortable.
- Rotate sample sites and fingers.
- Ensure the lancet is set to the correct depth otherwise the sample may be too shallow to test, or may bleed excessively if it's too deep.
- Reduce the depth of the lancet during exercise. Increased body temperature and blood flow to the hands (especially during lifting) allow blood to flow more easily.

ESSENTIAL TIPS

- Make sure your hands are hygienic and residue free. Do bear in mind using alcohol gels can influence the reading on some meters. Hands must be dry.
- If in doubt, test again.
- Ensure you calibrate your machine as instructed.
- Always keep a spare meter, set of batteries, lancets.
- Always have enough supply of test strips – order in advance.
- Replace your lancets regularly to avoid infection and injury.
- Keep your device away from the sun and extreme heat.

CONTINUOUS GLUCOSE MONITORING DEVICES (CGM)

A CGM is a small compact device that tracks glucose continuously throughout day and night, notifying when blood glucose levels run high or low so you can take necessary action. They may not change as rapidly as a finger prick test, as some systems have a 'lag-time' of 15-20 minutes. If in doubt, it is best to use the finger prick to double check.

A CGM can be used effectively to overcome guesswork and the hassle of regular finger pricking.

A discreet sensor applied to the skin transmits blood glucose data wirelessly to a receiver and display screen. Glucose activity shows in real time and it is easy to see when it's trending high, low or staying within range.

Depending on the software, CGMs can provide informative feedback for healthcare professionals and dedicated fitness enthusiasts. They can accurately identify problematic trends with glucose, which allows you to refine whatever lifestyle, diet, exercise or medication variables are causing the issue. This ensures better diabetes management.

CGMS ARE USEFUL FOR ANALYSING AND ANTICIPATING TRENDS IN BLOOD GLUCOSE LEVELS RATHER THAN SINGLE SNAPSHOT READINGS.

THERE ARE VARIOUS SUPPLIERS OF CGMS

- Medtronic
- Animas
- Abbot
- Dexcom

Anyone can use a CGM. However, high-risk patients may have a greater need than well-controlled patients.

High-risk individuals include:

- Young children.
- Pregnant females.
- Patients with frequent, severe hypoglycemia.
- Patients with impaired ability to deal with the consequences of hypoglycemia (e.g. people suffering seizures or panic attacks).
- People who work stressful jobs.

CGMs are available on prescription for high-risk individuals. If you're interested discuss it with your diabetes specialist, the next time you're in clinic.

COST

If your health service won't prescribe a CGM, you can purchase your own. However, they are extremely expensive. The equipment initially costs in the hundreds or thousands of pounds and sensors are an additional, ongoing cost.

You need to do a cost-to-benefit assessment of using these devices. I personally work well with a simple blood glucose meter and have no intention of changing. However, I have exceptionally good control and understanding of my diabetes.

Others may benefit greatly from investing in a CGM device. To invest in oneself is the best thing you can do.

BE CAREFUL NOT TO RIP OFF THE ATTACHED SENSOR WHEN CHANGING CLOTHES OR DURING EXERCISE.

THINK WHERE YOU PUT THE SENSOR, BASED ON THE TYPE OF EXERCISE YOU ARE PLANNING.

ENSURE THE SAMPLE SITE IS HYGIENIC AND RESIDUE-FREE BEFORE APPLYING THE SENSOR.

DIABETES MEDICATION

I appreciate many readers rely on different brand names of diabetes medication. To avoid confusion, I will refer predominately to the generic names rather than the brand or proprietary name (examples of which are in brackets) of all currently established and upcoming drugs.

Depending on the type of diabetes you have, a wide class of drugs are involved in its management.

Insulin is the most effective treatment for directly lowering high blood glucose. Other medications lower blood glucose indirectly, by assisting the pancreas to produce more insulin, increasing the sensitivity of the body's cells to insulin itself and even delaying digestion so carbohydrates enter the blood stream slower than normal.

Examples of these medications include:

- Biguanides (Metformin)
- Sulphonylurea
- Alpha-glucosidase inhibitor (Acarbose)
- Prandial glucose regulators
- Thiazolidinediones (Pioglitazone)
- Incretin mimetics
- DPP-4 inhibitors (gliptins).
- SGLT2D inhibitors

Other novel (experimental) therapies like gene therapy and islet transplantation also exist.

I don't discuss individual dosing protocols for each medication as this is such a highly personalised matter. Regardless, standard dosing patterns and formulas are only to be used as starting points for insulin therapy. Adjustments are inevitable, especially as you acquire more muscle mass and train harder from year-to-year.

What is important is understanding the pharmacology behind how the drugs work and how they can mimic a healthy, fully functioning pancreas In someone without diabetes.

WHAT WORKS FOR ONE INDIVIDUAL WON'T ALWAYS WORK FOR YOU!

THE ROLE OF INJECTABLE INSULIN

Insulin's primary job in diabetes management is to prevent the buildup of glucose in the bloodstream and transport it into the body's cells for energy. Insulin clears glucose out of the blood stream from external sources (the diet) and blocks its production from internal sources (the liver and muscles.)

People with T1D require insulin from the outset due to the complete loss of insulin-producing beta cells.

People living with T2D or LADA may still produce some of their own insulin.

As previously discussed, a C-peptide blood test can be performed to find out how much insulin your pancreas is producing. This is important to know as certain individuals require different amounts of insulin depending on their body's degree of insulin resistance.

For example, someone who weights 100 kg (220 lbs) and is completely insulin resistant may require hundreds of units of insulin.

INSULINS DISCOVERY

The discovery of insulin in Canada in 1920-1921 is one of the greatest medical discoveries of all time.

Surgeon Frederick Banting and his student Charles Best observed injections of pancreatic cell extracts were able to relieve diabetic symptoms in dogs whose pancreases had been removed.

The pancreatic extracts contained the hormone insulin, which was eventually isolated and purified.

As scientists learn more about the human body, diabetes and blood glucose metabolism, new and innovative treatments are becoming more and more available.

CLASSES OF INSULIN

There are three classes of insulin – animal (derived from pancreases of pigs or cattle), human (produced genetically from bacteria or yeast) and analogues (genetically altered variations of human insulin).

There is no evidence that human insulins are superior to animal insulin [1], or that insulin analogues are superior to human insulin for the majority of people [2].

Nevertheless, human insulin and insulin analogues are the most popular insulin medication, although a small number of people still prefer to use animal insulin.

SIDE EFFECTS

Problems can occur when insulin administered doesn't match the body's needs precisely. Taking too much insulin can cause low blood sugar or hypoglycemia. This can easily be treated by reducing meal time insulin or by consuming a fast acting carbohydrate snack. Extreme cases of hypoglycemia may need to be treated with an injection of glucagon or an intravenous infusion of dextrose.

The use of injectable insulin can lead to unnecessary weight gain by increasing calorie intake to treat hypoglycemia. Also some individuals may overeat calories as a means of protecting themselves from hypoglycemia.

ANYONE TAKING INSULIN IS AT SEVERE RISK OF HYPOGLYCEMIA. IT IS ESSENTIAL TO CARRY A MEDICAL IDENTIFICATION TAG AT ALL TIMES.

On the contrary, taking too little insulin, can result in high blood glucose or hyperglycemia. This can be corrected by administering additional insulin, commonly known as a corrective dose. The amount to take depends entirely on the level of blood glucose at the time of testing.

CHOOSING YOUR INSULIN: ANIMAL VS. GENETICALLY MODIFIED

The decision about what type of insulin to use should be based on personal need, potential side effects and personal preference.

Information about the availability and properties of synthetic insulin treatments should be available from your healthcare professional. On the contrary, information about natural animal insulin is not readily available. Consequently, many patients with diabetes are unable to make an informed choice of treatment between natural animal vs. genetically modified insulin.

WHAT ARE THE RISKS?

The long-term safety of insulin analogues has not been established.

The Cochrane Reviews, which are considered the highest standard of evidence-based health care, caution against the use of insulin analogues because of the lack of evidence of long-term safety [3].

Nevertheless, human insulin and insulin analogues are the most popular insulin medication, although a small number of people still prefer to use animal insulin

Exercise your choice.

It is important that people with diabetes are actively involved in deciding their treatment options and can ask for evidence to support any recommendations, especially if they wish to change their current insulin regime.

DIFFERENT TYPES OF INSULIN

The action of insulin will vary depend on the type of insulin used, its rate of absorption into the blood stream and also the sensitivity of the body's cells to insulin.

In order to resemble the natural insulin production of the pancreas, an effective insulin program must include both Basal and Bolus Insulin.

BASAL (BACKGROUND) INSULIN

Basal insulin is the foundation to every person's insulin regime. It can be administered via a pump, injection of medium or long acting insulin.

As previously discussed, one of the major roles of the liver is to store glucose as glycogen. Over the day, stored glucose is released steadily into the blood stream to provide the body's vital organs and tissues with a constant source of fuel.

In order for secreted glucose to make it into cells for energy and prevent the liver from dumping too much at once, the pancreas secretes an appropriate amount of insulin every few minutes into the bloodstream.

This is known as basal insulin and regulates blood glucose levels 24 hours a day. Basal insulin should be able to balance blood glucose levels in the absence of food, exercise and mealtime (fast acting) insulin.

In people with T1D or extreme cases of T2D, the pancreas loses its ability to produce insulin. Consequently, the liver continues to dump glucose without breaking, leading to chronic hyperglycemia.

BASAL INSULIN MUST BE IN EQUILIBRIUM WITH THE LIVER'S SECRETION OF GLUCOSE 24 HOURS A DAY.

Basal insulin needs are usually greatest during the night. This is due to an increase in counter-insulin hormones, such as growth hormone, and cortisol. Commonly, known as the 'dawn phenomenon', which results in an increase in blood glucose levels between the hours of 2am-8am.

Basal needs tend to be lower during the day due to increase insulin sensitivity that comes with day time physical activity, exercise and use of faster-acting bolus insulin. On the contrary basal needs can increase during the day with heightened levels of stress and illness.

BASAL INSULIN NEEDS ARE INFLUENCED BY THE BODY'S PRODUCTION OF OTHER HORMONES THAT INFLUENCE THE LIVER'S SECRETION OF GLUCOSE INTO THE BLOODSTREAM.

Basal Insulins come in a number of different forms, most notably Intermediate and long acting forms.

Different types of insulin can be used to stimulate the body's normal basal insulin secretion.

Before I outline the different types of basal insulin medication, it's important to understand the onset, peak and duration of insulin action.

Onset: When insulin starts to lower blood glucose.

Peak: When insulin has its greatest effect on blood glucose.

Duration: For how long the insulin has a blood glucose lowering effect.

Let's discuss the different types of basal insulin.

INTERMEDIATE ACTING INSULIN

- Taken once or twice a day to provide background insulin or alongside rapid-acting insulin.
- Sometimes used by carers to treat patients who have limited access to nursing facilities. For example, injecting intermediate insulin 4-6 hours prior to a meal or snack could eliminate the need to inject fasting acting insulin at the specific mealtime.
- Cloudy in appearance, and needs mixing to re-suspend.

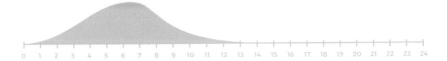

INTERMEDIATE ACTING INSULLIN (NPH OR ISOPHANE)

STARTS 1-2 HRS   PEAKS 4-8 HRS   LASTS 12-16 HRS

If you are using an NPH or any other pre-mixed insulin solution, ensure you have mixed the solution properly prior to administration. Since it's a peptide hormone, avoid shaking vigorously in case you damage the hormone. Instead, roll the premixed vial/pen gently until the solution appears evenly mixed.

Avoid contaminating vials of fast acting insulin with intermediate acting insulin.

LONG ACTING INSULIN

- Usually injected once a day and doesn't have a peak period of action.
- Many athletes and active gym goers actually inject this form of insulin twice a day for greater flexibility and blood glucose control.
- Doesn't have to be taken with food.
- Clear in appearance.
- Avoid mixing the two Insulins detemir (Levemir) and glargine (Lantus) together.

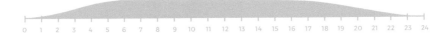

LONG ACTING BASAL INSULIN (DETEMIR/LEVEMIR)

STARTS 1-3 HRS   PEAKS MILDLY 6-12 HRS   LASTS 18-24 HRS

Use of basal insulin has minimal risk of hypoglycemia, due to its consistent absorption and lack of exact peak time.

Insulin pump users have the greatest degree of flexibility, as pump users can use small pulses of rapid acting insulin to stimulate the body's basal insulin needs. As a result, peak action times are less of an issue.

Changes can be made to basal dosing as and when needed, for situations like exercise, increased levels of stress and illness. More on this later.

BOLUS (MEALTIME) INSULIN

In response to meals, larger amounts of insulin are secreted to match the rise in blood glucose from the food that is eaten.

Carbohydrates have the most significant impact, compared to protein and fat, with protein having a mild effect.

In people without diabetes, bolus insulin is secreted in a number of phases. The first phase occurs with the first bite of food, additional phases occur over the next hour to three and a half hours. The amount of insulin released from the pancreas matches the rise in blood glucose from the food eaten.

Let's discuss the different types of bolus insulin available for diabetes treatment.

RAPID ACTING INSULIN

- Can be injected before, during or after food.
- Clear in appearance.
- Particularly useful when eating foods that spike blood glucose quickly, such as rapidly digesting sugars and starches.
- Also useful for quickly rectifying hyperglycemia.

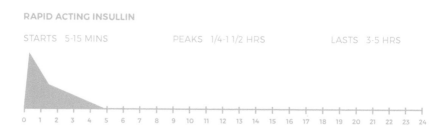

RAPID ACTING INSULLIN

STARTS 5-15 MINS   PEAKS 1/4-1 1/2 HRS   LASTS 3-5 HRS

0 1 2 3 4 5 6 7 8 9 10 11 12 13 14 15 16 17 18 19 20 21 22 23 24

SHORT ACTING (REGULAR) INSULIN

- Injected 15–30 minutes before a meal.
- Not usually the most practical insulin for meal times, due to its slower mode of action.
- Suitable for those with certain medical conditions associated with delayed gastric emptying.
- Clear in appearance.

SHORT ACTING INSULLIN (REGULAR)

STARTS 15-30 MINS   PEAKS 2-3 HRS   LASTS 4-6 HRS

0 1 2 3 4 5 6 7 8 9 10 11 12 13 14 15 16 17 18 19 20 21 22 23 24

Mixed analogues – These typically provide a 70/25 or 70/30 combination of intermediate and either short or rapid acting insulin.

HOW IS INSULIN DOSED?

Insulin is measured in units. Every unit will lower blood sugar the same amount irrelevant of what type of insulin used.

The only exceptions are:

- The long acting insulin known as detemir (Levemir), which is 25% less potent than normal insulin.
- Whether or not the insulin concentration has been diluted. Some people dilute their insulin to accommodate certain types of syringe. It can also be diluted for treating children who are very sensitive to insulin's effects.

INSULIN DELIVERY

Taking insulin is incredibly easy and safe nowadays. It can be administered with disposable, super thin needles or super convenient pre filled pens and automated pumps.

STRATEGIES FOR INJECTING INSULIN

Air Bubbles

If you use an injectable pen, syringe or pump, air bubbles are Inevitable. Miniscule bubbles aren't really an issue, however, larger bubbles can be a problem and jeopardize your ability to dose accurately.

Getting rid of large bubbles is important. If your using a pen or syringe:

- Position the needle upwards.
- Tap the device to bring the air bubble to the tip of the needle (or just below).
- Slowly press the plunger with your thumb or base of your hand and expel the trapped air into the atmosphere.
- You'll know it's been removed when insulin comes to the tip of the needle.

For pump users, large air bubbles in the reservoir are a problem if they enter the infusion line and replace insulin. You can get rid of these air bubbles by following a similar approach. Simply, hold the reservoir and position the needle upwards with the air bubble facing toward you. The plunger should be further away than the needle.

Tap the reservoir until the air bubble enters the neck of the reservoir, then squirt insulin to get rid of the air bubble.

Insulin at room temperature is less likely to cause bubbles.

Injection Site

The American Diabetes Association recommends Insulin is injected into the subcutaneous tissue of the upper arm and the front and side aspects of the thigh, buttocks, and abdomen (with the exception of a circle with a 2-inch radius around the navel) (4).

Intramuscular injection is not recommended for routine injections. However, individuals who are incredibly lean may have trouble accessing these recommended sites of subcutaneous tissue. They must find other suitable areas to administer under the guidance of their healthcare professional.

Problems with injection sites

One of the biggest problems I've seen with people using injectable insulin is the development of a condition called lipodystrophy, a problem relating to how the body produces, uses, and stores body fat.

Repeated injections and infusions (via pump) into the same area of skin can be responsible, resulting in fat beneath the skin swelling and going hard, almost like scar tissue. This can negatively affect the absorption of insulin, which inevitably leads to problems with blood glucose control.

Be mindful that different injection sites will result in different speeds of action. How fast you need your insulin to act is entirely dependent on your individual circumstances.

Think before injecting, not after.

Injecting insulin into a trained or pre-trained muscle group will increase its speed of action, regardless of insulin type. This is a result of increased blood flow around the area.

For individuals that are incredibly lean, such as completive level bodybuilders. Injecting into subcutaneous fat tissue may be difficult, especially If sub 10 % body fat. I've been in this scenario a number of times.

The only solution I found was to pinch as much skin as possible in areas like the thigh or buttocks, where the last remaining bits of body fat tend to lie. Shooting in the abdominals was nothing but painful especially if you nabbed a vein close to the surface of the skin, which tend to surface more the leaner you get.

There were many times I simply had to inject into muscle.

I don't recommend this unless you have discussed a valid strategy and reasoning with your healthcare professional. Great care and consideration must be taken especially if you're an ultra-lean, well-muscled, highly trained person in a hypocaloric state.

Always keep your injection sites clean. I use a disinfectant soap daily during showering to keep my skin hygienically clean.

Storage

Insulin is a peptide-based hormone and must be stored in a cold, dry place (but not frozen).

Since insulin is a protein, excess heat and/or sunlight can de-nature the hormone, alerting its structure and rendering it less effective or in extreme cases ineffective. This can lead to hyperglycemia.

Generally speaking, most insulin can be kept at room temperature for up to 30 days. But, in order to keep it fresh, it's best to keep it cool and return to the fridge when not in use.

I've found the best place to store insulin is in the egg section of a fridge or pull out drawers. If you're on holiday, pop your device in a glass of ice (in a sealed zip up bag) and tuck it in the shade (under the sunbed or drinks table).

Do not use insulin that is out of date or strange looking in appearance. Also, bear in mind every time you pierce the rubber stopper, there is some chance germs may enter the vial or end up inside the needle. Keep your hands and injectable equipment as clean as possible.

Other Modes of Insulin Administration

Besides injection, there are many other ways to take insulin.

THE PUMP (CLOSED-LOOP ARTIFICIAL PANCREAS)

The convenience of intravenous blood glucose sensing and insulin delivery is the main concept behind the development of the closed-loop artificial pancreas.

The closed loop system includes a subcutaneous continuous glucose monitor (CGM), which senses blood glucose levels in real time.

This data is fed back to another device known as a continuous subcutaneous insulin infusion pump (CSII), which requires the insertion of a temporary thin tube into the subcutaneous tissue.

Insulin pumps, are battery powered devices that slowly infuse insulin into the body. They are well suited to patients who have trouble managing their blood glucose levels or don't like to use needles.

There are many benefits to using a pump including:

- **More flexible living**: Less hassle of injecting in public.
- **Precise dosing**: Pumps can dose insulin to the nearest .025, .05 or.1 of a unit – meaning less chance of overdosing and going low.
- **Finer tuned adjustment**: During periods of stress, illness, growth and menstruation
- **Measurement of data**: Pumps sync an abundance of blood glucose readings and behavior over smartphone and computer. This allows for accurate assessment and review of treatment strategies.

Invented at Guy's Hospital in London, the concept for the pumps is based on methods to infuse parathyroid hormone into dogs and other animals.

Insulin is delivered via a flexible plastic tube and an associated needle called an infusion set. Infusion sets must be changed every couple of days to prevent clogging and/or infection.

The infusion sets are typically worn on the abs, buttocks or upper thigh (around the hip). Most infusion sets have a disconnect feature that allows the pump device and tubes to be rapidly disconnected for life events like showering, sex or exercise. Most modern day pumps have built in safety features to prevent accidental dosing, if the device where to get knocked accidently. They are also water proof.

PUMP THERAPY ALLOWS INSULIN DOSES TO BE GIVEN AT THE TOUCH OF A BUTTON, WITHOUT THE NEED FOR A PHYSICAL INJECTION.

Depending on the type of insulin pump used, blood glucose data from a CGM can be fed to an external device such as a smart phone, read and used to determine insulin dosing either manually or automatically.

Automated (artificial pancreas) pumps with built in algorithms can automatically adjust the rate of insulin delivery based on the blood glucose data from the CGM.

Background insulin levels (basal) can be adjusted more easily than they can from multiple daily injections (MDI), as there is a variable infusion of both rapid and slow acting insulin compared to one large bolus of long acting insulin like that used in MDI.

During exercise, individuals need to make adjustments to their insulin dose so that it resembles normal physiological conditions. I discuss this in greater detail in the exercise section of the book.

Low-intensity exercise is renowned for lowering blood glucose. Therefore, a reduction in insulin infusion may be required. On the contrary, high-intensity exercise such as weight lifting is well known to increase blood glucose levels, which justifies an increase in insulin infusion during training sessions.

The practicality, usability and simplicity of the closed-loop artificial pancreas make it a promising investment to a large segment of the T1D population and those living with T2D who require insulin.

However, the closed-loop artificial pancreas does have problems. The ever-changing fluctuations in blood glucose pose a challenge for these devices to work flawlessly. A user must be prepared to make a lot of adjustments until they find a schedule that works.

The causes of rising and falling blood glucose levels in T1D vary according to circumstances.

One of the biggest problems with pump users is mechanical fault or the pump being physically ripped off. I tell all my pump wearing clients to be careful in the gym, especially if they are wearing a weight lifting or dipping belt. The obvious side effects of this are hyperglycemia and ketoacidosis. They rarely occur in those using long or intermediate acting insulins as there is always insulin in the blood stream.

Insulin Patches are at an early stage of research. They aim to painlessly infuse insulin through the skin and into the bloodstream, similar to how nicotine patches work.

Prometheon, a US company, is currently developing the TruePatch.
The patch, which is about the size of a small coin, is covered with hundreds of tiny micro needles pre-loaded with insulin and glucose-sensing enzymes that sense increases in blood glucose, and then release insulin into the blood stream.

The patches have already been shown to lower blood glucose in mice with T1D for up to nine hours (5). More pre-clinical tests and subsequent clinical trials in humans will be required before the patch can be administered to patients, but this approach shows great promise. (5)

Inhaled insulin delivers insulin in a dry powder. It is inhaled through the mouth directly into the lungs, where it passes into the bloodstream.

A 2007 review concluded that an inhaled brand of insulin called Exubera appeared to be as effective, but no better than injected short-acting insulin. That inhaled brands cost more means they are unlikely to become cost-effective treatments (6) and there is currently no inhaled insulin available on prescription just yet.

ARTIFICIAL PANCREAS IMPLANTS

Development and pre-clinical trials on an artificial pancreas are currently taking place.

The device, made from a unique form of metal would contain a few weeks supply of insulin and be implanted into the body between the lowest rib and hip.

A layer of special glucose-sensing gel around the casing of the device controls the release of stored insulin into the blood supply around the gut and then into the vein to the liver, mimicking the normal process for a person with a healthy pancreas.

As the insulin lowers the glucose level in the body, the gel reacts by hardening again and stopping the supply.

The device requires no electronics, meaning the risk of rejection by the body is minimised.

Professor Joan Taylor from Leicester's De Montfort University (DMU) is the leading scientist behind the device. She claims the artificial pancreas will help all people living with T1D and some T2D sufferers who require insulin.

TAKE HOME MESSAGE

The optimal dosing strategy for insulin has not been identified and will likely vary from person to person.

Consequently, any mode of insulin therapy used must be modified carefully.

Key factors that influence insulin dosage:

Body Composition Change
- Recent muscle gain/loss
- Recent fat gain/fat loss

Day to Day Living
- Dietary intake
- Gastrointestinal dysmotility
- Work days vs. non-work days
- Night shift work - sleep deprivation
- Training days vs. non-training days
- Alcohol ingestion
- Illness
- Other medications
- Stress

Life Cycle Related Events
- Puberty
- Menstruation
- Pregnancy
- Menopause
- Post-Menopause

Other Factors
- Body temperature especially injection site
- Environment temperature

METFORMIN (GLUCOPHAGE/GLUMETZA)

Metformin is a diabetic medication that is considered the first and best line of treatment for T2D. It makes your body more sensitive to insulin while at the same time telling your liver to suppress glucose production.

It is considered cheap and safe and is linked to having a modest impact on weight loss (7) or is at least weight-neutral. It has also been shown to increase ovulation in those suffering from PCOS and can, therefore, help with fertility (8).

It is available in different forms depending on the country you live in. The options include tablets for immediate release (up to three times a day) or prolonged release (usually once a day), and as an oral solution for those who cannot swallow.

Metformin is also sometimes combined with other diabetes medicines to treat the disease in two different ways. The combinations include: metformin + pioglitazone, metformin + vildagliptin and metformin + sitagliptin

Metformin is taken with a meal. Many people forget their tablets and often end up consuming an extra meal to take their tablets.

Side Effects

Diarrhoea is a common side effect of metformin. Some people find taking it with or after food helps to reduce the chances of this happening.

SULFONYLUREAS/MEGLITINIDES/SECRETAGOGUES

These medicines stimulate the pancreas to release insulin. They are only useful in people with T2D whose beta cells still produce insulin.

Although sulfonylureas stimulate the release of insulin, they do not reduce insulin resistance, which is a common feature of T2D.

Sulfonylureas medication is known to cause weight gain in patients.

Side Effects

Weight gain is the most noticeable side effect of sulfonylureas.

The drugs can also cause hypoglycemia, which can be severe and long-lasting.

Sulfonylureas are excreted from the body by the kidneys. If kidney function decreases, this may lead to increased levels of the medicine in the blood, which can increase the risk of side effects.

Other drugs such as fluconazole (Diflucan) may interfere with the breakdown of sulfonylureas, which can lead to increased levels of sulfonylureas in the blood and therefore increase the chances of hypoglycemia and weight gain.

ALPHA-GLUCOSIDASE INHIBITOR

This comes in a tablet form called Acarbose and is used in the treatment of T2D.

Acarbose works by slowing down the absorption of starchy foods from the intestine. Consequently, blood glucose levels rise more slowly after a meal.

It is critical to take each dose with the first bite of each main meal. It is usually taken three times a day.

Side Effects

When used in conjunction with insulin and other diabetes medicines, Acarbose can cause excessive lowering of blood glucose and hypoglycemia. The drug can also cause bloating and wind.

PRANDIAL GLUCOSE REGULATORS

This medication stimulates cells in the pancreas to secrete more insulin. Their rapid onset and short duration mean they need to be taken prior to eating.

If you miss a meal, the dose must be omitted. Prandial glucose regulators can be taken up to three times daily.

Two generic forms are Repaglinide and Nateglinide.

Side Effects

When used in conjunction with insulin and other diabetes medicines, this particular class of drug can cause excessive lowering of blood glucose and hypoglycemia.

THIAZOLIDINEDIONES (PIOGLITAZONE)

The only version of this class of drug is a tablet called Pioglitazone, which improves the sensitivity of cells to insulin. This reduces the burden on cells in the pancreas and allows them to carry on producing insulin.

Pioglitazone can be taken once or twice daily with or without food.

Side Effects

Thiazolidinediones can cause weight gain due to excessive water retention. This may pose problems for people with cardiovascular conditions.

When used in conjunction with insulin and other diabetes medicines this particular class of drug can cause excessive lowering of blood glucose and hypoglycemia.

INCRETIN MIMETICS

Incretin mimetics are a group of medications that increase levels of hormones called incretins. These metabolic hormones help the body produce more insulin and stimulate a decrease in blood glucose levels.

They can influence appetite and the rate at which the stomach digests food and empties. Incretin mimetics are only used to treat T2D.

GLUCAGON-LIKE-PEPTIDE 1(GLP-1)

GLP-1 is an injectable medication that provides benefits to those with T2D.

GLP-1 is a hormone produced in the gastrointestinal tract. It encourages the pancreas to produce more insulin and suppress the counter-regulatory hormone glucagon, which opposes insulin action and increases blood sugar. GLP-1 has also been shown to suppress hunger levels in the brain and how quickly food leaves your stomach (gastric emptying) to make you feel fuller (more satiated).

When you have T2D your body produces less GLP-1. Medication is, therefore, a tactical replacement. There are various types of GLP-1 medication available on the market.

The drug liraglutide (brand name Victoza) is injected once daily and has been shown to aid weight loss. Alternatively, if you want to avoid the hassle of daily injections you can have a weekly injection of dulaglutide (brand name Trulicity). Earlier forms of the drug involved twice-daily injections.

Side Effects

Transient nausea has been the most frequently reported adverse effect [9].

DPP-4 INHIBITORS (DIPEPTIDYL PEPTIDASE-4)

DPP-4 inhibitors are another relatively new class of diabetes medication. As the name implies, they inhibit an enzyme called DPP-4, which breaks down the hormone GLP-1, which helps your pancreas produce more insulin and less glucagon. GLP-1 also slows gastric emptying, which leaves you feeling fuller for longer. Taking a DPP-4 inhibitor means the naturally occurring GLP-1 your body produces will last for longer, thus increasing its effects.

A meta-analysis of 13 studies into the treatment of all three DPP-4 inhibitors found the effect of this group of drugs on weight to be neutral [10,11].

The names of this class of drug include Sitagliptin, Januvia, Janumet, Vildagliptin, Galvus, Eucreas, Saxagliptin, Onglyza, Alogliptin, Vipidia, Vipdomet, Linagliptin, Trajenta, Jentadueto. There are also combined versions of the drug available with metformin (as mentioned above).

Side Effects

Nasopharyngitis (inflamed nasal passages), nausea, heart failure, joint pain and skin reactions have all been observed in clinical studies [12].

SGLT2D INHIBITORS (SODIUM-GLUCOSE COTRANSPORTER-2)

SGLT2D inhibitors are a relatively new class of drugs in the management of T2D. They decrease the amount of glucose absorbed in the kidneys and encourage excretion via urine.

Generic names for this class of drug include Dapagliflozin, Canagliflozin and Empagliflozin. There are also combined versions of the drug available with metformin.

Side Effects

Your urine will test positive for glucose while you are on this medication. There is also a risk of genital and urinary tract infections. People with T2D have also reported cases of diabetes ketoacidosis.

TZDS (THIAZOLIDINEDIONES)

These medicines reduce insulin resistance in muscle and fat. They also decrease levels of glucose produced by the liver. The two medicines in this class are pioglitazone (Actos) and rosiglitazone (Avandia), which has been withdrawn from the market due to links with heart problems.

Side Effects

These medications can lead to weight gain, often due to excess fluid retention, which may result in further health complications. Other studies have suggested increased risk of coronary heart disease and osteoporosis with rosiglitazone [13]. The drug is currently withdrawn for diabetes treatment.

NEWER (EXPERIMENTAL) TREATMENTS

ISLET TRANSPLANTATION

Islet cell transplantation involves the transfer of specific islet cells from an organ donor into the body of someone else.

Once the cells are transplanted, the islets begin to produce insulin, actively regulating the level of glucose in the blood. If this procedure proves successful, a person living with T1D may be able to live without daily insulin injections

Experimental research carried out in rats, dogs, monkeys and humans is promising. The main implication of treatment is the requirement to take immunosuppressant drugs to prevent the rejection of the implanted cells. Also, in many human studies, the transplants continued functioning for longer when some insulin continued to be injected.

GENE THERAPY

Experimental gene therapy research has been successful in animal research.

Although in its infancy, scientists anticipate gene therapy will one day free people from the ill effects and hassle of managing diabetes.

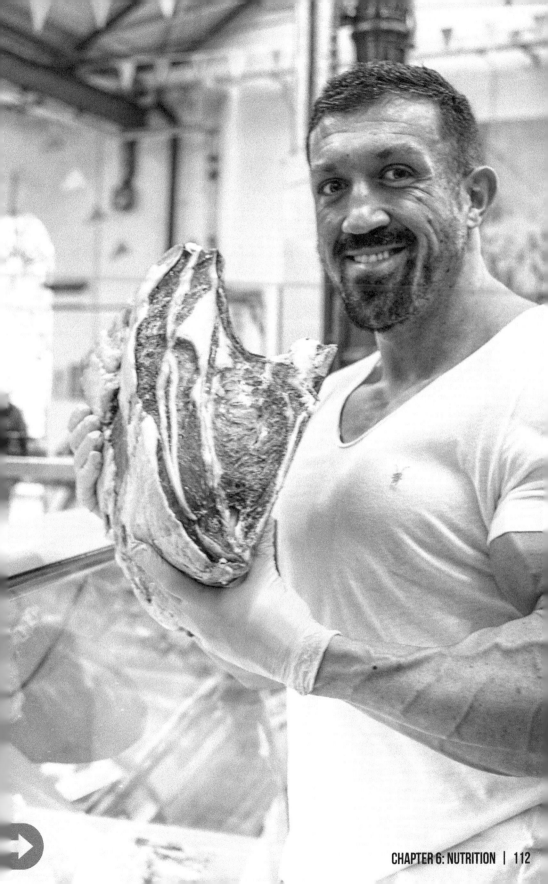

CHAPTER 6: NUTRITION

DIABETIC NUTRITION

The weight of evidence supporting the key role nutrition plays in good health, growth, reproduction and disease is overwhelming.

We live in a time of mass information and mega confusion around what to eat and what not to eat. Nutrition is a hugely debated subject rife with conflicting advice and misinformation.

At the same time there's a tremendous amount of suffering and ill health as a result of our relationship with food. Nutrition-related diseases, such as obesity and T2D are on the rise, along with increased concerns about body image and eating disorders.

Every week you hear about a new diet plan, app or supplement that promises the world but fails to deliver.

The problem is, many of our dietary strategies are unsustainable. They force restriction, over-exercise and under-eating, driving our bodies into emotional and physical submission.

This chapter is all about food and how to eat for a healthier, stronger and better-looking body. Make no mistake, I won't bombard you with another dull diet plan that dictates what and when to eat. Nor will I encourage you to follow a dietary fad or system that's impossible to stick to.

I'll be showing you how to build your own diet from the plate up, assess its effectiveness and fine-tune it to your exact goals and personal lifestyle. Most importantly, every nutritional aspect will be discussed in the context of T1D and T2D diabetes, which is often overlooked in mainstream media.

There is zero fluff and zero gimmicks over the course of this chapter. I have incorporated as much scientific evidence as possible, instead of doing what most do in the fitness industry: make bold claims using my imagination and thin air. I've also tied in my own personal experiences of eating and living with diabetes.

AS PREVIOUSLY MENTIONED, NONE OF THE ADVICE CONTAINED WITHIN THIS RESOURCE IS INDENTED TO REPLACE THAT OF YOUR MEDICAL PROFESSIONAL. IT IS MERELY OPINION BASED ON THE CURRENT BODY OF SCIENTIFIC EVIDENCE.

DIABETES AND NUTRITION: KEY GOALS

Before we get into the nuts and bolts of nutrition, let's review the fundamental goals of diabetic nutrition, many of which are shared by T1D and T2D diabetes.

- Promote glycemic control short and long term.
- Ensure the necessary medication is taken for specific quantities of food.
- Consider pre-existing medical conditions that may influence food intake, and make the necessary adjustments or exclusions.
- Promote healthy body composition.
- Meet essential nutrient requirements and prevent deficiencies.
- Promote long term dietary adherence by taking into account personal food preference, cultural beliefs, food accessibility/storage, cooking skills and affordability.

A nutrition strategy that accomplishes these goals will undoubtedly improve your quality of life.

This chapter covers pretty much everything you need to know about diabetic muscle building and fat loss nutrition.

We'll look at the following areas:

- What is nutrition?
- Why most diets fail.
- Adherence – the secret to dietary success
- Energy balance.
- Macronutrients – foods, facts and functions.
- Nutrient timing
- A step-by-step guide on how to build your diet from the plate up.
- Supplements.

UNDERSTANDING NUTRITION

You Are What You Eat, Breakdown, Absorb and Don't Excrete

You could say the second process of digestion (after chewing) is nutrition.

Every time we consume food, our bodies undertake a wide range of physical and chemical processes to extract nutrients and utilise them properly.

These key processes include:

- **Nutrient Absorption & Assimilation**

How much of the food you eat ends up being used by the body? The answer depends on two processes.

Absorption of key (macro)nutrients, vitamins, minerals and other chemicals from food within the gastrointestinal tract (the gut). This is achieved by both chemical (enzymes, acids) and physical (chewing/stomach churning) breakdown.

Once absorbed, some nutrients can either be utilised straight away or undergo processing in the liver for more effective use. This process is known as assimilation.

A HEALTHY GUT IS ESSENTIAL WHEN IT COMES TO GETTING THE MOST OUT OF YOUR FOOD.

- **Anabolism (Building Processes)**

This complex process, which is also known as biosynthesis, occurs when specific building block substrates like glucose and amino acids are converted into more complex products within the body.

This process includes the growth of new proteins, cells, substances and energy stores within the body.

Nutrition plays a vital role in providing the building blocks for such anabolic processes to occur.

Individuals looking to improve the look of their body should strongly focus on promoting anabolism (growth and repair) of muscle tissue. At the same time they should also seek to guard against the muscle breakdown effects of catabolism.

- **Catabolism (Breakdown Processes)**

Catabolism relates to specific processes within the body that are responsible for the breakdown of molecules, cells and tissues into smaller units for energy or other reactions. This can include muscle mass, fat tissue and bone.

Most people consider catabolism as an unwanted or unhealthy process. However, it depends entirely on the context.

Catabolism involves the breakdown of body fuel stores, including stored carbohydrate (glycogen) and stored body fat. It is also vital in muscle tissue remodelling, an important adaptation to resistance training.

Muscle breakdown is an unfavourable catabolic scenario hard training individuals seek to avoid.

Besides improving aesthetics and performance, enhanced muscle mass elevates your metabolic rate, increases glucose uptake, and reduces the risk of obesity, which are all of particular interest to a person living with diabetes.

Muscle loss is the result of prolonged energy deficit, the absence of resistance training and poorly controlled diabetes, as discussed earlier.

- **Excretion**

Every human body rids itself of waste, including the harmful and non-harmful products of digestion and other bodily processes.

Regarding nutrition, you lose and don't reabsorb what you excrete.

Individuals with poorly controlled diabetes will excrete key nutrients through their urine, including glucose and vital minerals like magnesium, calcium, potassium, zinc, chromium and selenium.

Kidney disease, an unfortunate complication caused by poorly controlled diabetes, can cause the loss of other nutrients, such as protein, through urine.

You could say diabetes is a disease of undernutrition.

FOOD IS INFORMATION

Food provides information to our bodies. This information depends on two key factors:

- **Quantity** – The total amount of food you consume, but especially energy (calories).

Our bodies need a specific amount of energy to function on a day-to-day basis. The amount needed varies from person to person. Our bodies don't respond well to massive quantities of food and excess energy, which can lead to obesity and all its nasty complications.

On the contrary, too little food can result in malnutrition, starvation and eventually death.

The balance of energy must be just right for our bodies to thrive.

- **Source** – The composition of the food sources you consume.

Where energy comes from is just as important as how much you consume. Every food you eat has a unique profile of nutrients, all of which serve different roles within the body. These include everything from the growth of muscle tissue right through to the production of hormones.

Some nutrients are essential; some are not. But they all provide a unique message to the body.

Let's look at this in detail.

UNDERSTANDING FOOD QUANTITY

Quantity in this context refers to the amount of energy you take in via food and drink.

The energy obtained from food is measured in calories (or, in some countries, kilojoules). Calories are often written as kcal/Cal on food packaging.

We've all heard the saying: a calorie is a calorie.

Is this really true?

Well, it depends. Let me explain...

In food science, yes, a calorie is a calorie.

Calories provide energy in the form of heat.

A calorie is defined as the amount of energy needed to raise 1 gram of water by 1 °C.

Scientists measure the amount of heat produced by completely incinerating food in a small airtight oven submerged in water. This device is known as a bomb calorimeter. The only variable is the type of food being burnt. Higher calorie foods burn more energy and give off more heat.

Each macronutrient yields its own unique amount of energy. Fat is the most energetic.

- Protein   4 kcals/gram
- Carbohydrate *   4 kcals/gram
- Fat   9 kcals/gram
- Alcohol   7 kcals/gram

It has been suggested that soluble fibre provides 2.75 kcal/g.

HUMAN BODIES AREN'T AS EFFICIENT AT USING ENERGY AS A BOMB CALORIMETER.

Human bodies aren't as efficient at using energy as a bomb calorimeter.

A variety of factors determine how food calories are processed by our bodies, including the source of calories (macronutrients), the timing of food, glycemic control and many other factors outside of our control.

We use energy for various functions ranging from moving and thinking to producing hormones and building muscle.

Some calories yield energy more efficiently than others, whilst other calories fill us up and reduce the desire to eat more calories, consequently lowering energy intake.

Individually each factor may not account for much but when added up over time they can have a huge impact on energy balance and your ability to get lean, build muscle and perform your best.

NOT ALL CALORIES ARE THE SAME.

I talk in greater detail about this throughout the chapter and highlight key strategies you can use to manipulate macronutrients in your favor, especially when it comes to building muscle and maximising fat loss.

ENERGY BALANCE - WHY CALORIES MATTER

Before you select the exact amounts, formulas and ratios of macronutrients you consume, you must first understand the concept of energy balance.

This refers to the balance of energy consumed from food against the energy burned from physical activity and other bodily processes.

Energy balance influences body composition management and your ability to perform work, especially exercise.

Energy balance is said to be at a steady state if you are neither gaining nor losing weight over prolonged periods of time.

Weight loss or gain is a result of days, weeks and months of being in a positive or negative energy balance.

There is a big difference between weight loss vs fat loss and weight gain vs. muscle gain.

It's amazing to see so many people chasing the single goal of weight loss or weight gain with no clear interest in what is lost or gained.

To gain weight, you must consume more energy (calories) than you burn (to create an energy surplus).

The size of the surplus will influence the rate and also the quality of weight gained.

Generally speaking, weight gain comes in the form of fat, glycogen (stored carbohydrate), water retention and muscle protein (if an adequate training stimulus is provided).

The primary focus of any weight gain strategy should be lean muscle. Fat gain is inevitable when an energy surplus occurs but should be kept to an absolute minimum for health and aesthetic reasons except in people who are extremely underweight.

FOCUS ON MUSCLE GAIN NOT WEIGHT GAIN.

DIABETES AND WEIGHT GAIN

Not everyone living with diabetes needs to lose weight. Some people have the opposite problem: being underweight and having little muscle mass. Eating calorie-dense food, like cakes, buns and crisps may seem like a good idea to fill out your frame but it isn't the best or healthiest option, especially if you have diabetes.

WHEN TRYING TO GAIN WEIGHT BLOOD GLUCOSE LEVELS MUST BE CONTROLLED.

No matter how many calories you eat, if blood glucose levels are always running high, as a result of poor food choices or not being able to match insulin doses with dietary carbohydrate, your body will fail to hold on to what you feed it. As hyperglycemia progresses, the body perceives it's starving. The cells cannot use the glucose that is building up in the bloodstream – glucose and its calories are wasted via the urine. And hyperglycemia is catabolic to both fat and protein tissues so instead of storing weight, you end up losing weight.

To Lose Weight you must burn more calories than you consume.

This creates an energy deficit, which promotes the use of stored body energy for fuel, notably fat and stored carbohydrates in the liver and muscles.

Calorie deficits must never be too extreme or else they will result in muscle loss, a reduction in performance and undesirable changes in body chemistry.

Focus on fat loss not weight loss.

ALL POPULAR FAT LOSS DIETS INVOLVE CALORIE RESTRICTION

All popular fat loss diets get you to the same place – negative energy balance.

They all help you lose weight. However, you must always question their sustainability over the long term.

Let's review some of the most popular diets and see how they go about achieving caloric restriction.

LOW CARB DIETS

Low carb diets are a broad category and there is no universal agreement on what characterises them. The Institute of Medicine describes 45-65% of total energy as the appropriate carbohydrate intake for adults [1]. Therefore anything below 45% may be considered a low carb diet, although many advocate much lower carbohydrate intakes of less than 140g per day, or even 25-50g or less.

Regardless, reducing the amount of food consumed from carbohydrates will automatically lower calorie intake.

The calories lost from carbohydrate may be replaced by calories from protein. Protein has the greatest effect on fullness (satiety), meaning it reduces hunger and you eat less. Protein also requires more metabolic energy from the body to digest and use via the thermic effect of feeding, which means merely eating it instead of carbohydrate increases calorie expenditure.

KETOGENIC DIETS

Ketogenic diets have been shown to better suppress appetite than low-energy diets [2]. They involve eating fewer carbs, which leads to an energy deficit that is hard to make up even with the consumption of extra fat and protein, hence weight loss.

The efficacy of low carb/ketogenic diets at reversing and controlling T2D has divided the nutrition community. A recent critical review of low carbohydrate diets in people with T2D found no significant difference between low carbohydrate diets and high carbohydrate diets at improving metabolic markers and glycemic control. [3] Ultimately it seems that whatever diet is best for a person to achieve their goal is the one that counts.

We also need to question the sustainability of low carbohydrate/ketogenic diets over the medium and long-term. Failing to adhere to it beyond the short-term will undermine the ability to treat obesity and T2D and may render this approach more of a hindrance than an aid, especially if there is a rebound in eating habits and weight gain on cessation.

It's almost impossible to have a person with T1D follow a ketogenic diet because of the unpredictable fluctuations in blood sugar, episodes of hypoglycemia (that need to be treated with carbohydrate) and lack of biological feedback on the liver's rate of glucose production.

THE PALEO DIET

Paleo diets are associated with a high amount of fibre and protein, which reduces hunger and elevates the metabolism through the consumption of protein. This can be a sensible approach, as it can mean an increase in fresh foods, especially vegetables. However, some versions of paleo diets exclude an unhelpful amount of foods and food groups.

The word paleo, has also been played upon by food marketers, amplifying the price of common food products two or three times the norm. When was the last time you found a paleo brownie lying in the forest? My guess, never. Oh, and paleo protein powder, really?

LOW FAT DIETS

Reducing fat, the most calorific macronutrient at 9 kcal per gram, will undoubtedly result in lower energy intake.

Add exercise to any of the above approaches and the deficit gets even deeper.

Take Home: Energy Intake Matters

Regardless of what type of diet you follow, there is a myriad of evidence to support the idea that total energy intake is a far more important predictor of bodyweight.

Because not all calories are equal it is important to consider their individual roles in boosting the metabolism via the thermogenic effect of feeding, increasing metabolically active muscle tissue and influencing appetite.

METABOLIC RATE

Before we get into establishing a ballpark level of maintenance calories let's first review the key metabolic processes that use energy within the body.

Let's also highlight how certain macronutrients can influence these processes, which reinforces my earlier point that a calorie is not just a calorie in respect of nutrition.

The key processes that govern our total daily energy expenditure include:

- **Basal Metabolic Rate (BMR)**

This is the minimal energy requirement of the body at complete rest before eating, moving or exercising (bed bound) at room temperature.

At rest, the body requires fuel to run all its essential systems, which include the central nervous system, the reproductive system and everything else in between.

One of the most significant factors influencing resting metabolic rate is body composition, notably lean body mass [4].

Firstly, muscle tissue is more metabolically active than fat tissue, burning an additional 6kcals per day for every 1lb gained compared to 2kcals per day per 1lb of fat [5].

More importantly, increased muscle mass leads to increased force production and performance, which leads to increased calorie expenditure both during and after exercise when recovering.

Just think of the energy requirements needed to train with and recover from 100kg for x1 rep compared to 100kg for x10 reps. Ten times as much.

The extra muscle tissue is also more metabolically advantageous, since it will act as a larger reservoir to store glucose in the form of glycogen. The average person can store around 300-500g of muscle glycogen (females lower end). The more muscle though, the greater capacity for storage.

This is one of the main reasons why adding muscle mass via strength training and elevated intake of protein is favorable for fat loss.

A number of other factors influence metabolic rate, including:

- **Age** – Metabolic rate has been shown to decline with age. A large factor here is reduced muscle mass and hormones that drive metabolic rate.
- **Gender** – Males tend to have naturally higher levels of muscle than females.
- **Weight Gain** – Sudden weight gain increases energy expenditure.
- **Stress & Anxiety** – Can cause a rapid increase in stress hormones that influence energy expenditure.
- **Hormones** – A rise in certain hormones can elevate metabolic rate. Key examples include thyroid hormone and testosterone.
- **Temperature** – A colder environment can lead to increased energy expenditure.
- **Hereditary factors** – Differences in genes can affect metabolic rate. Diabetes is an example of this.

Most moderately active individuals will burn about 60%-75% of their total energy intake from their basal metabolic rate (6).

Once you have established your BMR you then need to consider all the other variables that influence how energy is used and expended throughout the body. This includes everything from the digestion of food to the decision to enter the gym.

- **The Thermogenic Effect of Feeding (TEF)**

This relates to the amount of energy burned during the digestion and metabolism of food. It usually equates to around 10% of total calories consumed daily by individuals who eat a well balanced mixed macronutrient diet including carbohydrate, fats and protein (7). Practically speaking, if you eat on average 2500 kcals per day (from mixed macros), around 250 kcal will be burned off via the TEF.

Protein alone requires significantly more energy to process compared to carbohydrate and fat at 15-25% of total energy, compared to 5% from fat and carbs.

- **Thermic Effect of Activity (TEA).**

One of the main factors in determining energy expenditure is your level of physical activity.

There is Exercise-associated thermogenesis (EAT) and Non-exercise activity thermogenesis (NEAT)

THE MORE YOU MOVE THROUGHOUT THE DAY, THE MORE ENERGY YOU WILL BURN.

EXERCISE-ASSOCIATED THERMOGENESIS (EAT)

People who exercise burn off increasingly more energy than those who don't. Exercise type, duration and frequency determine how much energy is used.

Certain types of exercise, like weight training and high intensity cardio have the ability to burn energy even after they're been completed.

DAILY ACTIVITY - NON-EXERCISE ACTIVITY THERMOGENESIS (NEAT)

Someone who is desk-bound for 8-10 hours a day will burn significantly less energy than someone who does manual work. It has been suggested that the obesity epidemic may be a reflection of our recently emerged and growing seated culture. A sitting body does not expend as much energy. The signals and calorie demand of a moving body literally turn off.

OBESITY AND SEDENTARY BEHAVIOR (SITTING) GO HAND IN HAND.

A highly active, heavier individual will burn more energy than a highly active lighter individual who performs the same level of activity. You are moving the entirety of your bodyweight, after all.

PEOPLE WITH LOW LEVELS OF NON-EXERCISE ACTIVITY ARE PREDISPOSED TO OBESITY.

A simple way to assess your day-to-day activity is to use a pedometer. Someone who moves 2,000 steps will burn less energy than someone who performs 10,000 steps.

NEAT also includes subconscious activities like fidgeting, coughing and other random movements throughout the day (8). They can differ greatly from individual to individual – think lazy vs. hyperactive.

IF YOU SIT FOR MOST OF THE DAY AND EXERCISE 4-5 TIMES A WEEK YOU ARE NOT PHYSICALLY ACTIVE OUTSIDE OF TRAINING.

- Non-Exercise Physical Activity (NEPA) – (Inclusive of TEA)

This refers to the amount of energy or calories burned through intentional movements, such as carrying the shopping or helping move furniture.

IS THERE SUCH A THING AS A 'SLOW METABOLISM'?

"I can't lose weight, because I have a slow metabolism".

Is there really any truth to this?

While there may be an element of truth to 'slow metabolisms' in those suffering from hypothyroidism, most people merely use it as a scape goat for poor results.

An interesting review by Donahoo and colleagues investigated the 'slow metabolism' myth and found that at a given body weight, the difference in energy burnt from person to person for vital day to day body functions is around 100-300kcal per day [9].

As I'm sure you'll agree this is only a small factor at play with regards resting metabolic rate and demonstrates that having a "slow metabolism" is at the most part, a poor excuse for ones lack of fat loss.

More important factors like 'non-exercise activity thermogenesis (NEAT)', frequency of hypoglycemia (need to eat), are more reliable predictors for ones predisposition to weight gain and slow rates of fat loss.

CALCULATING INDIVIDUAL ENERGY NEEDS

Trying to match your calorie expenditure to your actual calorie intake is extremely hard due to daily variations in health, mood, behavior, and changes in bodyweight over time.

You will always be estimating how many calories you burn off on a day-to-day basis, no matter what the most expensive Fitbit or Apple watch may tell you.

The only true way to measure resting metabolic rate and daily energy expenditure is by sitting in a direct calorimeter. Similar to a bomb calorimeter, but modelled like a bedroom.

The subject sits inside the chamber for a period of time, and the amount of heat they give off is measured. They can be sitting, running or performing any activity they like, but it must be within the chamber.

Although accurate, this procedure is limited to a testing environment and is not practical to body weight management. In all my years I have never come across anyone who is willing to live in one of these small chambers during the duration of a fat loss or muscle building goal. The chambers also cost a fortune, and are often difficult for the general public to get hold of.

Indirect calorimetry is another option. Although it doesn't measure energy expenditure directly, it gives an indication of how much energy somebody uses based on the proportion of air (O_2 & CO_2) breathed in and out.

I'll stop there, as not many of you will be have access to equipment that measures gaseous exchange 24 hours a day.

ARE CALORIE PREDICTION EQUATIONS ACCURATE?

Not entirely, however they do provide a great place to start when determining calorie intake.

Not everyone realises that popular calorie prediction tools, such as the Mifflin-St Jeor or Harris-Benedict formulas are based on set population samples measured using direct calorimetry in isolated experiments.

Their use has been scaled to the real world, but they fail to take into account the ever-changing calorie demands of day-to-day life.

Once a set calorie intake has been trialed, it can be adjusted accordingly to better suit individual needs and rate of progress. I provide step-by-step instructions on structuring calories and macronutrients in the building your diet section of the text and the online calculator found at

www.diabeticmuscleandfitness.com

GENERAL STAGES OF BUILDING A DIET

1. Estimate Total Calories

2. Set Protein Intake

3. Set Fat Intake

4. Fill Remaining Calories with Carbs

5. Adjust Based on Response

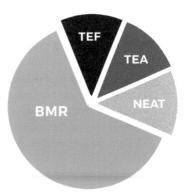

SO WHERE DO I START WITH MY CALORIES?

To save you a ton of stress, I've created a free downloadable calorie and macronutrient calculator for readers of this book. It can be found in the online resources section of www.diabeticmuscleandfitness.com

What does it do?

- Works out starting calories
- Accurately monitors rate of bodyweight and body composition change over time.
- Actively adjusts calorie intake in relation to progress, changes in bodyweight, training frequency and level of physical activity.

HIGH VS. LOW QUALITY FOOD

Let's take a closer look at the difference between high and low quality foods.

HIGH QUALITY FOOD

1,   For the purposes of this book, high quality foods are considered to be:
   - Generally lower in calories.
   - Higher in protein, essential fats and fibre.
   - Better sources of vitamin and minerals.
   - Palatable (depending on cooking method)

2,   However, they can take longer to prepare.

These foods tend to fill us up more due to their higher protein and fibre content. This can help reduce appetite and reduce calorie intake across the day, which in turn supports fat loss.

The higher protein content of these foods requires the body to process significantly more energy. This boosts metabolic rate, which supports fat loss.

These foods also provide essential nutrients (fat and protein) that cannot be produced by the body alone and therefore play a major role in human health.

Typical Examples

- Unprocessed meats, fish, eggs
- Wholegrain and vegetables
- Fruit

Implications:

Eat too much and you will gain weight. However, I am yet to hear of anyone who has gained a tremendous amount of body fat by eating too much fish and broccoli.

LOW QUALITY FOOD

- Typically higher in calories.
- Lower in protein, essential fats and fibre.
- Lower vitamin and mineral content.
- Very palatable.
- Convenient – Quick prep time.

UNDERSTANDING FOOD SOURCE
NUTRIENTS

Every food you consume has a unique composition of nutrients that provide materials and information to the body. This information can serve purposes as diverse as providing energy for movement to the production of key hormones.

Certain nutrients can also influence appetite and yield different levels of energy. This brings me back to the point about all calories not being equal.

When it comes to nutrition, we need to understand the key functions nutrients play in the body, the foods they are contained within and how the diabetic body deals with them differently

Let's review the following factors:

- Macronutrients - Foods, functions and intakes
- Micronutrients - Foods, functions and intakes
- Hydration
- High Vs. low quality food sources

MACRONUTRIENTS

Macronutrients provide energy for growth, repair and other important bodily processes. There are four main macronutrients:

- Carbohydrate provides 4 calories per gram.
- Fat provides 9 calories per gram.
- Protein provides 4 calories per gram.
- Alcohol provides 7 calories per gram.

There are essential and non-essential nutrients. In total there are eight essential protein-based amino acids and two essential fatty acids that must be obtained from the diet.

The body can produce its own carbohydrate non-essential amino acids and fatty acids. Alcohol is not essential for survival. (sorry guys)

JUST BECAUSE A GIVEN NUTRIENT ISN'T 'ESSENTIAL' DOESN'T MEAN IT'S NOT POTENTIALLY BENEFICIAL – THAT'S AN IMPORTANT DISTINCTION.

The body processes carbohydrates, protein and fat to make a compound called adenosine triphosphate (ATP). ATP is considered the main energy source for the majority of cellular functions within the human body.

The majority of differences between recommendations for people with T1D and T2D and those living without diabetes revolve around:

- Overall calorie intake (Fat loss vs. mass gain)
- Carbohydrate intake (due to its significant influence on glycemic control)
- Underlying medical conditions that influence nutrient intake, such as renal disease, food allergies and intolerances.

Over the course of this chapter I'll be giving you an insight into the roles of each macronutrient and how they can be tailored to your end goal.

MICRONUTRIENTS – VITAMINS & MINERALS

Vitamins and minerals play a number of key roles within the body, including energy metabolism, immune function, antioxidant supply, bone growth, muscle contraction and much more.

If energy requirements are being met through a varied balanced diet, the micronutrient intake is likely to be adequate. But a restricted calorie diet poses the risk of micronutrient deficiency. The extent of such a deficiency will be directly proportionate to the severity of the energy deficit imposed, and longer-term deficits pose an even greater risk.

The standard Recommended Daily Allowances can be used to assess if macronutrient needs are being met. However, the following people should pay particular attention to their vitamin and mineral intake:

- Individuals with poorly controlled diabetes.
- Athletes or individuals who exercise regularly.
- Individuals competing in sports where energy intake is restricted to meet weight or achieve an ultra low level of body fat conditioning.
- Female athletes during menstruation.
- Individuals who restrict dairy products due to lactose intolerance or those that unnecessarily remove dairy products as a strategy for reducing calories for fat loss.

Supplementation can be used to eradicate deficiencies and promote a sound nutritional status. I talk about supplements in greater detail towards the end of this chapter.

Other useful substances, such as phytonutrients, anthocyanins and tannins are also classified as micronutrients and are needed in small quantities.

Typical Examples

- Confectionery
- Fizzy drinks
- Takeaways and certain ready meals

Implications:

These foods taste great, pack a lot of energy and require little preparation but they don't fill you up and increase your potential to eat more calories.

They are quite possibly your worst nightmare when it comes to improving body composition and getting lean if relied upon as a sole source of nutrition.

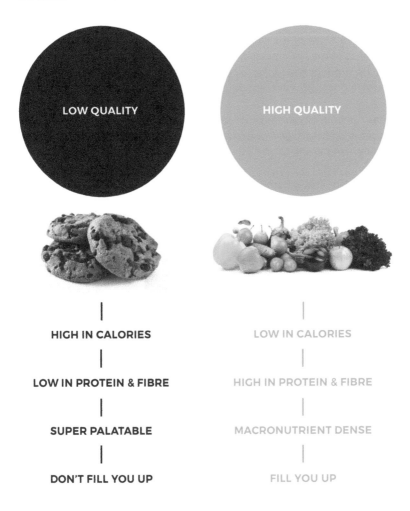

LOW QUALITY	HIGH QUALITY
HIGH IN CALORIES	LOW IN CALORIES
LOW IN PROTEIN & FIBRE	HIGH IN PROTEIN & FIBRE
SUPER PALATABLE	MACRONUTRIENT DENSE
DON'T FILL YOU UP	FILL YOU UP

IS "CLEAN EATING" REALLY THE BEST WAY TO LOSE WEIGHT.?

The term "clean eating" has no real definition.

If it can't be defined, how do you know what you're eating is 'clean'?

That's right; you can't.

Some people claim 'clean eating' refers to "real" or "unprocessed" foods, yet these people also consume whey protein, protein bars, shop bought food and fizzy diet drinks; all of which ARE highly processed. And, 'real' food, unless you're eating a polystyrene model of the food, I don't quite see the context of 'real'

Even if 'clean eating' excluded junk food, it still wouldn't necessarily be better for fat loss than a diet of the same macronutrients containing these foods. In fact the opposite may be true as the flexible dieting approach has been shown to be superior than a more rigid-type approach (e.g. clean eating) for long term weight loss/maintenance (10,11).

As long as the bulk of your nutrition comes from high quality foods, you keep your diabetes well managed, your body fat in check, avoid chronic stress, get enough sleep and are regularly active.

If the bulk of your diet is comprised of low quality food you will inevitably look and feel like crap. Always consider the dose and frequency of the type of food you eat.

MACRONUTRIENTS: **PROTEIN**

"Life goes faster on protein" ~
Martin H Fischer (German-American physician and writer.)

Protein is a massive buzzword in the fitness world, whether the subject is fat loss or lean mass gain. Protein drinks, protein bars and convenience food dominate our lives. But the reality is most people don't understand what protein actually is, and what its role in the body is besides building muscle. Protein has also received a lot of bad press for causing everything from kidney disease to cancer. But is this really the case?

FUNCTIONS

Proteins are the building blocks of life. Every cell in the human body contains protein. They do most of the work in cells and are required for the structure, function and regulation of the body's tissues and organs.

Key roles include:
- Growth (especially important for children, teens, and pregnant women).
- Tissue repair.
- Immune function.
- Making essential hormones and enzymes.
- Energy when carbohydrate is not available.
- Preserving lean muscle mass.

FACTS

The basic building block of protein is a chain of amino acids.

Proteins are made up of hundreds or thousands of smaller units called amino acids, which are attached to each another in long chains held together by peptide bonds.

Proteins differ according to the amount, type and sequence of amino acids found within their chains. For example, the protein found in steak has a completely different amino acid profile to the protein found in human hair. Every source of protein found in the body and food is unique.

PROTEIN NUTRITION

During digestion, whole proteins (found in food) are broken down into their smaller amino acid counterparts though the action of hydrochloric acid in the stomach and specific digestive enzymes along the digestive tract. They are absorbed as they pass through the liver for processing and metabolism.

In total, there are 20 naturally occurring amino acids, but the unlimited combinations and lengths of these amino acids allow for the vast variety of proteins that exist. These are classified into different sub-groups, including:

- Essential Amino Acids.
- Non-Essential Amino Acids.
- Conditionally Essential Amino Acids.

ESSENTIAL AMINO ACIDS

There are nine essential amino acids . The body must obtain them from the diet in order to prevent protein-related malnutrition. There is strong evidence to support the role of these amino acids in the muscle building process, particularly three of the nine amino acids that are termed branched-chain amino acids (BCAAs).

The quality of a protein source is determined not only by its digestibility but also by its essential amino acid content. Animal-based proteins, including dairy, are higher in protein quality compared to plant sources due to their greater bioavailability and higher amounts of essential amino acids and BCAA content.

A lot of plant-based sources of protein do not contain all the essential amino acids in the right quantities. Most vegetarians are well aware of this, which is why they often eat multiple plant sources at meals to ensure they obtain a broad spectrum of amino acids for health and muscle growth.

Essential Amino Acids
- Phenylalanine
- Threonine
- Tryptophan
- Methionine
- Lysine
- Histidine
- Valine *
- Leucine *
- Isoleucine *

* Branched-chain amino acids

Non-Essential

There are five dispensable amino acids, which humans are capable of synthesizing themselves.

- Alanine
- Aspartic acid
- Asparagine
- Glutamic acid
- Serine

Conditionally Essential

There are six of these amino acids, which must be supplied to the body only under special conditions, such as stress, illness, or ageing. They include:

- Arginine
- Cysteine
- Glycine
- Glutamine
- Proline
- Tyrosine

ADDITIONAL NUTRITIONAL PROPERTIES

Two notable properties of protein include its metabolic cost to digest, known as the thermogenic effect of feeding. A mixed diet consumed at energy balance results in a diet-induced energy expenditure of 5% to 15% of daily energy expenditure. Values are higher at relatively high protein and alcohol consumption and lower at high fat consumption.

PROTEIN REQUIRES THE MOST ENERGY OF ALL MACRONUTRIENTS TO DIGEST, ABSORB AND UTILISE.

Roughly 15% to 25% of the calories consumed as protein are burned off by the metabolism during digestion. Although the thermogenic effect of feeding is a small component of daily energy expenditure, it could play a role in the development and/or maintenance of obesity.

Not only is protein needed for health, but it also builds muscle, elevates the metabolism and satisfies appetite easily. Protein is a much more satiating (filling) macronutrient (compared to fat and carbs) and thus proves very beneficial to any fat loss protocol. If you feel full, you are less likely to graze on additional food.

Just think how awesome this nutrient is when it comes to losing fat. Think of it as nature's fat burner.

DIABETES AND PROTEIN INTAKE – HOW MUCH?

This debate has been going on for quite some time. It continues to rage because research has not provided conclusive answers and health professionals are unaware of much of the evidence. The biggest controversy surrounding protein intake and diabetes is kidney health.

Does eating too much protein damage the kidneys in those suffering from diabetes?

Let me cut to the chase:

1. Dietary protein DOES NOT CAUSE KIDNEY DAMAGE in those with healthy kidney function [1].

2. Chronically elevated BLOOD GLUCOSE levels can cause kidney damage. As such, people with poorly controlled diabetes are much more susceptible to damaging their kidneys.

3. Those with severely damaged kidneys may benefit from consuming a lower protein intake.

Before I review the current research, it's important to gain a solid background understanding of the role the kidneys play in the body and why people with diabetes are at increased risk of kidney disease.

WHAT THE KIDNEYS DO

The kidneys are powerful filtration units that filter over 220 litres of blood every 24 hours [2].

They perform a great deal of important functions:

*   Remove waste products from the body, including urea, a waste product of protein metabolism. Higher protein intakes induce measurable changes in kidney function [3]. These changes aren't necessarily bad; the kidneys simply have more to process.
*   Remove drugs from the body.
*   Regulate the body's salt, potassium and acid/base balance (the body's pH).
*   Release hormones that regulate blood pressure.
*   Produce an active form of vitamin D that promotes strong, healthy bones.
*   Control the production of red blood cells.
*   Maintain blood pressure and blood volume.

If the kidneys fail, our bodies would soon do the same.

Kidney function is measured by the following markers:

- Glomerular filtration rate (GFR).
- Blood urea nitrogen (BUN).
- Creatinine levels.
- The presence or absence of the protein albumin in the urine.

WHAT ARE THE WARNING SIGNS OF KIDNEY DISEASE?

Chronic kidney disease can be defined by having abnormalities in any (if not all) of the above markers for three months or more.

Key signs of kidney dysfunction include:

- Excess levels of protein in urine. Protein molecules should stay in the vascular system. The kidney acts as a sieve so the larger the holes, the greater the protein loss.
- Elevations in blood urea nitrogen (BUN), which highlight the accumulation of unwanted toxic by-products in the blood.

It's important to note, however, that elevations in certain kidney markers, such as creatinine levels can result from prolonged heavy exercise and cannot solely be relied upon to diagnose.

WHAT ARE THE MAIN CAUSES OF KIDNEY DISEASE?

The National Kidney Foundation has coined diabetes as one of the main causes of kidney disease, accounting for 44% of new cases [2].

The United States Renal Data System stated that in 2013 diabetes led to more than 51,000 new cases of kidney failure, and over 247,000 people are currently living with kidney failure resulting from diabetes [4].

Diabetic nephropathy is kidney damage caused by diabetes. In severe cases it can lead to kidney failure. But not everyone with diabetes has kidney damage.

The kidneys have many tiny blood vessels that filter waste from blood. High blood sugar from diabetes can destroy these blood vessels.

Other contributing factors include:

- Age
- Genetic predisposition (family history)
- High blood pressure
- Drugs and toxins
- Glomerulonephritis
- Kidney stones
- Injury

Myth: A high protein diet will damage your kidneys.

There is plenty of evidence to show that individuals who suffer from kidney disease have improved their health considerably with the aid of a reduced protein but nutritionally adequate diet.

This has led many to believe that high protein diets could be the main cause of renal disease in the first place.

This is completely flawed.

A review in the Journal of Nutrition and Metabolism examined the effects of protein intake on kidney function, with a particular emphasis on kidney disease.

The researchers concluded:
'Although excessive protein intake remains a health concern in individuals with pre-existing renal disease, the literature lacks significant research demonstrating a link between protein intake and the initiation or progression of renal disease in healthy individuals (5).'

In addition, the researchers highlighted there isn't sufficient evidence to justify public health directives aimed at restricting dietary protein intake in healthy adults for the purpose of preserving kidney function.

If protein was really that big of a deal for kidney health, there should be a lot more lifters with kidney disease needing dialysis. Where are they? We're not hearing about them? Hint: It's not happening...

WHAT ABOUT DIABETES AND PROTEIN?

First of all, let's look at the facts:

- Higher protein intakes increase the workload on the kidneys.
- Diabetics are at increased risk of kidney disease (nephropathy) especially if their diabetes is poorly managed.

IS IT WISE FOR PEOPLE LIVING WITH DIABETES TO CONSUME MORE PROTEIN?

In poorly controlled individuals with signs of kidney trouble, maybe not.

On the contrary, what about the person with well controlled diabetes who exercises regularly?

Should or could they consume more than the recommended protein allowance of 0.8g/kg body weight per day?

First things first.

- Exercise, especially weight training, increases the demand for protein for growth and repair.
- Hyperglycaemia increases protein breakdown (catabolism).

We must also take into account the well noted benefits and effect of protein on human metabolism and body composition.

First of all it promotes the growth of muscle tissue in response to strength training, which serves a number of highly useful health benefits.

- Increased functional strength.
- Increased glucose uptake (independent of insulin).
- Elevation in metabolic rate (an assistance to fat loss).
- Improvements in body image and self-confidence (stress lowering).

There may also be other unique benefits of strength training and its ability to improve glycaemic control independently of these changes that science is yet to unfold.

From a fat loss perspective protein is the most satiating macronutrient. It keeps us full and reduces the potential to overeat. Protein has a higher thermic effect of feeding, much more so than carbs and fats. Also, if carbohydrates are reduced in the diet they must be replaced with an alternative form of energy, replacing them with protein calories may be a good strategy to maintain glycaemic control.

WHAT'S THE DEAL?

There is substantial evidence to suggest high protein diets do not harm a set of healthy kidneys. Although people living with diabetes may have healthy kidney function, they are at increased risk of kidney complications, which may caution against higher intakes of protein. Further research is needed to investigate protein intake in people living with diabetes who have healthy kidney function.

Myth: A high protein diet is bad for your bones.

The myth stems from data published in 1982 by researchers Robert Heaney et al [6].

Middle-aged women were confined to a metabolic ward and consumed a set diet that matched their everyday intake of protein and phosphorous.

It was observed that calcium losses were positively correlated with protein intake, and calcium balance was negatively correlated. With calcium being one of the main minerals in bone the study contributed to the common belief that protein intake is harmful to bone health.

Since the study, an increasing amount of conflicting evidence has shown that protein intake is actually beneficial for bone health. After 20 years, in an editorial for the American Journal of Nutrition, Heaney critiqued his own research, and highlighted the women involved in the study were receiving abnormally low amounts of calcium and therefore the body was compensating by releasing stored calcium to compensate. He also highlighted how some groups had a conflict of interest in the evidence.

Heaney concluded:

"Human physiology evolved in the context of diets with high amounts of animal protein. There is no evidence that primitive humans had low intakes of either total protein or animal protein. That coupled with the generally very robust skeletons of our hominid forbears, makes it difficult to sustain a case, either evidential or deductive, for overall skeletal harm, related either to protein intake or to animal protein. Indeed, the balance of the evidence seems to indicate the opposite."

Further evidence to dispel the much believed claim is supported by a review published in the Journal of American College of Nutrition [7] which set out to investigate the claim that animal proteins cause an increased incidence of bone fractures.

The review concluded:

"Selective deficiency in dietary proteins causes marked deterioration in bone mass, micro architecture and strength, the hallmark of osteoporosis."

"Dietary proteins are as essential as calcium and vitamin D for bone health and osteoporosis prevention. Furthermore, there is no consistent evidence for superiority of vegetal over animal proteins on calcium metabolism, bone loss prevention and risk reduction of fragility fractures."

WHAT'S THE DEAL?

The claim that consuming a high protein diet leads to negative impacts on bone health is unfounded. The opposite is actually true, with a deficiency in protein proving detrimental to bone health.

Besides protein, the subject of bone health is a complicated multifactorial issue influenced by a range of other notable factors, including overall energy intake, nutritional status, age, genetic factors, illness and medication use.

DO YOU NEED TO CONSUME PROTEIN AT EVERY MEAL?

Consuming protein at every meal is a valid strategy for curbing appetite, supplying a constant stream of amino acids for muscle recovery and slowing the release of glucose into the blood, which may aid glycaemic management.

However, there is no hard rule to have protein every time you eat - exceptions do exist, especially when it comes to diabetes nutrition.

For example, if I were to have an unexpected episode of hypoglycaemia. I'd have to consume extra 'unplanned' energy from carbohydrate to treat it.

Now, when you take into account it's very easy to over treat a hypoglycaemic event by either eating too much carbohydrate or consuming mixed macronutrient based foods, particularly high in fat (chocolate for example).

It's easy to see how unplanned energy can sneak into the diet and influence energy balance and increase the chances of gaining fat.

My point is this: when you consume extra energy to treat a hypoglycaemic event, you will need to adjust your caloric intake from the other macronutrients in order to maintain caloric balance with the caveat that your protein and fat intake still meet your essential needs.

Here's the take home message: relax and be prepared to pull back your protein intake when you consume unplanned carbohydrates and fats to treat hypoglycaemia.

SUPER CHARGE YOUR PROTEIN INTAKE WITH LEUCINE

Out of all the amino acids, leucine possesses the most anabolic properties. Leucine is a potent activator of muscle protein synthesis (MPS) in isolation, and sufficient leucine can enhance the MPS response to a meal that is suboptimal for protein [8].

Poorly managed T1D can result in reduced muscle mass and weakness. Physical activity (especially resistance training) and targeted protein nutrition (in particular leucine) for individuals that can't consume adequate sources of quality protein, such as those with a poor appetite or those on a strict vegetarian/vegan diet. 'Spiking' meals with leucine supplementation could play a crucial role in protecting and supporting the growth of muscle mass in these populations.

HOW MUCH?

2-3 g of Leucine per meal has been shown to maximise protein synthesis outside of training – this is equivalent to 25-35 g of high quality protein per Post-workout leucine requirements are greater. Opt for 5 g if consuming a sub optimal source of protein or appetite has been poor all day.

BASED ON PERSONAL EXPERIENCE LEUCINE DOES INCREASE BLOOD GLUCOSE. HOWEVER, ITS RESPONSE MAY DIFFER FROM INDIVIDUAL TO INDIVIDUAL.

HOW MUCH PROTEIN?

GENERAL POPULATION

According to the European Food Safety Authority (EFSA) Panel on Dietetic Products, Nutrition and Allergies (NDA) 0.83 g/kg of body weight per day [9] is sufficient for all individuals, including those living with diabetes, with healthy kidney function.

However, it has been suggested that intakes up to twice this are regularly consumed from mixed diets by some physically active and healthy adults in Europe and are generally considered safe [9].

SPECIFIC POPULATIONS

Protein needs are generally higher in children and women who are pregnant or lactating [10].

EXERCISING INDIVIDUALS

There is an abundance of research indicating those who engage in physical activity/exercise require higher levels of protein than the aforementioned 0.8g/kg body weight per day, regardless of the type of exercise (i.e. endurance, resistance etc.) or training state (recreational, moderately or well trained [11, 12, 13, 14, 15, 16, 17]).

Needless to say, consuming protein above and beyond the standard recommendation may be considered 'high' in government nutrition eyes [18]. However, in the field of sports nutrition, there is ongoing debate as to what 'high protein' actually entails, with research investigating suggesting intakes as high as 4.4g/kg/day [19] in resistance trained men and women offer no deleterious effects [20] on health or body composition in healthy individuals.

Athletes or highly active individuals looking to build muscle and lose body fat could opt for a daily intake of (1.4-2.0g/kg bodyweight/0.45-1g/lb bodyweight [21])

Sedentary people and those looking to maintain body composition should aim for a daily target of (0.8g/kg bodyweight/0.36g/lb bodyweight [21]) and upwards.

TAKE HOME MESSAGE

Individuals wishing to consume higher intakes of protein should only do so under medical supervision. This will entail regular monitor blood work, and close monitoring of kidney function.

Those with existing kidney disease would be wise to reduce their protein intake and seek medical supervision with regards to a suitable intake of protein.

GENERAL KEY NOTES

1. Consume a range of 1.4-2.0g protein per kg bodyweight (22).

2. The bulk of your protein intake should come from high quality animal sources, unless you have unique dietary requirements. Animal sources like meat, dairy and eggs are superior for stimulating protein synthesis compared to plant sources.

3. Consume a minimum of 20g of high quality protein per meal and especially after training. If performing whole body workouts it may be wise to consume up to 40g (22).

4. 2-3 grams of Leucine maximises protein synthesis, which is equivalent to 25-35g of high quality protein per meal. People with low appetite or those who consume little animal protein may benefit from spiking meals with supplemental leucine.

5. Frequently consume protein at least every three hours, especially after a weight training session.

6. Timing. Although not essential, it is probably wise to consume protein shortly after a workout.

7. Monitor blood glucose and administer appropriate medication in response to dietary protein intake.

TO EAT OR NOT TO EAT?

Fat has received considerable attention over recent years. Newspapers, books, online articles and TV programmes have given many mixed and confusing messages about fat.

One week we hear that fat is bad, contains too many calories and causes heart disease. The next week fat is good, helps with fat loss and protects against heart disease.

The problem is, information about fat is often delivered by food journalists with no scientific training or understanding of fat.

Also, most scientific research in this area has been poorly interpreted, or the studies have been too short to give conclusive recommendations.

These mistakes get repeated and discussed over time and soon create a false dogma that misleads and frightens people into changing their food choices. A prime example would be the scare stories surrounding saturated fat and heart disease. However, a recent meta-analysis by the British Heart Foundation found little correlation between the saturated fat content of a diet and the risk of heart disease. Nevertheless, this shouldn't be interpreted as 'saturated fat is good for you'. Like all fats, it should be consumed within an acceptable macronutrient distribution range and within your calorie limits (if your aim is to maintain a stable weight).

In fact, there is solid evidence to support that butter, a rich source of saturated fat, has hardly any link with death, CVD and diabetes [24]. But this does not automatically mean we should start eating more butter.

For the general layperson, it can be really hard to differentiate truth from fallacy.

There is undeniable proof that certain forms of dietary fat are indispensable to good human health and nutrition whilst others are potentially harmful. Let's consider the evidence and look at how a highly active person living with diabetes can incorporate this essential macronutrient into their muscle building and fat loss nutrition efforts.

WHAT IS FAT?

Generally speaking, when you hear the word fat, you think of two things:

1.   The fats in food: oil, butter, and the white stuff coated around a good steak.

2.   The fat on your body.

Fat has many different roles within the diet and the body.

Dietary fat, which is technically known as triglycerides (TG) are made up of one molecule of glycerol and three fatty acids. There are other fats, most notably cholesterol and other minor lipids, which we will touch on in due course.

Triglyceride is formed from three fatty acids attached to a molecule of glycerol (a sugar alcohol).

3 FATTY ACIDS + GLYCEROL

The functional properties of each molecule depend on the specific types of fatty acids found in it.

Fatty acids can be long, medium or short in length. These important structural factors determine the effects of the fat on health and metabolism.

FATE OF FAT

The fate of fat is mostly determined by the liver. Some fat gets stored within the liver; some are burned immediately as fuel, and some are stored in muscle. The remainder is carried in the blood to specialised fat cells called adipocytes.

A typical human has tens of billions of these cells and each contains a single droplet of fat.

Like muscle cells, fat cells can increase in volume and number.

Fat cell hypertrophy occurs when the fat cell increases in size (volume) by storing fatty acids as triglyceride.

Fat cell hyperplasia, involves an increase in the number of fat cells, which contrary to old-fashioned beliefs does occur in adults.

Many of these fat cells lie beneath the skin as subcutaneous fat stores. Some cells are found in the muscle and organs and some lie around the organs of the abdomen, where they are known as visceral fat (belly fat).

The distinction between visceral and subcutaneous fat is important. Visceral fat behaves differently to subcutaneous fat, and is directly linked to numerous health problems (25). It is well known that excess internal organ or visceral fat of the liver and pancreas are strongly linked to T2D.

KNOW YOUR FATS

Fat - a much-maligned macronutrient that has been subject to a lot of abuse over the years.

The reality is certain aspects of dietary fat can be harmful to human health, whilst others are essential for life.

Let's discuss the various elements of what makes up fat from the cholesterol in your blood through to the monounsaturated fat in your Brazil nuts.

CHOLESTEROL – IT'S INVOLVED IN PRETTY MUCH EVERYTHING.

Cholesterol is a small, waxy, fat like substance that serves many biological roles in the body, which include:

- Being an iImportant component of cell membranes:
- Being a building block for many important hormones.
- Tissue repair.

THE HUMAN BODY HAS THE ABILITY TO PRODUCE AND REGULATE ITS OWN CHOLESTEROL.

To make up for the difference between what is consumed in the diet and what is needed by our bodies to function, the liver has the capacity to synthesize cholesterol from carbohydrate, protein and fatty acids.

The more cholesterol we consume from our diets, the less we produce. On the flip side, when no cholesterol is consumed from the diet (for instance a vegetarian diet) the body's cholesterol production increases to compensate.

In fact, the amount of cholesterol absorbed by the intestinal walls generally amounts to much less than 50% of the amount consumed [26]. It could be argued that it simply isn't possible for humans to eat enough cholesterol containing foods to supply enough cholesterol for human needs.

CHOLESTEROL IS ESSENTIAL TO HUMAN LIFE. WITHOUT CHOLESTEROL THE BODY WOULD NOT FUNCTION, HOWEVER IT IS NOT CONSIDERED AN ESSENTIAL NUTRIENT AS THE BODY CAN MAKE IT ENDOGENOUSLY.

Since neither cholesterol nor triglycerides are soluble (dissolve) in water, they need to be transported around the blood stream to their end destination by special proteins known as lipoproteins (comprised of protein and fat)

This transport system is complex, and well beyond the scope of this text. But there are a few important facts worth knowing.

Low Density Lipoproteins (LDLs), which is often-termed bad cholesterol, transport cholesterol and triglycerides from the liver to other organs, but they differ in size and density. LDLs that transport triglycerides are denser and smaller than those that transport mostly cholesterol, which are larger and more buoyant.

High Density Lipoproteins (HDLs) transport cholesterol back to the liver so that it can be excreted mainly via bile.

FATS AND OILS

There are three major categories of naturally occurring fat and oils: saturated, monounsaturated and polyunsaturated. There is a fourth category known as trans-fat (also called hydrogenated fats), which is generally not considered a natural form of fat, with the exception of one naturally occurring trans-fat, conjugated linoleic acid, which is also a popular sports nutrition supplement.

Each category of fat is comprised of different fatty acids, all with different structural and nutritional properties.

ESSENTIAL VS. NON-ESSENTIAL FATTY ACIDS

The majority of fat can be synthesised from ingested protein and carbohydrate. However, some fats cannot. These are termed 'essential fats' and need to be consumed in the diet.

Let's take a closer look at each category of fat and consider which forms are essential and which are not.

Saturated Fats

The type of fat many of us will be familiar with, saturated fat, comes in many different forms (short, medium and long chains) depending on the source and is solid at room temperature.

The main source of saturated fatty acids is animal foods, such as meat, eggs and dairy products.

Many people mistakenly coin such animal fats as entirely saturated. This is wrong as many animal meats contain mixed ratios of saturated, mono and polyunsaturated fat. For example, beef is 46% saturated and lard is 40% saturated.

The body uses saturated fat for a number of different biological roles including:

- Energy
- Hormone production
- Organ padding
- Cell Signalling

Although saturated fat isn't essential, there are important reasons to include reasonable quantities of coconut oil, butter and lard in our diets.

The 2015-2020 Dietary Guidelines for Americans recommends people limit saturated fat to less than 10% of calories a day (27).

DO CHOLESTEROL & SATURATED FAT CAUSE HEART DISEASE?

Let's discuss 'The Lipid Hypothesis'

In the 1950s a biochemist named Ancel Keys published a study that compared heart disease and fat consumption across half a dozen countries.

Keys observed that the countries that ate more fat had a greater prevalence of heart disease.

His findings, along with other studies, including the popular Minnesota Business and Professional Men's Study were used to form the famous lipid hypothesis, which claimed:

1. Eating foods high in saturated fat and cholesterol raises the cholesterol level in your blood.
2. High cholesterol, particularly LDL plays a key role in the development of atherosclerosis and coronary heart disease.
3. Decreasing saturated fat and cholesterol intake reduces blood cholesterol levels, which significantly reduces coronary heart disease (28).

Contradictory evidence failed to surface, and the infamous lipid hypothesis became universally accepted for more than 50 years. It influenced a wide range of public health and nutrition polices.

CONTRADICTIONS

Keys' observations overlooked data from countries that consumed a lot of fat but had little heart disease, like Holland and Norway. He also omitted data from countries like Chile where fat intake was low but incidence of heart disease was high.

The findings from these countries did not support the lipid hypothesis.

Also, the research used to support Keys' observations, such as the Minnesota Business and Professional Men's Study, contained flaws. For starters, its small sample size, which was based on a high socioeconomic sample of men who were successful in business and professional life could never be applied to the general population.

TIMES HAVE CHANGED

There is now a substantial body of evidence dispelling the lipidhypothesis [29, 30, 31, 32, 33] and changes to nutritional guidelines are already in place.

It is now accepted that the effect of particular foods on cardiovascular disease cannot be predicted solely by their content of saturated fatty acids.

The Dietary Guidelines for Americans 2015-2020 states that dietary cholesterol is no longer a 'nutrient of concern', which has been accepted in the UK and many other countries for well over a decade. I discuss cholesterol more in the next section.

SATURATED FAT INTAKE

Since the recommended limit for saturated fat intake is less than 10% of an individual's total daily calories [27], manipulations in dietary intake are required.

Where should the remainder of calories and macronutrients come from?

CARBS

Evidence from epidemiologic and intervention studies has shown no clear benefit of substituting carbohydrates for saturated fat, although there may be benefits, especially for those managing diabetes, if the carbohydrate is unrefined and has a low glycaemic index [34].

If blood glucose levels are well managed, increasing carbohydrate intake over saturated fat may be highly beneficial for those participating in regular weight training, which relies heavily on carbohydrate as a source of fuel.

OTHER TYPES OF FATS

I go into greater detail on the different types of dietary fat in the next few pages.

But as we are on the topic of saturated fat, let's see how other forms of fat can be manipulated to accommodate a lower, healthier intake of saturated fat.

Interesting research has shown that populations who eat a typical western diet can lower their risk of heart disease by ≥2-3% by replacing 1% of their energy from saturated fats with polyunsaturated fats (35). However, this figure is most likely underestimated due to the fact it is only based on a single measure in a predicated analysis. We also need to consider the fact there may be high amounts of unhealthy trans fatty acids found in many popular food products rich in polyunsaturated fat, for example margarine.

Saturated fats can also be replaced by monounsaturated fatty acids, which are considered health-neutral provided they are consumed within an individual's energy needs and consumed as part of a diet that provides all the necessary essential nutrients. This is often considered to be a Mediterranean diet.

FOOD VS. NUTRIENT-BASED RECOMMENDATIONS

Food-based recommendations are always going to be more practical for the everyday lay person over nutrient-based dietary advice. However, with the growing number of calorie tracking apps, building a diet based on macronutrient ratios is relatively easy nowadays.

Also, the effect of a specific food (e.g. meat and dairy products) on the risk of cardiovascular disease cannot be determined simply on the basis of its fatty acid profile. There may be other important components within the food that are highly beneficial to health. A prime example would be milk and its associated calcium intake, or dark chocolate, which is loaded with different types of saturated fatty acids and health-promoting polyphenols that have been shown to reduce the risk of coronary heart disease (36).

The only exception to this may be highly processed meat products, which are typically stripped of their naturally occurring health promoting elements and loaded with other high calorie ingredients, artificial preservatives and stabilisers.

ATHEROSCLEROSIS

When a blood vessel is damaged, cholesterol is called upon to repair it. Depending on the extent of the damage fatty deposits can appear on the walls of the blood vessels (known as plaque). These plaques (or atheromas) are known as atherosclerosis and cause the arteries to harden and narrow, restricting the blood flow and oxygen supply to vital organs.

High blood pressure causes the plaque to rupture, resulting in bleeding of the artery wall. Chips of the clot can become lodged within the body, resulting in strokes and heart attacks depending on where they end up. It could be the brain, heart or even a limb.

However, just because cholesterol is correlated to the formation of plaque and furrowing of the arteries does not mean it caused the damage in the first place.

Damage to blood vessels is increased by a number of risk factors, including:

- Obesity (metabolic syndrome and T2D)
- Poor glycemic control
- Genetic predisposition
- Excessive intake of man-made trans-fat
- Smoking
- Oxidative stress,
- Low grade inflammation
- Chronic stress

CHOLESTEROL – CORRELATION DOESN'T EQUAL CAUSATION

DIABETES AND CARDIOVASCULAR RISK

It is well established that people living with all forms of diabetes are more susceptible to cardiovascular disease (CVD), stroke and other heart diseases.

High blood pressure along with elevated levels of oxidative stress and glycation that result from hyperglycemia, are thought to be big players in causing major damage to the cardiovascular system. However, the current body of evidence is unclear.

Damage to the cardiovascular system is not ideal for an individual looking to maximise their muscle building and performance potential. It is imperative to take every measure possible to prevent it.

PREDICTING HEART DISEASE RISK

A lipid profile is a blood test that measures the amount of cholesterol and fat in your blood. These measurements are used internationally by doctors and health care professionals to predict cardiovascular disease (CVD).

YOUR LIPID PROFILE

A report typically contains the following items, in this order:

Total cholesterol: A number giving all the cholesterol in the blood (good HDL plus bad LDL). A higher total cholesterol may be due to high levels of HDL, which is good, or high levels of LDL, which is bad. So knowing the breakdown is important.

Triglycerides: A type of blood fat.

High-density lipoprotein (HDL): Good cholesterol that helps protect against CVD.

Low-density lipoprotein (LDL): Bad cholesterol and a major contributor to CVD.

Total cholesterol to HDL ratio: The amount of total cholesterol divided by HDL. This number is useful in helping doctors predict the risk of developing atherosclerosis.

Diabetes UK provides the following guideline cholesterol levels to aim for:

Total cholesterol: under 4.0 mmol/l (155 mg/dl)

Levels over this may mean you are at risk of CVD although as previously mentioned, you would need to look at the HDL/LDL breakdown to make a better decision.

LDL levels: below 2.0 mmol/l (77 mg/dl)

LDL goals vary depending on your medical history but generally speaking for people with diabetes it is considered optimal if it is less than the above. Anything higher will require a lifestyle change including both dietary and physical exercise is advisable. This may also include such medication as statins.

HDL levels: at least 1.0 mmol/l / 39 mg/dl (men) or 1.2 mmol/l / 46mg/dl (women)

HDL helps transport bad cholesterol out of the blood and so higher levels are considered good..

Women tend to have higher HDL levels and are therefore protected somewhat from CVD more than men due to their levels of naturally occurring Oestrogen.

Triglyceride levels: less than (or equal to) 1.7 mmol/l (151 mg/dl)

Triglycerides have been linked to CVD and Diabetes and are closely related to total cholesterol levels.

LIFESTYLE CHOICE AND CHOLESTEROL

Besides genetics, lifestyle can negatively affect your cholesterol levels. The most prominent influencers include: diet, smoking, drinking, uncontrolled diabetes, other health conditions like hypothyroidism and the use of certain medication.

It's wise to monitor cholesterol readings after prolonged use of medication, particularly exogenous (manually administered) insulin and anabolic steroids.

IN SUMMARY

Even if you do accept the role of good or bad readings of cholesterol, there is a broad range depending on age, gender, lifestyle, diet etc. It's best to monitor those mentioned above to ensure you are at a low risk of CVD and other vascular complications linked to diabetes and high cholesterol.

Unsaturated Fats
Unsaturated fatty acids can be further divided into:

- Polyunsaturated fatty acids
- Monounsaturated fatty acids

Polyunsaturated Fatty Acids
Polyunsaturated fats are liquid at room temperature and have multiple double bonds. The two primary classes of these fats are the essential omega-3 and omega-6 fatty acids.

The body cannot produce omega-3 and omega-6 fatty acids. For this reason they are known as essential fats, or EFAs.

EFA Omega 3
Omega-3 fatty acids (n-3 polyunsaturated fatty acids) are dietary nutrients that play a key role in human health and disease prevention/management.

Their list of functions is extensive, and they're particularly useful to anyone living with diabetes who wants to enhance wellness, muscle building, fat loss and performance.

Key functions of omega-3 in the body include:

- Anti-Inflammatory roles (may be more beneficial to NSAID's, which can impair muscular adaptions from training if abused or used over prolonged periods of time)
- Cardiovascular protective
- Brain-mood supportive
- Recovery-pain, tissue remodelling and repair
- Insulin sensitivity
- Body composition
- Anabolic/anti-Catabolic Properties

Omega-3 fatty acids can be found in animal and plant sources.

Plant sources such as flaxseed, chia, hempseed, canola oil, walnuts and certain vegetable oils contain significant amounts of the plant-based omega-3 fatty acid A-linolenic acid (ALA) and stearidonic acid (SDA).

Animal sources, particularly fish/krill oil and oily fish contain the omega-3 fatty acids eicosapentaenoic acid (EPA) and docosahexaenoic acid (DHA)

Researchers now believe that the majority of health benefits we get from dietary omega-3 fats come from EPA/DHA, particularly DHA

DHA is recognised as one of, if not the most important, nutrients for brain function (cognitive performance, learning ability, memory etc) and also for visual sharpness in the retina of the eye.

Most of the favourable effects of DHA/EPA ingestion on various risk factors for cardiovascular disease are not matched by consuming equivalent intakes of ALA, A-linolenic acid, the plant-based form of omega-3

Studies have shown higher intakes of ALA (1,200 mg/day) can reduce the risk of heart disease by approximately 20% (37). Whereas, higher intakes of fish (up to five servings a week, providing approximately 650 mg DHA/EPA combined/day) have been shown to reduce heart disease mortality by 40% based on epidemiological studies.

WHICH SOURCE IS BEST?

Generally speaking, the richest and most available sources of omega-3 fatty acids are found in oily fish and fish oil. Flaxseed and other plant-derived oils are totally lacking in DHA/EPA combined whereas DHA/EPA are found in fish/fish oils, which contain very minor amounts of ALA.

The Body Can Convert ALA to EPA/DHA, although not efficiently.

The body has the capacity to synthesize EPA & DHA from the short-chain omega-3 alpha-linolenic acid (ALA) found in plant sources like flaxseed and walnuts. The body can also generate EPA from stearidonic acid, another plant-based omega-3 (naturally found in soy and canola oils, and hemp).

A common misconception, especially amongst vegetarian and vegans, is that essential needs for EPA and DHA can be met by consuming plant-based food sources of ALA.

However, what they don't take into account is the conversion of ALA from plant sources like flaxseed oil to DHA is relatively poor in healthy people and even worse in people deficient in certain nutrients.

RISK OF DEFICIENCY

This raises concern for people who may be deficient in a range of nutrients. They include people living with chronic illnesses, such as diabetes, and vegans and vegetarians, who tend to eliminate entire food groups from their diet. And, end up in many cases being deficient in iron, a key intermediate in the conversion of ALA to EPA/DHA. The bioavailability of iron is poor from plant sources compared to animal sources.

Studies have shown that ALA supplements (like flaxseed oil) fail to raise blood plasma levels of DHA in vegans, despite low DHA levels at baseline [38]. Although there may be exceptions for those supplementing with an algae-derived source of DHA, more research is needed.

OMEGA-3 IDEALLY SHOULD COME FROM A MIX OF SOLID FOOD AND SUPPLEMENTS.

Most people don't eat enough omega-3 compared to other forms of dietary fat.

The current American dietary guidelines recommend consuming eight or more ounces (226g) a week (less for young children) from a variety of seafood, which provides on average 'the total package' of 250 mg per day of EPA and DHA [27]. Women who are pregnant or breastfeeding should consume between 8 and 12 ounces (226-340g)

EFA OMEGA-6

Omega-6 is another essential fatty acid necessary for human health. The body cannot produce it so it must be eaten.

Like omega-3, omega-6 plays an essential role in various bodily processes, including brain function, growth and development, immune function, metabolism and reproduction.

Omega-3 helps to reduce inflammation; omega-6 promotes inflammation, which at times is healthy and essential for human growth, development and repair.

Too much omega-6, in conjunction with excess calories and limited omega-3, is an area of concern. It has been shown to promote inflammation and contribute to modern diseases, such as heart disease, obesity and diabetes.

Unfortunately, omega-6 fats are ubiquitous in the modern diet. They're found in nearly all processed, refined and restaurant-cooked foods, and recent statistics suggest they may constitute as much as 20% of calories in the average American's diet.

Vegetable oil is one of the most popular sources of omega-6 fatty acids. Unfortunately most vegetable oil has been industrially modified, resulting in a host of unfavourable structural changes that are detrimental to health, especially when the product is consumed in excess.

A 1:1 ratio between omega-3 and omega-6 is associated with healthier blood vessels, lower lipid counts and a reduced risk of plaque build-up.

Fish oil is a great addition to the diet for balancing the ratio of omega-3 and omega-6 fatty acids in the blood.

MONOUNSATURATED FATTY ACIDS

Monounsaturated fats are also liquid at room temperature. Key sources include:
- Olive oil
- Avocados
- Nuts – macadamia, almonds, cashew and pecans

In terms of health, monounsaturated fats are neutral-to-beneficial because they reduce levels of LDL in the blood. Therefore, this type of fat could serve as one of the main sources of fat within the diet.

TRANS FATS

Man-made trans-fatty acids are derived from partial hydrogenation of vegetable oils.

This industrial process involves pumping hydrogen gas into liquid vegetable oil. This changes vegetable oil into a solid or semi-solid fat. These structural changes are important for food manufacturing: for instance they help to hold a cupcake together and increase the shelf life of junk food.

The consumption of industrially produced, partially hydrogenated vegetable oils (trans fat) is associated with an increased risk of cardiovascular disease, infertility, endometriosis, gallstones, Alzheimer's disease, diabetes and some cancers [39].

The intake of trans fat is relatively low in the UK and northern Europe. It tends to be consumed in greater quantities in other countries, particularly the United States. Be mindful of this when travelling.

The 2015-2020 Dietary Guidelines for Americans recommends trans fat should be avoided [27].

Thankfully, many fast food and supermarket chains have considerably reduced or eliminated the use of these types of man-made fats in their food.

Interestingly, the removal of trans fatty acids from food supply has been identified as a 'best-buy' public health intervention in low- and middle-income countries, where healthy eating education and reliance on home cooked produce may be low [41].

NATURALLY OCCURRING TRANS FAT (AN EXCEPTION)

CLA (conjugated linoleic acid) is a naturally occurring trans fatty acid produced in the digestive systems of ruminant animals, such as cows, sheep and goats. It is found in small quantities of grass-fed meat and milk.

Human consumption of naturally occurring trans fatty acids is generally low. There is evidence to suggest that it does not adversely affect health, compared to industrially produced trans fatty acids.

FAT COMPOSTION OF COMMON COOKING OILS

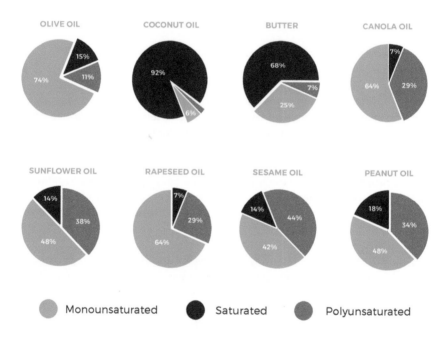

RECENT CHANGES IN DIETARY FAT RECOMMENDATIONS

There is no scientific basis for placing a limit on fat intake, and it can result in poor dietary choices. For example, many foods rich in healthy fats, such as salmon, olive oil and avocadoes pack significantly more nutritional value than artificially processed dressings, deli meats, confectionery and ready meals that claim they're fat-free.

Just recently the U.S. Department of Health and Human Services Dietary Guidelines Advisory Committee made a game-changing edit to its recommend amount of fat we should eat.

It used to advise that fat be kept below 35% of total calories (not bodyweight). It no longer has a recommended upper limit for total fat intake (27), which means no more freaking out about the total fat content of your food. People need to focus more on food choice.

FOOD CHOICE MATTERS, NOT THE FAT CONTENT.

DOES THIS MEAN I CAN EAT AS MUCH FAT AS I WANT?

No. Just because fat and cholesterol have been given nutritional exoneration doesn't mean it's OK to swap your steel-cut oatmeal for a six-egg, bacon-loaded omelette every day of the week.

Long term overconsumption of calories from fat or any other macronutrient will inevitably lead to obesity and a host of other health implications that will jeopardize diabetes prevention and management.

DIABETES AND LIPID METABOLISM

TYPE 1 DIABETES

The main macronutrient focus for T1D management is carbohydrate.

However, there is strong evidence that dietary fat and free fatty acids (FFAs) also play a significant role by impairing insulin sensitivity and enhancing glucose production in the liver (42).

In America, the Diabetes Control and Complications Trial conducted research that found strong links between long-term dietary fat intake and blood glucose control (independent of BMI).

Patients who consumed the lowest range of fat (circa 62 g fat per day) had an average A1C of 7.14% compared with A1C 7.47% in those consuming a higher intake of fat (circa 120 g fat per day (43)). However, these results may have been influenced by personal diabetes management.

BE MINDFUL THAT DIETARY FAT HAS THE POTENTIAL TO INFLUENCE BLOOD GLUCOSE LEVELS.

Interestingly, additional research by Ahern et al found that T1D subjects required more insulin to cover a higher fat pizza meal than a lower-fat pizza with identical carbohydrate content (44, 45).

These findings highlight limitations to the current carbohydrate-focused approach to insulin bolus dose calculation and make us reconsider the effects of dietary fat, especially saturated fat as an important nutritional consideration for glycaemic control in people living with T1D.

However, these findings are limited to a small population of people who don't strength train on a regular basis. Due to the effects of resistance training on insulin sensitivity, the glycaemic response to a high fat meal will inevitably differ between trained and non-trained individuals.

Further work is needed to determine whether body composition, training status, age, BMI, diabetes duration, or gender underlies the differential susceptibility of individuals to dietary fat-induced insulin resistance.

TYPE 2 DIABETES

In T2D, increased levels of visceral fat are thought to negatively impact metabolic function, leading to the accumulation of triglycerides in muscles, liver and pancreatic beta cells. This interferes with insulin signalling and insulin secretion, which results in insulin resistance and beta cell dysfunction.

DEFINING DIETARY FAT NEEDS

At present, there are no recommendations on dietary fat intake for people living with diabetes who exercise regularly.

KEY CONSIDERATIONS

Considering the essential role played by fats in human health, we must be able to define minimal, excessive and optimal intakes, especially for people living with diabetes.

Once a minimum intake of essential fat has been met, it becomes far less important than protein and carbohydrate.

Fat doesn't provide the main source of fuel for hard weight training sessions, nor does it directly support recovery by increasing protein synthesis or restoring muscle glycogen stores.

Dietary fat intake can be manipulated to a large degree, provided its essential needs are covered.

Eating too little fat can interfere with the muscle building pathways, which rely heavily on fat-based steroid hormones like testosterone as well as other intracellular signalling molecules. There really is no need to go lower than 15% of total calories unless you're in the final week or two of preparation for a bodybuilding show or photo shoot.

Eating too much fat will quickly create an energy surplus due to its high calorific content and increase the potential for obesity, which carries a host of implications for health, physical appearance and performance.

Provided calorie intake is balanced, and necessary amounts of carbohydrate and essential protein have been consumed, dietary fat has no scientifically proven 'excessive' intake.

IT IS POSSIBLE TO CONSUME ENERGY FROM DIETARY FAT IN LARGER QUANTITIES THAN PROTEIN AND CARBS, WITHOUT POSING A RISK TO HEALTH OR BODY COMPOSITION.

HOW MUCH FAT DO I REALLY NEED?

Once overall calories and essential protein have been calculated, dietary fat should be based on a relative percentage of total calorie intake, instead of set grams per lb.

The reason for working to a relative percentage is because as bodyweight decreases, fat intake will also decrease proportionally, which increases the potential of not getting enough dietary fat.

GOAL	FAT
FAT LOSS	15-25%
MASS GAIN	15-30%

The percentage of fat you choose to consume is entirely down to personal dietary choice.

Some individuals may feel and work better on a higher fat, lower carbohydrate diet, whilst others work better on a higher carb, lower fat diet. It's a matter of testing various intakes of carbohydrate and fat and seeing how they feel. There is no one-size-fits-all.

Staying above the minimum intake of 15% should be easy for almost all individuals under almost all circumstances, as you will see in the case study example below.

This case study is based on the previous example I used for calculating protein and fat.

I discuss the percentages and calculations in greater detail in the 'building your diet' section of this chapter.

Goal: Fat Loss
Age: 23
Height: 5ft 11
Gender: Male
Body Weight: 90kg
Maintenance Calories: 2800 kcal
Calories adjusted for fat loss goal (-20%): 2240 kcal

Step 1
Protein Intake (1.4 to 2.0 g/kg/day)   90 x 1.4g = 126g protein

N.B. The protein recommendation here is not a minimum – it's based on weight loss studies showing that protein within this range retains lean mass when compared to the standard minimum (0.8g/kg for instance).

Step 2
Fat Intake (Min 15%-25% of intake)
25% of 2240 kcal = 560 kcals/9 kcals (per 1g Fat) = 62g fat

Step 3
Carbs (remainder of calories)
2240 kcals – 504 kcal from 126g protein – 560 kcals from 62g fat
= kcal 1176/ 4 kcal (per 1g carb) = 294g carbs

2240 kcal   126g Protein (23%)   294g Carbs (52%)   62g Fat (25%)

This calorie and macronutrient example has been developed using the minimum recommended intakes for protein and maximum recommended intakes for fat.

WHAT PROPORTIONS OF DIETARY FAT DO I NEED TO CONSUME?

The 2015-2020 Dietary Guidelines for Americans offers the following recommendations about dietary fat:

- Avoid trans fat.
- Replace saturated fat with healthier monounsaturated and polyunsaturated fats.
- Dietary cholesterol is no longer a nutrient of concern.

THE NEGATIVE EFFECTS OF EXCESS BODY FAT ON HEALTH AND MUSCLE BUILDING POTENTIAL

BODY FAT STORAGE

Most people see fat cells simply as storage units for excess energy.

However, since the 1980s medical research has continued to demonstrate that fat tissue is an on demand 24/7 metabolic factory that secretes a variety of hormones and chemical signals, including some implicated with cancer and diabetes.

Excess body fat, particularly visceral fat, which is stored around your midsection, tends to play a greater role in promoting abnormal signals than subcutaneous fat (the fat padding underneath the skin)

It was recently discovered that fat cells secrete leptin, a molecule considered to be satiety signal. The lower your body fat, the higher the leptin levels, and therefore the more satisfied you feel after a meal.

But as body fat increases, leptin decreases and so you always have that lingering desire to nibble at food, which can lead to a vicious cycle whereby your body thinks you need to consume more and more.

Excess body fat increases oestrogen production (in both sexes). Oestrogen promotes female characteristics in girls, such as widening of the hips and growth of breasts. The aromatase enzyme (within fat cells) is responsible for converting valuable muscle building testosterone into oestrogen – hardly an ideal scenario for building a rock hard muscular physique.

Surplus oestrogen can contribute to an array of unsightly and unhealthy consequences, including female fat distribution (man boobs/gynecomastia) and accelerated cancer growth.

Excess body fat also results in other abnormal signals, including the over-production of naturally occurring inflammatory molecules.

High body fat, particularly visceral fat brings other complications, including cardiovascular problems, some cancers and T2D.

As cases of obesity are increasing in adults, so are cases of diabetes. The reason for the strong relationship between obesity and T2D is still largely unknown and is subject to a great deal of research. However, most research involving animals does not translate to humans.

So at last, fat is no longer considered just an energy store, the ugly culprit who gets blamed when the clothes you wore last summer are annoyingly tight in the wrong places. Instead, it's regarded as a highly active cell that tries its best to maintain the body's energy homoeostasis. Many other molecules have been identified that are secreted by fat cells but they're beyond the scope of this book.

BODY FAT IS A FULLY FUNCTIONAL ENDOCRINE GLAND, MUCH LIKE YOUR THYROID OR PANCREAS THAT OPERATES TO ITS OWN SET OF RULES. YOUR CURRENT LEVEL OF FAT DETERMINES ITS ACTIVITY, WHICH IS YET MORE REASON TO KEEP YOUR WAIST IN CHECK.

Gaining too much fat too quickly can also permanently increase the number of new fat cells in the body, which makes it harder for you to get leaner when you diet. This process is called adipogenesis, and occurs during periods of intense weight gain and calorie surplus.

TAKE HOME MESSAGE

Fat tastes great and certain types are essential to human health.
It's advisable to consume the bulk of your dietary fat from non-processed food sources. Processed food products can be incredibly tasty, but they don't fill you up. This makes them easier to overeat, resulting in excess energy intake and the addition of unwanted body fat.

Consume the majority of your dietary fat from monounsaturated sources.

Limit saturated fat to less than 10% of total daily calories and divide the rest between polyunsaturated fats, with as few as possible (if any) coming from man-made trans fatty acids.

Though the quantity and type of fat you consume on a daily basis are important in optimising health, there are many other important dietary and lifestyle factors to respect.

High levels of body fat, especially visceral fat are unhealthy and will wreak havoc with your health, diabetes management and muscle building potential.

Maintain only a healthy layer of body fat so that everything works as it should.

MACRONUTRIENTS: **CARBS**

- Carbohydrates, or carbs, provide 4 kcal of energy per gram.

- Glucose is the primary sugar circulating in our blood and the central sugar in human energy metabolism.

- Carbs are moved around the body in the blood as blood glucose and stored in the liver and muscles as glycogen.

- Foods containing carbs can also be an important source of fibre, which can help promote a healthy gut.

- Excess calories from carbs, just like any other macronutrient will lead to unwanted fat gain.

- Carb sources low on fibre don't tend to fill us up as much as protein and fat and can easily be overeaten.

- Carbs can taste great and can be part of a healthy sustainable diet provided the laws of energy balance are respected.

CARBOHYDRATE AND DIABETES

- Carb consumption causes a rise in blood glucose (sugar), far more than the other macronutrients.

- Low carb diets can work well for fat loss, reducing diabetes medication and improving glycemic control, especially in people who are inactive.

- Highly active people who under eat carbohydrate run the risk of reducing exercise performance and experiencing hypoglycemia.

- Many athletes were traditionally encouraged to have a high carb diet all the time. Modern advice focuses more on varying or tapering the amounts according to exercise workload and aims of the session. This is called perioidisation.

- Carbohydrate counting is an essential strategy for people living with diabetes, especially those with T1D.

WHAT ARE CARBOHYDRATES?

Carbohydrates provide the body with glucose (and other sugars), which is the body's preferred use of energy to support everyday bodily functions and physical activity. This means that if carbohydrate is available, the body will preferentially utilise it as a fuel source over protein and fat.

For body composition and training purposes carbohydrates are incredibly important after protein. If protein resembled the parts of a car, carbohydrates would resemble the fuel to drive it.

Carbs are found in a wide variety of foods and come in a variety of different forms, including sugars, fibre and starches.

CARBOHYDRATES (EXCEPT ARGUABLY FIBRE) ARE CONSIDERED NON-ESSENTIAL BECAUSE THE BODY CAN SYNTHESISE THEM. TECHNICALLY WE CAN LIVE WITHOUT CARBOHYDRATE FOR RELATIVELY LONG PERIODS OF TIME.

In nutrition, carbohydrates are typically divided into two categories, simple and complex, both of which contain different forms of carbohydrate.

SIMPLE CARBS

Simple carbohydrates include two distinct groups: monosaccharide (single sugars) and disaccharides (double sugars).

Both groups of sugar are digested quickly and provide the body with a rapid source of energy.

MONOSACCHARIDES

Glucose is the most important simple sugar in human metabolism. It is the primary energy source for every cell in the human body. Cells use glucose either by aerobic respiration, anaerobic respiration or fermentation.

Other examples of simple sugars include:

- Fructose in fruit
- Galactose in milk
- Ribose is a component of DNA/RNA

DISACCHARIDES

Simple single sugars can be combined with other simple sugars to make disaccharides. Simple sugars can be found in many everyday food products.

- Sucrose (glucose and fructose) - table sugar.
- Lactose (glucose and galactose) - milk sugar.
- Maltose (glucose and glucose) - typically found in beer.

Any carbohydrate that contains more than two simple sugars is said to be a complex carbohydrate or polysaccharide.

COMPLEX CARBOHYDRATES

Complex carbohydrates are made up of individual simple sugar molecules strung together in long, complex chains.

They play various roles, including

- Energy storage (muscle and liver glycogen).
- Starches and fibre found in foods.
- A structural component in plants (cellulose) and certain insects.

FIBRE

The UK government's Scientific Advisory Committee on Nutrition (SACN) defines dietary fibre as any substance:

'Resistant to digestion and absorption in the small intestine and has a demonstrable physiological effect potentially associated with health benefits in the body, such as increasing stool bulk, decreasing intestinal transit time or decreasing post prandial glycaemia.`(rise in blood glucose)'

Evidence indicates that a diet rich in dietary fibre reduces the risk of T2D, cardiovascular disease and colo-rectal cancer [12].

DIETARY FIBRE HAS A NUTRITIONAL VALUE OF 2 KCAL/G, WHICH IS MUCH LOWER THAN THE NUTRITIONAL VALUE OF DIGESTIBLE CARBOHYDRATES AT 4 KCAL/G.

SIMPLE VS. COMPLEX – WHICH IS SUPERIOR?

The distinction between simple and complex carbohydrates is mistakenly used to distinguish nutritional quality, with complex carbohydrates being deemed nutritionally superior.

There may be fair arguments for this. However, fearing their consumption is unreasonable - some simple carbohydrates provide an excellent source of vital nutrients, especially fruits and dairy.

There is a time and place for both types of carbohydrate in our diets, like during exercise or to treat an episode of hypoglycemia. I talk about this in more detail later.

WHAT HAPPENS WHEN YOU CONSUME CARBS?

Digestible, absorbable carbohydrates like sugars and most starches from foods like bread, pasta, potatoes and cereal are digested in the gut, absorbed and transported to the cells of the body and used for energy or stored for future use.

However, dietary fibre is neither digested nor absorbed in the small intestine and remains in the intestines relatively intact, ready to be devoured by the bacteria within our gut.

The potential benefits of gut bacteria would require an entire chapter and is beyond the scope of this text. Their role is highly complex but useful in the synthesis of nutrients, vitamins and other compounds.

Certain short-chain fatty acids obtained from fibre are of particular interest to scientists, as they have shown to play a role in immunity [13], inflammation [14] and protection against obesity [15].

Insoluble fibre also plays a mechanical role and keeps you regular by adding bulk to your faeces. It is found in seeds and the skins of fruit as well as whole-wheat products and brown rice.

Digestible (soluble) fibre attracts water, and turns to a gel during digestion, slowing the digestion of food. Soluble fibre is found in oatmeal, nuts, beans and certain fruits. It is also found in psyllium, a common fibre supplement.

For most people, it's good to have a range of insoluble and soluble fibre in your diet. One exception would be individuals suffering from bowel disorders irritated by fibre.

STORAGE

Once you eat carbohydrate, insulin is (normally) produced in proportion to the amount of carbohydrate (sugar) that appears in the blood after digestion. The more carbohydrates eaten, the more insulin secreted, and vice versa.

As previously discussed people living with diabetes have derangements in insulin production, with T1D individuals being completely deficient and T2D being resistant to its actions.

Insulin's primary role is to bind to the target receptors on the surface of the muscle cells and signal the uptake of glucose from the blood for storage or use. Insulin also acts on adipose (fat) and liver tissue. The way in which glucose is stored depends entirely on the type of cell doing the storing.

Muscle cells store glucose as muscle glycogen.

Liver cells can store glucose as liver glycogen and during times of calorific excess convert glucose into fat via a process called de novo lipogenesis.

Fat cells store glucose as fat, especially during periods of calorific excess. This process is known as lipogenesis.

INSULIN AND MUSCLE BUILDING

INSULIN IS AN ANABOLIC AND ANTI-CATABOLIC HORMONE FOR PROTEIN METABOLISM. PHYSIOLOGICAL CHANGES IN CIRCULATING INSULIN ARE SUFFICIENT TO INHIBIT MUSCLE PROTEIN BREAKDOWN AND A CERTAIN AMOUNT OF INSULIN IS THOUGHT TO FACILITATE MUSCLE PROTEIN SYNTHESIS.

However, it seems that exogenous (injectable) insulin above what is required to maintain homoeostasis is ineffective at modifying muscle protein metabolism.

The fact carbohydrate consumption stimulates insulin secretion significantly more than other macronutrients (fat, protein) makes carbohydrates anti-catabolic to muscle tissue, especially when amino acids (from protein sources) are available as well.

Unfortunately, insulin is anabolic to fat tissue as well when excess calories are consumed.

When you over-consume calories from carbohydrate beyond your body's needs, you initiate unwanted fat gain. Additional carbohydrate also poses an additional challenge for blood glucose control.

FRUCTOSE (FRUIT SUGAR) - AN OUTLIER

Fructose, a simple sugar found in fruit and other food products we eat regularly is dealt with slightly differently than glucose.

The liver is pretty much the only organ that metabolises fructose due to the fact it has a specific transporter for it [16]. The liver preferentially utilises fructose as fuel, leaving glucose to be utilised as fuel across the rest of the body.

The liver has limited storage capacity for fructose, especially when you take into account its role in glucose storage also.

FRUCTOSE HAS GAINED A BAD REPUTATION

Fructose can bypass the need for insulin, and be converted to fat via the process of de novo lipogenesis. This can also occur when muscle glycogen stores are full and excess carbohydrate, including fructose is converted to fat. This concept is the reason for fructose earning a bad rep as one of the leading causes of obesity, fatty liver disease and insulin resistance.

DO I HAVE TO AVOID FRUCTOSE?

The majority of research surrounding this unique carbohydrate is conducted in rodents using unrealistically high amounts of fructose that would be extremely hard to consume in a real life human diet.

It is fair to say the food additive high fructose corn syrup, which is found in confectionery and other food products increases the potential to over-consume fructose compared to just eating fruit alone.

Yet the research doses would still be difficult to achieve. Additionally, when fructose is supplemented to the diet of people in caloric balance, there is no evidence of it causing liver damage [17].

Instead of pointing the finger at small factors like fructose, it's important to consider the bigger picture when it comes to health and nutrition.

There is no denying the fact that obesity is much more likely a result of excess calorie intake from poor quality food choices combined with reduced energy expenditure as a result of modern culture.

While 'excess' energy from fructose may adversely affect health, it should not be given sole blame for this as its role has not been dissected out from excess calories from other sources. There are much bigger, more important factors to consider.

The danger is in the dose.

It is misleading to rely on fructose overfeeding studies or the media scaremongering to term fructose as 'evil'...

There is no proven reason to avoid natural, whole fruit especially when calorie intake and blood glucose levels are well managed and other essential nutrient needs are met.

Potential Benefits of Fructose Consumption.

Fructose is not glycaemic, meaning that consuming it does not tend to raise blood glucose levels. Additionally, fructose is much sweeter than glucose so satisfying a sweet tooth with high fibre fruit or the occasional fructose sweet is much easier to manage than satisfying a sweet tooth with alternative sources of sugar.

CARBOHYDRATE REQUIREMENTS

Carbohydrate intake in people living with diabetes is a hotly debated topic.

Researchers, diabetic patients and health gurus actively debate which type of intake is best. Many advocate low carbohydrate diets whilst others support higher or more moderate carb diets.

'Are low carb diets really the best way to eat for everyone living with diabetes?'

'In what context would low carb not be suitable?'

Low carbohydrate diets have always been considered the primary dietary therapy for diabetes. In fact severe, carbohydrate restriction was prescribed for people living with T1D until 1922, when the discovery of exogenous insulin made it possible to consume carbohydrate-containing foods, although often with less than ideal glycemic control.

The benefits of low carb diets are immediate and well documented for controlling blood glucose and promoting weight loss [18].

However, the majority of research on low carb diets is limited to non-trained individuals looking to lose fat and/or improve their glycaemic control.

Firstly, It is well established that the dietary needs of highly active people are different to those who are sedentary. This questions the value of the current body of evidence and highlights the need for more research in this area.

Secondly, not everyone living with diabetes wants or needs to lose weight. Certain individuals may want to maintain their current body weight or, in some cases increase body mass.

Over the next few pages, I want to discuss carbohydrate needs for exercise and body composition goals in highly active people living with T1D and T2D. I will also outline the pros and cons of low carbohydrate nutrition as well as dispel common myths and fallacies.

PROPOSED BENEFITS OF LOW CARBOHYDRATE DIETS IN DIABETES MANAGEMENT

- **Reducing carbohydrate intake will reduce blood glucose and risk of hyperglycaemia.**

Glycaemic control is the main focus of diabetes management. It is universally accepted that carbohydrate has the greatest effect on blood glucose, and its restriction provides the most significant reduction in post-meal glucose and HbA1c [19,20,21,22,23] (average glucose control)

- **Reducing carbohydrate reduces calorie intake, which reduces the likelihood of obesity. Obesity is strongly linked to the progression of insulin resistance and T2D.**

Refined carbohydrate is less filling than other macronutrients, or carbohydrate sources high in fibre.

Carbs can be very easy to overeat and have the potential to drive us into a calorie surplus, especially when they're in a refined form and/or consumed alongside protein and fat. Just think of a delicious cheese loaded meat feast pizza.

This is one of the reasons why popular low-carb diets, such as the Atkins diet [24] don't account for calories. They assume that the greater satiety of protein and fat will automatically control calorie intake.

- **Eating a low carb diet can still lead to improvements in glycaemic control even without weight loss.**

As previously mentioned many people living with diabetes do not need to lose weight. Research has shown low carb diets (up to 20% of total intake) are suitable for maintaining current body weight whilst also improving glycaemic control and key hormonal and lipid biomarkers [25, 26, 27, 28, 29].

- **During carbohydrate restriction, people with T2D can reduce and in some cases eliminate their medication. While, people with T1D diabetes may be able to lower their medication requirements.**

A reduction in carbohydrate intake will lead to a reduction in blood glucose levels, which reduces the need for medication in both T1D and T2D, particularly injectable insulin [30], glucose disposal agents [31] and other forms of diabetes medication.

Lower carb diets theoretically require less insulin, meaning there should be less chance of hypoglycaemia, which requires the consumption of unnecessary calories, increasing the potential for fat gain.

Medication is expensive especially in countries where you have to pay for your health care. Low carb diets could ease the burden on the wallet.

Reducing carbohydrate intake also reduces the potential for hyperglycaemia, especially post mealtime. For example, if I didn't eat 20g of carbohydrate in one meal but instead consumed 10g of protein and 10g fat, which meal would have a greater effect on my blood glucose level? Of course, it would be the carbohydrate meal.

The resultant hyperglycaemia (if left uncontrolled) is the main underlying factor behind diabetic health problems. Therefore one could argue a pretty strong case for managing diabetes by promoting a lower carb way of eating.

PEOPLE LIVING WITH T2D WHO REDUCE THEIR CARBOHYDRATE COULD POTENTIALLY REDUCE THE DEMAND ON THE INSULIN-PRODUCING CELLS OF THE PANCREAS AND, AS A RESULT, IMPROVE THEIR BODY'S SENSITIVITY TO INSULIN. HOWEVER, THIS EFFECT IS LIKELY TO BE MORE SIGNIFICANT VIA FAT LOSS AND GENERAL CALORIC RESTRICTION AS OPPOSED TO CARBOHYDRATE RESTRICTION ALONE.

The Flip Side: Carbohydrate's Beneficial Role In Body Composition and Performance

How would these findings apply to individuals who weight train 4-6 times a week? Especially when you take into account the physiological benefits weight training has on metabolic rate and blood glucose control, which would otherwise be unchanged in an inactive person living with diabetes.

You also need to ask whether you can you stick to a low carb diet.

It is increasingly clear that the 'best' diet is simply the one you can stick to over the long-term [32]. No matter what a diet contains, adherence determines if you benefit.

CARBOHYDRATE CAN ALSO PLAY A HUGELY BENEFICIAL ROLE IN SUPPORTING BODY COMPOSITION, PERFORMANCE AND BLOOD GLUCOSE MANAGEMENT.

From a body composition and performance standpoint glucose plays a pretty big role, including:

- Supplying the Body with its Preferred Fuel Source.

- Replenishing Muscle and Liver Glycogen.

- The anti-catabolic effect of Insulin on Muscle.

- Treating Hypoglycaemia.

- The ability to stimulate metabolic rate during prolonged periods of caloric restriction.

DEFINING CARBOHYDRATE NEED - MINIMAL, EXCESSIVE AND OPTIMAL INTAKES

Carbohydrates are a non-essential dietary nutrient, meaning your body can synthesise them from other sources. Nevertheless, there are minimal, excessive and optimal intakes.

Eating too little carbohydrates can potentially:

- Increase risk of hypoglycaemia, especially in those living with T1D.
- Decrease training performance and motivation due to low muscle glycogen.
- Reduce the potential for muscle growth due to the anti-catabolic effect of insulin and chronically low muscle glycogen.
- Promote feelings of dietary restriction, potentially limiting adherence and increasing the chances of dietary blowout.
- Limit body composition improvements and performance

THE INITIAL WEIGHT DROP WHEN FOLLOWING A LOW CARBOHYDRATE DIET IS PRIMARILY A RESULT OF FLUID LOSS. THIS MAY BE A GREAT START TO A FAT LOSS JOURNEY BUT SHOULDN'T BE EXPECTED WEEK AFTER WEEK.

Consuming too many carbohydrates can:

- Increase risk of hyperglycaemia and hyperinsulinemia, both of which are highly detrimental to health, body composition and performance.
- Facilitate fat growth and decrease the insulin sensitivity of muscle tissue (jeopardising muscle growth)
- Increase appetite due to its low satiety value, which increases the potential to over-consume calories and the chances of unwanted fat gain.

ATHLETES WITH DIABETES ENGAGING IN HIGH VOLUME ENDURANCE EXERCISE HAVE SIGNIFICANTLY HIGHER NEEDS FOR CARBOHYDRATE.

INCREDIBLY LEAN INDIVIDUALS WHO PERFORM A LOT OF TRAINING, OR WANT TO INCREASE BODY MASS MAY NEED TO EAT MORE CARBOHYDRATE THAN NORMAL.

Optimal Carbohydrate Intake should:

1. Provide enough carbohydrate to enhance physical performance and regenerate energy stores post exercise.

2. Support blood sugar management by providing adequate availability of carbohydrate to treat hypos.

3. Be covered with adequate amounts of injectable insulin and other medication.

4. Obtain adequate amounts of fibre to promote a healthy gut.

5. Be tweaked and adjusted to match changes in body composition and performance outcomes.

6. Suit personal preference, e.g. taste and mood.

THE PUMP

In weightlifting and bodybuilding circles, many people seek 'the pump', a phrase popularised by Arnold Schwarzenegger in the film Pumping Iron. Arnold actually described the pump as a better feeling than sexual intercourse.

The pump describes a well-fed and hydrated muscle that becomes engorged quickly with blood during training.

Anecdotal reports suggest that carbs are crucial for achieving muscle fullness and the much sought after pump. Sorry, I don't have scientific research to support this, but after performing thousands of gym sessions, I can safely say that training on ultra low carbs generates a pathetic pump. It is an unfortunate trade off when you're dieting down to ultra low levels of body fat.

CARBOHYDRATE MYTHS AND FALLACIES

Myth: High carb diet leads to chronically high insulin levels. Carbohydrate drives insulin, which drives fat gain.

Fact: Your body can store fat even when insulin levels are low. Total energy intake matters more when it comes to rate of fat gain.

Carbohydrates and insulin have been given a bad name and are often viewed as the reason behind why we get fat.

Firstly, let me explain in very simple terms the underlying theory behind insulin, carbohydrates and fat gain.

There is an enzyme in your fat cells called hormone-sensitive lipase (HSL), which is responsible for breaking down fat. Insulin suppresses the actions of this hormone, meaning you break down less fat.

Since carbohydrate has the greatest influence on insulin secretion over other macronutrients, it is the main reason why this nutrient is demonized. But this is a very narrow view of the body's ability to process food and burn and store fat.

Although insulin secretion may go up during meal times and suppress fat burning temporarily, it's important to consider what goes on for the remaining 24 hours across the day.

People alternate between fed and unfed states across the day. The net balance between what is stored vs. what is burnt off ultimately dictates how much fat we gain, regardless of the type of macronutrients consumed.

Carbohydrates and insulin aren't needed for fat storage; your body can store fat even when insulin is low.

If carbohydrate and high insulin levels were to blame for making people fat, how can you explain the increased levels of obesity in the USA compared to populations that consume the majority of their diet from carbohydrate, such as Italy, France and Japan?

Adding to that, recent data from the U.S. Department of Agriculture has estimated consumption of sugar has dropped by nearly 14% from its peak in 1999, when the average American consumed nearly 422 calories per day in sugar and other sweeteners (33).

So if carbohydrate and sugar intake have gone down in the American population yet obesity levels have gone up, what gives?

Simple – Americans eat more calories and burn off fewer. Energy balance matters a great deal, not the insulin fairy.

HOW MANY CARBS DO I REALLY NEED?

Carbohydrates are a non-essential dietary nutrient, meaning your body can synthesise them from other sources. Nevertheless, there are minimal, excessive and optimal intakes.

Carbohydrate intake varies between individuals and is usually dictated by the following factors:

Body Composition
Individuals with greater levels of muscle mass have a greater metabolic need for carbohydrate due to increased storage for muscle glycogen. Needless to say, carbohydrate provides the perfect source of fuel for the type of training required to sustain high levels of muscle mass.

Training Volume
Greater training volume and intensity can justify a higher intake of carbohydrate for performance needs.

Training Goal – Fat Loss Vs Muscle Gain
If your goal is fat loss you might want to start by consuming greater amounts of protein (provided your kidney function is healthy) due to its ability to suppress appetite.

During a mass gain phase, you may want to consider eating slightly less protein due to the fact it can reduce appetite and hinder your ability to meet higher calorie needs.

Respect the fact protein pales in comparison to carbs as a fuel source. Your training performance may be better off with more carbs. If you try to fuel your training with protein, it will also prove very expensive.

Glycemic Control
As previously discussed, low blood sugar can be solved with additional carbohydrate whereas high blood glucose justifies a lower intake of carbohydrate until blood sugar has been corrected with insulin.

Personal Preference
The amount, type and frequency of carbohydrate consumed in someone's diet will depend on their personal preference for carbohydrate-based food. If someone doesn't like the taste of carbohydrate food, they do have the capacity to reduce intake indefinitely.

Intra Workout Carbohydrate
Generally speaking, total carbohydrate intake across the day matters more than what you consume during training. The only exception to this is during double or triple day training sessions.

During training, I've found 30-60g of carbs per hour to suffice. However, if you are trying to lose body fat, you may want to eat your carbohydrates from whole food sources for appetite control rather than in liquid form during training. Liquid form would be the most suitable option during a weight training session to protect against bloating and discomfort. Nevertheless bloating and discomfort remains a possibility with intra workout supplementation.

It is essential to monitor blood glucose levels closely in and around exercise. The idea of purposely reducing bolus insulin prior to training may prove useful when performing low intensity training, such as cardio, but maybe not for high intensity training or weight lifting, as it has the tendency to increase blood glucose.

Insulin availability (extreme cases, such as when you forget)
What happens if you forget your insulin? Or break your pump? Contacting your nearest doctor and chemist is a must. However, in the time between doing so you may have to make compromises with your food selection for obvious reasons.

WORKING OUT HOW MANY CARBS TO EAT?

Work out your essential nutrient requirements first.
Before working out your carb intake, establish the minimum requirements for essential nutrients, which are 1.4g of protein per kg of body weight and 15% of total calories for fat. Higher protein intakes up to 2g may be more beneficial for those trying to lose weight.

CONSUMING THE LOWER LIMITS OF FAT AND PROTEIN WILL ALLOW FOR A HIGHER CARB INTAKE, WHILST CONSUMING THE HIGHER INTAKES WILL RESTRICT CARBOHYDRATE INTAKE.

ONCE CALORIES FOR ENERGY BALANCE HAVE BEEN ESTABLISHED ALONG WITH ESSENTIAL PROTEIN AND FATTY ACID NEEDS, CARBOHYDRATE CAN MAKE UP YOUR REMAINING CALORIES.

There is always flexibility to adjust carbohydrate intake depending on how much you play about with protein and fat ranges. Whether you go high or low is entirely based on your personal feedback.

THERE ARE CURRENTLY NO RECOMMENDATIONS FOR CARBOHYDRATE INTAKE IN HIGHLY TRAINED INDIVIDUALS LIVING WITH DIABETES, ESPECIALLY T1D.

WHAT IS THE BEST TIME TO EAT CARBOHYDRATE?

Interestingly, the timing of carbs isn't worth fussing about because it only makes marginal differences to muscle vs. fat gains.

The only major time to be concerned with carbohydrate timing is when treating hypoglycaemia/ hyperglycaemia or when refuelling between training sessions that are within close proximity.

WHAT ABOUT DURING TRAINING?

The timing of carbohydrate in and around exercise, along with current blood glucose levels will influence what fuels are burned during workouts. When people without diabetes consume carbohydrates prior to exercise there is a, marked reduction in fat burning compared to when carbohydrates are taken 30 minutes into the training (34).

Commencing training with a blood glucose of 6-10 mmol/L (108-180mg/dL) and delaying eating carbohydrate until 20-30 minutes into training could optimize the rate of fat burning. However, this focuses on the training window alone and doesn't take into account the major effects of food intake, physical activity and blood glucose control across the day.

It has also been suggested that exercising in a hyperglycaemic state increases reliance on carbohydrate as fuel compared to exercising in a normal blood glucose range (35). This results in more rapid depletion of muscle glycogen and increase the chances of fatigue, leading to poor performance.

CASE STUDY

I discuss the percentages and calculations in greater detail in the 'building your diet' section of this chapter.

Goal: Fat Loss
Age: 23
Height: 5ft 11
Gender: Male
Body Weight: 90kg
Maintenance Calories: 2800 kcal
Calories adjusted for fat loss goal (-20%): 2240 kcal

Step 1
Protein Intake (1.4 to 2.0 g/kg/day)   90 x 1.4g = 126g Protein

N.B. The protein recommendation here is not a minimum – it's based on weight loss studies showing that protein within that range retains lean mass when compared to the standard minimum of 0.8g/kg.

Step 2
Fat Intake (Min 15%-25% of intake)
25% of 2240 kcal = 560 kcals/9 kcals (per 1g fat) = 62g fat

Step 3
Carbs (remainder of calories)
2240 kcals – 504 kcal from 126g protein – 560 kcals from 62g fat
= kcal 1176/ 4 kcal (per 1g carb) = 294g carbs

2240 kcal   126g Protein (23%)   294g Carbs (52%)   62g Fat (25%)

This calorie and macronutrient example has been developed using the minimum recommended intakes for protein and maximum intakes for fat.

On the contrary, if I wanted to eat more protein and fat, purely based on personal preference or if I found difficulty in managing my blood glucose due to consuming higher amounts of carbohydrate, I would re-work my macros and strive to eat a higher intake of protein. This would leave fewer calories available to use for carbohydrate.

THE DEMAND FOR CARBOHYDRATES IS GENERALLY HIGHER ON TRAINING DAYS COMPARED TO NON-TRAINING DAYS. TRAINING PERFORMANCE MAY BE IMPROVED BY ADJUSTING ACCORDINGLY.

WHAT ABOUT FIBRE INTAKE?

According to the 2015 The Scientific Advisory Committee on Nutrition (SCAN), we should eat at least 30g per day of fibre because this is the minimum amount associated with reduced risk of disease.

There is evidence to show that certain isolated fibres have positive health effects on blood lipids and digestive function but due to the small body of evidence, it is debatable whether these components confer the full range of health benefits associated with consuming a mix of dietary fibre rich foods. Consume your fibre intake from a variety of food sources.

CARBOHYDRATE GRAM COUNTING

Measuring carbohydrate intake is crucial for blood glucose management, especially with T1D. Once you know how many carbohydrates are in a particular meal, you can adjust your insulin and other medications in proportion.

If you haven't already, I highly recommend going on a carbohydrate counting course. These courses are delivered by local healthcare professionals and are usually free to attend. Carbohydrate counting courses have different names depending on where you live. In the UK and Ireland, there are a number of education courses, including BERTIE and DAFNE (Dose Adjustment For Normal Eating).

Bear in mind the generic dosing protocols (grams per carbs to units of insulin) promoted in these courses are merely a rough starting point and their accuracy will vary greatly from individual to individual.

HOW TO COUNT CARBOHYDRATES

All food manufacturers are required to list product ingredients. If you look on a food label, you will see everything from portion size, calories, carbohydrates right through to sweeteners, preservatives and everything else in between.

One of the simplest ways to count carbs is to look at the total carbohydrate content and breakdown on a food label. You can also use popular online food databases like MyFitness Pal or Calorie King.

The label will list the following:

- Sugars (simple carbohydrates)
- Starch (+ other forms of carbohydrate)
- Fibre

Added together they tell you the total amount of carbohydrate.

Although different sources of carbohydrate digest quicker than others, it is generally best to count the total amount of carbohydrates on a food packet, as most carbohydrates eventually convert to glucose.

For example 20g of carbs from sweet potato will raise blood glucose slower than 20g of carbohydrate from sugar loaded confectionary, but after several hours the total rise in blood glucose will be the same.

FIBRE

Fibre is a carbohydrate that is resistant to digestion and does not tend to raise blood glucose levels. When reviewing the nutrition information of a label, subtract grams of fibre away from the total amount of carbohydrate to calculate the proportion.

ARTIFICIAL SWEETENERS

There are only a select few artificial sweeteners that have no significant effect on blood glucose levels.

These include:
- Acesulfame K
- Sucralose
- Aspartame
- Stevia

ARE ARTIFICIAL SWEETENERS SAFE?

Generally speaking yes.

The most recent evidence from epidemiological studies suggests that they don't cause cancer or weight gain (37). Nor are they toxic in the doses consumed in food.

Despite what many scaremongering health gurus may say there is very little evidence to indicate any long-term health risks in humans from consuming artificial sweeteners (38, 39), which are typically found in diet soft drinks.

Some studies have actually shown that artificial sweeteners may even improve weight loss and long-term control of body weight (37).

However, diet soft drinks are still bad for your dental health (40). This makes dental hygiene a priority for those who consume carbonated soda regularly. Drinking your fizzy drinks through a straw is a valid strategy to avoid acid damage.

Poor dental hygiene is a major barrier to eating the nutrients you need for muscle growth and recovery.

SUGAR-FREE FOODS

Food marketers will do anything to sell their products, even if it means pulling the wool over your eyes. This especially applies to the carbohydrate content of fancy new 'sugar-free' foods. A prime example of these claims can be found on most 'low carb/sugar-free' protein bars.

Remember sucrose, the simple carbohydrate we talked about earlier? It's most popularly known as table sugar and contains a combination of glucose and fructose.

If a food product doesn't contain a gram of sucrose (table sugar) it can claim on the label to be sugar-free – sneaky, eh?

JUST BECAUSE FOOD SAYS IT'S SUGAR-FREE DOES NOT MEAN IT WON'T AFFECT YOUR BLOOD GLUCOSE LEVELS.

Sugar-free foods can contain a variety of carbohydrate fillers and substitutes that escape this loophole, such as xylitol, mannitol, lactitol, isomalt and sorbitol (sugar alcohols)

Calculate for the carbohydrate content of these products but realise these kinds of fillers won't have as strong an effect on blood glucose levels as normal carbohydrate sources.

TAKE HOME MESSAGE

Low carbohydrate diets can be beneficial to fat loss and diabetes management in sedentary individuals. However, they may be counterproductive to a highly active person living with diabetes who has muscle building, fat loss and performance goals.

If you're highly active and enjoy carbohydrate-based foods, eat them. There is no need to restrict an entire food group if you're going to end up driving yourself mad craving your favourite carb-based foods 24/7. Just ensure you respect your overall calorie intake and administer the necessary medication to control your blood glucose.

For people living with T1D, regular blood glucose testing and carbohydrate counting are useful to maintaining glycaemic control.

If you don't tolerate carbs well, consume fewer of them and get more of your calories from fat and protein but again, remember to respect your overall energy intake.

YOUR BODY CAN STORE FAT EVEN WHEN INSULIN AND CARB LEVELS ARE LOW. TOTAL ENERGY INTAKE MATTERS MORE WHEN IT COMES TO FAT BALANCE.

Alcohol, along with carbohydrate, protein and fat, is a macronutrient. It contains seven calories per gram and is found in different quantities across a range of beverages, ranging from spirits and wine to beer and shots.

ALCOHOL AND DIABETES

Alcohol in its purest form has the tendency to lower blood glucose levels because it hinders the liver from secreting glucose into the bloodstream. This means hypoglycaemia is a real possibility when consuming alcohol, especially spirits, or when taken with low calorie, sugar-free soft drinks.

PREVENTING HYPOGLYCAEMIA IS OF PARAMOUNT IMPORTANCE WHEN DRINKING.

When drinking, firstly assess the carbohydrate content of the beverage. For things like cider, beer and spirits with sugary mixers you will need to inject a bolus to cover the carbohydrate content. However, you need to be mindful of how much alcohol is contained within each drink and how much you plan to drink in total. Over the course of a night you may need to taper off your bolus to prevent a delayed drop in blood glucose that results from the alcohol.

Most people tend to stick to the same alcoholic beverages every time they go out. This consistency can allow you to predict patterns in the way your blood glucose behaves.

Be incredibly mindful that being drunk can often be mistaken for a hypo. I have made this mistake many times and ended up super-high on social occasions.

ALCOHOL AND BODY COMPOSITION

Alcoholic drinks can be incredibly calorie dense. A typical pint of 5% beer is approximately 170 kcal. This is due to the high carbohydrate content of some alcoholic drinks. Remember too that a gram of alcohol is 7 kcal as opposed to 4 kcal from carbohydrate or protein.

Also, when you're intoxicated your food choices tend to go out the window, especially on the trip home or when you return home and raid the cupboards. This links back to my point earlier on about food environment – don't keep crap in the house. Make it as hard as possible to overeat junk food.

When drunk you are nowhere near as mindful of food choice or counting calories. A week's effort of eating and training can easily be flushed down the toilet by a midnight alcohol-fuelled binge. Never mind waking up the next day with an awful blood glucose reading.

You also dramatically increase your chances of injury. Whether that be falling over, getting knocked down by a car or starting an argument. An injury will wreak havoc with any muscle building and fat loss efforts.

ALCOHOL AND EXERCISE RECOVERY

There are a number of problems with drinking alcohol after exercise.

First of all, you will most likely be dehydrated. Alcohol consumption has a diuretic (water loss) effect, which can result in further dehydration. Although it contains fluid, the alcohol component of a drink inhibits the release of the hormone AVP (arginine vasopressin) or argipressin, an anti-diuretic hormone produced in the kidneys that allows you to retain water and regulate fluid balance.

Additionally, alcohol has vasodilation properties, meaning blood flow is re-directed to the body's surface. i.e. the skin, causing further sweat loss and dehydration. This is the reason for those rosy cheeks when you're drinking.

Alcohol may also suppress the body's ability to create and resynthesize glycogen (stored carbohydrate in muscle and liver), which will undoubtedly delay the recovery and restoration of muscle fuel stores. This is problematic if you're planning multiple training sessions.

Alcohol can reduce the rate of muscle protein synthesis (the process of muscle growth and repair) by blocking certain bio-chemical pathways that activate this process. The end result is delayed muscle repair and increased muscle soreness, which carries over into crappy performance in other training sessions.

If you are counting calories, and consume alcohol at the expense of other nutrients from the diet, notably protein, essential fats and carbohydrate, which are significantly more important for recovery then you will undoubtedly slow your progress.

TO DRINK OR NOT TO DRINK?

The occasional alcoholic beverage (or two) is absolutely fine and can be included as part of a healthy diet and training regime geared towards fat loss or mass gain in people living with diabetes. To prevent alcohol from interfering with your progress and health, consider the following.

- Monitor blood glucose behaviour as much as possible when drinking.
- Learn the difference between being drunk, and suffering a hypoglycaemic episode.
- Carry a fast acting source of carbohydrate with you when drinking as a hypo prevention strategy. I've found a tube shaped packet of hard chewy sweets (Mentos) best for nights out.
- Expect a delayed hypo when sleeping after a day or night of drinking – have precautionary measures in place.
- Consume a recovery meal or drink containing both carbohydrate and protein as soon as possible post exercise and before consuming alcohol.
- Rehydrate as soon as possible after a night of drinking.
- Rehydrate post-exercise, and attempt to establish fluid balance before consuming alcohol.
- Alternate alcoholic drinks with water to minimise the negative effects of alcohol on hydration status.
- Keep the cupboards low in junk food after a night of drinking, with the exception of hypo prevention foods.
- Be mindful that alcohol contains calories and can contribute to fat gain and obesity.
- Use common sense – getting drunk every night of the week is not healthy and highly detrimental to any of your health, muscle building, and fat loss progress

We're all human and enjoy social gatherings. Enjoy your alcohol, but remember the danger is in the dose and frequency. Enjoy in moderation and always prioritise exercise recovery.

WHY DIETS FAIL

Before I go into the nuts and bolts of calories, food choice and setting up your diet, I want to tackle the main reasons why most diets fail. The same principles hold true for those looking to gain weight.

So...

What exactly makes the perfect diet?

A quick Google search on 'The Perfect Diet' presents me with 124,000,000 results.

Great choice of diets, Right?

But with all this information why is obesity and T2D still a growing problem?

Surely there's more than enough information out there for people to use in their quest to become healthier, leaner, stronger and fitter?

What's the problem – is losing weight and getting in shape, not simply a matter of eating less and moving more?

And why do some people lose a ton of weight then put it back on again?

ARE PEOPLE JUST LAZY?

Common sayings like, 'get up of your ass' or, 'put the fork down' are not the most successful ways to treat obesity. Such advice has a very low success rate, which is why we need to shift the way we think.

The question of how to eat in order to maintain a healthy weight has never been more important. Too much attention is placed on which diet is best, which macro split is best, what super food is best and what supplement will do the most work for me.

The media spin their wheels comparing one diet to another, and we spin along with them, buying into so-called magic fixes only to be left no better off than when we started because we gave up half way or failed to keep the weight off after finishing the said diet.

The reality is, most people know what to do – they simply don't know how to stick to it. So the solution is to find something you can stick with that works – but sadly it's not that easy for many of us to do this.

A great piece of research conducted by The Journal of The American Medical Association (46) entitled 'A Call for an End to the Diet Debates' supports this view.

The study set out to review the body of research around studies that compared one diet to another. Lots of data was taken into account across a vast range of diet study comparisons. The study reviewed every type of diet imaginable from low fat, low carb, low GI and the Atkins diet through to the paleo diet and many others.

It found the diets debated the same old stuff, such as food choice, calories, carbs, proteins, fats, blood tests, supplements etc.

BOTTOM LINE?

There was no bottom line. No diet significantly outperformed the others. In fact, many produced similar weight loss results.

In other words – The diets worked!

SO WHY AREN'T THESE DIETS BEING PUT TO GOOD USE?

The reality is that although the diets work, most people don't stick with them long enough for sustainable fat loss.

The study concluded that those individuals who stuck to their diets the longest were the most successful at losing fat and keeping it off.

SO WHAT'S THE TAKE HOME MESSAGE?

Food intake is important when it comes to fat loss. But the conversation must shift away from 'the perfect diet' and focus more on the bigger picture of building long-term behavior and lifestyle habits that support fat loss efforts.

In other words, you are what you do on average. Regardless of what your diet is called or made up of, if you can't stick to it over the long haul, you won't reap the benefits, especially when it comes to maximising fat loss and body recomposition.

The same also applies to your exercise regime – it must also be sustainable and work in harmony (as much as practically possible) with your lifestyle and training ability. If it's too extreme, you simply won't last nor be able to sustain any form of result for long.

A CLOSER LOOK AT ADHERENCE ISSUES

Before I get into the nuts and bolts of calories, nutrients and supplements lets take a closer look at some of the common problems that make supposedly perfect diets not-so-perfect in the long run.

TRYING TO BE EXACT

Trying to be exact will stress you out. It's more important to develop mental flexibility than trying to work out your metabolic flexibility, which may not exist.

Remember, the calorie values you see on the back of a food packet are merely estimates. The calorie and nutrient content of an apple grown in your town will be slightly different to the calorie and nutrient content of an apple grown in another town.

As such trying to work your diet around exact calorie and calorie guidelines will prove difficult, especially as your food preferences change.

Different goals require different levels of accuracy. For example, a competitive bodybuilder who is in the final weeks of dialling in for competition will require a higher level of accuracy when measuring his or her caloric intake than a rugby player looking to maximise game performance.

SOLUTION

Aim to work on a rough rather than rigid template. Accept you will never be exact.

LACK OF CONSISTENCY

On the other hand: to state the obvious, if you're not reasonably accurate and are consistently off with your calorie intake you are destined to plateau and even regress your body composition and performance related goals.

This is simply a result of overindulging.

The odd slip-up isn't a problem so don't beat yourself up about it. However regular slip-ups become habit and should make you question your agenda.

Is my diet and training approach too extreme, increasing my hunger and driving me mad for high calorie foods?

Am I in the right state of mind mentally to pursue my goals of chasing a better body? Is my personal life in check, am I comfort eating? Am I in a bad environment?

SOLUTION

Realise you are what you do on average.

YOU DON'T ENJOY THE PROCESS

One of the most important aspects of getting (and staying) motivated to build a better body is enjoying the process.

You won't stick to a diet comprised of foods you dislike. Equally, you won't stick to a training programme that's too difficult.

We must look beyond simple vitamins, minerals, carbs, protein and fats and consider the entire eating experience. The aroma of food, the pleasure of cooking it and the social interaction at the dinner table all have the potential to nourish our body and mind.

How do you feel when sitting down to a delicious home-cooked meal with family and friends?

I get feelings of excitement, pleasure right through to utter fulfilment.

The problem is most people are afraid to eat foods they like. The common perception of eating tasty food doesn't correlate with getting in shape. And, no I'm not just referring to fast food and confectionery.

The general feeling is one must suffer in order to look good by eating a bland, restricted diet or training with the idiotic ethos of 'pain is weakness leaving the body'.

I don't blame people for thinking like this, especially when you take into account the vast amount of self shaming, food shaming, sacrifice-related messages that are portrayed across the media (especially social media) nowadays.

ANY OF THE FOLLOWING RING A BELL?

No carbs after 6.'

'Suck it up now, and you won't have to suck it up later'.

'Sore is the new sexy.'

No wonder people go crazy after their diet ends and binge eat the very foods they restricted in the first place.

Living between extremes of control and losing control is not healthy.

Don't develop a love-hate relationship with food.

SOLUTION

You'd be surprised just what kinds of foods you can consume in a fat loss 'diet' once you gain an understanding of basic nutrition, energy balance and how to cook properly.

Firstly, calories matter a great deal when it comes to losing or gaining weight. If you stick to your calorie limit and meet your minimum macronutrient targets for essential fats and protein across the day (not just in one meal) you'll give yourself a substantial amount of freedom, diet flexibility and mind space!

For example, people label certain foods good or bad regardless of dose and frequency.

The reality is we don't eat food in isolation. We eat diets so there are no good or bad foods, only good or bad diets.

Later in this chapter, I outline how you can build your diet choosing the very foods you love.

FAILURE TO MEASURE

How do you know your approach is optimal? How do you know it's even working?

If you aren't assessing, you just guess – simple!

It's amazing to see so many people jump head first into their diet journey with no clear plan or intention of assessing what they do. You can put a safe bet on that if you're not measuring you're going to fail or at least achieve mediocre results.

Measurements provide feedback as to the effectiveness of your approach.

SOLUTION

Two key areas must be measured:

1. The Variables that get you towards your end goal. They include nutrition, training and lifestyle.

Approximate calorie intake, how you respond to certain foods, how much weight you lifted in the gym and how many hours sleep you've had over the week all matter.

2. The End Goals of health, body composition and performance.

YOU WANT TO LOOK, FEEL AND PERFORM BETTER, RIGHT?

Keep a close eye on all of these goals and assess if you're happy with progress – if not, a variable needs changing! On the other hand, if your progressing at a steady rate, awesome. If it isn't broke – don't fix it!

Measurement is a fundamental principle of the Diabetic Muscle & Fitness Guide, especially when it comes to blood work. In fact, I've dedicated a complete chapter to the topic. I outline every factor you need to measure and how you can adjust your nutrition, training and lifestyle when things aren't going to plan.

You can read more about measurement and why it is so important in chapter 8.

EXTREMISM

This refers to radical adjustments to your diet (and training) in stark contrast to what you're comfortable with.

The more extreme the behaviour change, the poorer the adherence and the greater the likelihood of behavioural backlash over time.

Most dietary blunders start with an extrinsic goal. It could be anything from a hot date, the holiday to the beach, a wedding, a photo shoot for a local press article or even wanting to compete in a local fitness competition.

You look at yourself and realise you need to get in shape and drop some weight fast.

Based on everything you know, whether it's been from hearsay or what you've read in magazines and books over the years, your only understanding of how to lose weight is, 'eat less, move more'.

This holds some truth, however, like most people you think more is better. You slash your food intake, which also includes your favourite social vices of alcohol and chocolate. You also start going to the gym every day.

Based on how you lived before it's a radical change.

Initially, it works – weight falls off, and your willpower is at an all time high.

As time goes by your body and mind begin to struggle with what you've thrown at it. Willpower takes a blow, but you persist – only 3 weeks left, 2 weeks....

You finally get there, the day you've been finally waiting for. You look much better than you ever have. You did it!

But there's a problem: what do you do next?

You say to yourself it's over, let your hair down, relax, eat and drink up...

Fast forward 6 weeks – you're heavier than before you started, haven't set foot in the gym and feel and look like shit.

The problem? The plan wasn't sustainable.

All that work for nothing.

How many people do you know have started a diet, done well and kept the weight off?

Not many!

Don't get me wrong if you have a specific date you need to be in shape for, so be it.

SOLUTION

Generally speaking, fitness shouldn't have a time scale. Instead of looking for a 30-day abs challenge or a 20-day detox, think long-term. You must be prepared to put the work in for years; lots of years.

ANTI-LIFESTYLE

If you are a student and live on a limited budget, you'll struggle to buy expensive cuts of meat. And, if you live in shared accommodation you may struggle to store a week's worth of food using shared facilities.

If your cultural beliefs don't allow for the consumption of certain types of meat, so be it – you can't and won't eat them. If you have a demanding job, you can hardly eat a meal at your own leisure. You may have to wait and consume it at another time.

SOLUTION

The diet must fit your life, not the other way around.

This includes everything from shopping budget, your ability to eat during the day, culinary skills, right through to cultural beliefs.

ALL-OR-NOTHING APPROACH

Taking an all-or-nothing approach to diet is one sure way to stress out. Rigid meal plans are a sign of this approach.

The reality is:

- Food preference may change with mood.
- You might not always be able to eat at a particular time.
- Your supermarket might run out of a particular food.
- You might have to eat at an important social occasion.
- You will mistrack.

Don't get me wrong. Meal plans can be a great learning tool but long-term they are not sustainable. The minute most people go off plan, everything else goes out the window.

You must be flexible in your approach by adjusting food choices as you go. For example, if you go to a lunch party and fancy a treat that isn't outlined in your diet plan.

What do you do?

A.   Stick to the plan and stress yourself out all day thinking about the food.

B.   Eat everything you can at the lunch and spend the rest of the day eating crap. All just because you went off plan.

C.   Consume the food, tie it in with your overall energy intake and return to normal eating after.

Of course, C is the most sensible answer. But most people go with A and B. As outlined earlier there is no such thing as good or bad food. Provided you keep within your set calorie targets it is more than acceptable to adapt your diet as you go.

LACK OF VARIETY

Don't let good food go to waste! It was created for a purpose. And, no this doesn't relate to French fries. I'm talking about real deal, delicious, wholesome, minimally processed cuisine from all over the world.

Following a diet that contains a limited food selection may limit your intake of key nutrients and contribute to deficiencies. The benefits of fibre will depend on you eating a variety of different fibre sources. Varying your protein intake allows for a varied amino acid intake – each amino acid serves a unique purpose. Varying fat sources allows you to take advantage of the different health properties each fatty acid possesses. Sticking to a small list of foods may result in severe digestive and total body discomfort the very minute you step outside this list due to the down regulation of key digestive enzymes.

THERE IS NO MAGIC MACRO PLUG & PLAY FORMULA

Macros are important, especially the essential fats and amino acids.

However, fussing about the exact proportions of carbs, fats and protein in your diet will result in stress.

As long as you've met the minimum threshold for each nutrient, energy balance will always dominate as the number one player when it comes to promoting fat loss and body composition change.

As outlined earlier, your food preferences may change with mood, certain foods may be unavailable, and we need to avoid the all-or-nothing style approach that can often lead to crawling the walls the minute you go outside your set macro guideline.

I've outlined specific ranges for all the macronutrients in this chapter, but again remember: they are a guide and open to change.

TAKE HOME MESSAGE

Getting in shape is one thing, staying in shape is another.

The Diabetic Muscle and Fitness Guide doesn't provide you with an exact meal-by-meal diet plan. Instead, it presents a set of guidelines and knowledge to build a diet from the plate up.

This trumps working off a set plan any day.

BUILDING YOUR DIET FROM THE PLATE UP

This is the exact set up system I have used and refined from working with a wide range of clients over the last five years.

In this section I will cover:

- How to establish a calorie baseline.
- How to set calorie intake for fat loss.
- How to set calorie intake for mass gain.
- How to work out macro(nutrient) targets.
- How to measure the effectiveness of your approach.
- How and when to change things (for better progress).

People generally have one of two goals: lose fat or gain muscle mass. People with T1D may want to lose fat or gain body mass whilst in most cases T2D's need to lose weight.

You may be starting this programme as a complete beginner, or you may have a few years experience under your belt. Generally speaking, the more body fat you carry the less training experience you will have. On the contrary, you may have a few years training under your belt but are very unhappy with how you look and perform.

Let's fix that.

FAT LOSS AND MUSCLE GAIN FUNDAMENTALS

- **Untrained individuals with poor eating experience can make absolutely astonishing gains in a very short period of time.** This is known as 'newbie gains'. The sudden change in dietary intake and physical activity gives the body no option but to change. So, for those of you starting out, take advantage of this and realise your first year will yield your best results of all time. Make the most of it!

- **Fat can be lost quicker than muscle is gained.** So those losing fat will experience more obvious rapid changes to their physiques compared to those chasing mass gain.

- **Building new muscle takes time and aggressive patience.** No matter who you look up to on social media, building a great body takes years, plenty of years.

- **Most people diet and train too hard too soon.** Adjustments to any fat loss or mass gain programme must be slow, diligent and tactful to ensure high quality results and maximum adherence.

- **Fat loss requires an energy deficit.** It's easier and more effective to control the energy balance through diet, i.e. eating more or less rather than moving more or less.

- **Muscle gain requires an energy surplus.** However, the surplus mustn't be too excessive to cause excessive or unnecessary unhealthy fat gain.

- **Deficit phases for fat loss can and should be larger than surplus phases for mass gain.**

- **Too much training can run the system down and increase the chances of burning out, overreaching and overtraining.**

- **Cardio, while useful, should never be relied upon as your primary mode of exercise if your goal is to build a stronger, leaner more muscular body.**

- **The primary purpose of weight training is to build muscle, not burn calories.** You have 23 hours outside of the gym to manipulate your diet and burn off energy with activity.

- **Always strive to get maximum results from the minimum effective dose of effort.**

- **Slow tactful adjustments to energy balance (up or down) work better than extreme fluctuations.**

SETTING UP YOUR DIET – FIVE KEY STEPS

I've outlined everything you need to know about building your diet from the plate up in the next five steps.

You'll get to grips with setting your calorie base, macro split and how to tweak your intake for fat loss or mass gain. I'll also teach you how and when to adjust your diet if and when progress plateaus.

If you can be bothered doing it manually, head over to the members site and download my super handy diet building and tracking tool.

Simply answer a few questions about your goals and how quickly you want to achieve them, and the tool will calculate how many calories to eat, and what macro targets to work off.

You then track basic body measures on a daily or weekly basis, and the tool makes the relevant adjustments required to progress moving in the right direction. No guess work needed.

Download it at **www.diabeticmuscleandfitness.com/resources**

Before You Go Further (with or without the online tool)

The information presented is by no way intended as medical advice or as a substitute for medical counselling and is for information purposes only. The information should be used in conjunction with the guidance and care of your physician.

STEP 1: CALCULATE MAINTENANCE CALORIES

Whether your goal is to gain muscle, lose fat or boost sport/exercise performance, the most important aspect of setting up your diet is working out the amount of calories you need to maintain your weight. This dietary info is then used to determine an appropriate caloric intake for your goals, whether it's eating slightly less for fat loss or slightly more for weight gain.

There are a host of different calorie equations available. However, no equation should be considered the Holy Grail, they merely provide an estimate and do not account for:

- How our bodies react to calorie surplus and deficit circumstances. This includes individual changes in (NEAT) Non Exercise Activity Thermogenesis – fidgeting, moving around etc. discussed in the previous chapter.

- Body composition – those with higher levels of muscle mass will burn more calories than individuals carrying less muscle at the same body weight.

Medication use and its ability to speed/slow metabolic rate. Hormone replacement therapy, and insulin are two prime examples.

DIABETES AND ENERGY BALANCE

Since insulin is involved in the organisation and storage of fuels, poorly controlled diabetes can result in faulty issues with energy metabolism. This is a result of lack of insulin production and/or a loss of insulin action on target cells (insulin resistance).

The worse blood glucose control is, the less energy is absorbed by cells, after food has been consumed. And, the greater the breakdown of current cells for fuel.

This factor is not taken into account with any of the popular calorie equations.

I can't stress enough how important it is to master the control of your diabetes. Never purposely put yourself into hyperglycaemic state to lose fat. You'll lose muscle, which increases body fat percentage, jeopardize performance and put your health at risk.

A ROUGH STARTING POINT – NO MORE!

No matter what calorie calculator you use, its only purpose is to establish a rough calorie starting point, which can and should be adjusted over time.

1. Adjusting Calories To Your Goal

The next step is to adjust your maintenance calories to your goal of fat loss or lean gain.

FAT LOSS: START WITH A 20% DEFICIT IN OVERALL CALORIES.

People who are extremely active will have to be more cautious when creating deficits to avoid muscle loss and loss of adherence due to hunger pangs and dips in mood. On the flip side if someone is extremely inactive they may need to drop even lower to lose fat, even if they exercise daily.

HOW DO I CREATE THE DEFICIT?

To create an energy deficit, you can reduce your food calorie intake and/or increase energy expenditure by adding cardiovascular exercise.

However, there is a fine balance between manipulating the two. There should always be enough food in the diet to support performance, recovery, manage blood glucose levels and keep you full (adherence)
Cardio must be added in carefully to avoid interference with performance, recovery and adherence.

CARDIO FOR FAT LOSS

Cardio is a tool for burning off additional calories above what you would normally burn doing set activities in that same time period

How much and what type of cardio you do is highly dependent on your cardiovascular fitness, the amount of body fat you have to lose, your recovery capacity (nutrition, rest and stress management) and the time you have available.

WEIGHT TRAINING SHOULD ALWAYS BE YOUR PRIMARY MODE OF EXERCISE IF YOU WANT TO BUILD A STRONGER, MORE MUSCULAR LOOKING BODY.

HOW MUCH FAT CAN I EXPECT TO LOSE EACH WEEK

The rate at which you lose fat is highly dependent on your current body fat percentage rather than total bodyweight. If you're carrying more fat you will get away with greater rates of fat loss than leaner individuals.

On average males should strive for 0.5-1% of bodyweight per week (1-1.5 lbs) to minimise muscle and strength loss. This rate of loss will be somewhat lower if they're very lean to begin with and somewhat higher if they're fatter at the outset.

Females typically have to accept slower rates of fat loss, usually between 0.25-0.5 lbs per week due to their smaller physical size and less lean body mass.

Just because you can lose more doesn't mean you should, as the process might prove unsustainable and lead to dreaded backlash of hating exercise and eating everything around you.

Extreme deficits can result in muscle loss, reduced resting metabolic rate, reduced performance/ recovery potential, increased levels of hunger signalling hormones and poor dietary adherence.

FAT LOSS NUTRITION TIPS

I give a ton of fat loss tips throughout the course of this text. Here are a few of the key ones I've found useful during any fat loss phase.

- Consistency is key – keep detailed records of calorie intake, activity and assess how it influences your bodyweight over a prolonged period of time.

- Be mindful of low volume, high calorie foods. They don't fill you up, pack a lot of calories and are often hidden in many ready and convenience foods.

- Intermittent fasting, which involves prolonged periods of fasting between meals can be a great tool for fat loss if blood glucose levels are controlled. The increase in stress hormones during a fast can blunt appetite. Also, the psychological motivation of eating a calorie dense meal later in the day, when at home rested can prove extremely satisfying. Be mindful of blood glucose if you are taking long breaks between meals.

- Learn how to cook and flavour your food. No one is motivated to eat disgusting food. Check out local cooking courses, cookbooks and some of the delicious fat loss recipes on the members' site at **www.diabeticmuscleandfitness.com**

MASS GAIN: START WITH A 10% INCREASE IN CALORIES

The approach to gaining muscle mass and increasing strength is very different to losing fat.

I don't recommend the typical bulking approach to mass gain, where the quantity of weight gained matters more than the quality of weight gained. This old school bodybuilding approach to building muscle is unhealthy, unsightly and counter-productive to the idea of looking, feeling and performing better. It also creates a ton of work when it is time to get lean.

Progress during a mass gain phase is a lot slower and harder to judge than fat loss. Muscle mass takes a long time to grow, and physically may not look as impressive compared to what can be achieved over a similar time spent focused on fat loss.

BE CONSERVATIVE IN YOUR APPROACH TO MASS GAIN

I like to be slightly more conservative with mass gain nutrition by increasing calorie intake by only 10% above maintenance. It is easy to acquire fat along with muscle if you aren't careful.

HOW MUCH WEIGHT SHOULD I EXPECT TO GAIN EACH WEEK?

This is highly specific to the individual in question and all depends on your gaining capacity. The fresher you are to weight training the more weight you can expect to gain. Individuals who are more experienced and closer to their genetic potential for muscle mass are less likely to gain as much.

Extreme surpluses cause unwanted fat gain, which jeopardises health. They can also be hard to sustain over time.

Beginner	1-1.5% of bodyweight per/week *
Intermediate/Advanced	Up to 0.75% of bodyweight per/week

This rate of weight gain will inevitably slow down the more experienced you become.

WHAT ABOUT CARDIO?

There is little need to perform cardio during a mass gain phase as it uses up energy and defeats the purpose of eating more. Don't get me wrong: if you enjoy certain types of cardio, work away. Just understand the more energy you burn off, the more you will need to eat.

If you're concerned about losing your cardiovascular fitness, bear in mind weight resistance training can also be used for that purpose, especially when you train with shorter rest periods, modified strongman training or kettlebell/bodyweight complexes.

MASS GAIN NUTRITION TIPS

Poor appetite, busy lifestyles and anxiety can be a barrier to eating for mass gain. Here are a few eating tips I've found super useful when trying to pack on mass post-contest, when my bodyweight is at is lowest, leanest and weakest.

- Choose low volume, high calorie food sources like oils and nuts. They're easy eating, pack a lot of calories and carry the benefits of vitamins, minerals, antioxidants, fibre and many other health benefits.

- If you're struggling with appetite, try going for a short walk. This might stimulate appetite.

- Be wary of consuming too much caffeine. It can blunt appetite. Also, respect the timing of caffeine intake. Bear in mind the effects of caffeine peak after around 45 minutes so consuming it five minutes before training may result in it kicking in post-workout when you need to wind down. Also, taking it too close to bedtime will impair sleep quality.

- Low calorie high volume foods like sugar-free jelly, green vegetables and fibre supplements can fill you up and reduce eating capacity.

- Listen to your body, if you aren't hungry, don't eat. Wait until you're hungry.

- Again, learn how to cook and flavour your food. Check out some of the delicious muscle building recipes at **www.diabeticmuscleandfitness.com**

HOW DO I ADJUST CALORIES FOR LONG-TERM PROGRESS?

Once a set calorie intake has been given enough time to take effect, its effectiveness needs to be measured in relation to the rate of body weight change, improvements in physical appearance and also performance.

I provide a step-by-step guide on how to measure and fine tune your approach in the next chapter. But, for now, let's focus on getting started.

STEP 2: WORK OUT MACRONUTRIENT INTAKE

Once you've worked out how many calories you need for your goal, it's important to work out where these calories come from.

We've already highlighted the key foods, facts and functions of all the key macronutrients; protein, fat, carbohydrate and alcohol, which to no surprise won't be a primary fuel source...sorry, folks!

First and foremost there is no magic plug and play macro formula. Just like your calorie intake, it's up to you to find out what works best for your body, lifestyle and goals.

You may find a high carb/low fat diet works well for you, whilst a low carb/high fat diet leaves you feeling lethargic and weak. This involves paying close attention to how certain ratios of fuel make you feel and then tweaking up and down as needed.

Regardless of what macro split you choose, it must:

- Support life by providing adequate calories, essential amino acids and fatty acids
- Support glycemic control.
- Promote performance.
- Promote recovery.
- Stimulate mood.
- Keep you full (especially with fat loss).

It's up to you to trial test different macronutrient ranges and adjust accordingly to personal needs.

Fat loss requires caloric restriction and caloric restriction requires macronutrient restriction.

Mass Gain requires a tightly regulated calorie surplus.

I have summarized macronutrient targets according to specific goals below. These values are worked out in relation to the calorie targets you calculated in the previous steps.

GOAL	PROTEIN	FAT	CARBOHYDRATE
Fat loss	1.4-2.0g/kg *Higher end more suitable	15-25%	Remainder of calories
Mass Gain	1.4-2.0g/kg *Lower end more suitable	20-30%	Remainder of calories

WILL THESE TARGETS WORK FOR EVERYONE?

I have had great success using these values on myself and clients. However, they won't be suited to everyone. Self-trial and feedback is essential in finding out what ratios of macronutrients work best for you.

HOW DO I TRACK INTAKE?

Many calorie-counting apps are available. Long gone are the days of working out calorie intake using a calculator and good old pen and paper.

The apps are super easy to use and allow you to work out the calorie content of any food on the planet within seconds. You can track your daily eating habits and observe how many calories and grams of each macronutrient you are eating across the week, month or year.

You can also set calorie and macronutrient goals to see how far over or under your dietary intake is.

My favorite apps include My Fitness Pal, Lose It, Spark People and Fat Secret.

They are free to use, but also have more advanced paid options available. I've always used the free option on MyFitness Pal with zero issues.

There are also websites like www.eatthismuch.com, which work out your complete meal plan for you in line with your personal calorie needs.

STEP 3: FLEXIBILITY - WHAT & WHEN TO EAT

WHAT TO EAT?

Healthy, Sustainable yet Flexible Diet Breakdown

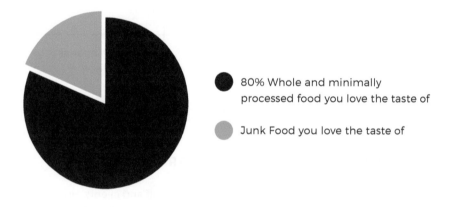

80% Whole and minimally processed food you love the taste of

Junk Food you love the taste of

AM I ALLOWED JUNK FOOD?

If you feel like the odd treat, eat away. Don't stress out and drown yourself in guilt thinking you'll turn fat overnight.

There is no such thing as a bad food, just good or bad diets.

Just remember to respect your overall calorie intake and administer the appropriate medication to control blood sugar levels.

TOO MUCH JUNK FOOD, ESPECIALLY SUGARY FOODS CAN JEOPARDISE BLOOD GLUCOSE CONTROL AND LEAVE YOU HUNGRY.

WHEN TO EAT?

Once you've established your total calorie intake, You need to work out when you are going to eat it all. Depending on your day-to-day job and lifestyle, you'll only be able to eat at certain times.

It's important to eat when and where you want. A fixed meal plan makes this difficult; often forcing you to suit the plan, not the other way round.

Generally speaking, you should only eat:

* When your body tells you to and not just for the sake of it.
* To control blood sugar levels.
* In a state of optimal digestion (non rushed eating).

HOW MANY MEALS PER DAY?

Generally speaking. 4-5 is a good number to work with.

If you eat too many meals, you'll end up thinking of food all day and annoy everyone around you with your constant lunch breaks and scoffing. If you eat too few meals, for instance by adopting an intermittent fast approach, you run the risk of going hungry or at worse hypoglycemic, which could increase the potential for you to consume unnecessary low quality high calorie convenience food over high quality nutrient dense food.

Nutrition should never be looked at on a meal by meal basis but as accumulative intake over time. The only exception to this is when treating low blood sugar or replenishing energy stores rapidly post-exercise as part of multiple session training splits.

POST-WORKOUT NUTRITION

General fitness heresy hearsay would have you believe you must slam a protein shake down within 30 seconds of finishing your last set in the gym.

But in reality the digested nutrients from your pre- workout meal, lunch and every other meal that day will be floating around your blood stream ready for use.

The need to prioritisze post workout nutrition exists under the following circumstances:

- Hypoglycemia
- Training whilst fasting
- Training two or three times per a day

STEP 4: ASSESSMENT

In order to assess the effectiveness of your approach, you must measure the following factors:

- Rate of body weight change
- Performance
- Mood/energy
- Blood sugar levels
- Medication dose

In **chapter 8** I provide a step-by-step guide on when and how to adjust your diet and training to ensure continual progress.

SUPPLEMENTATION

SUPPLEMENTS – WHERE DO YOU START?

WHAT WORKS? WHAT DOESN'T?

With all the vitamins, minerals, amino acids, fatty acids, fibre and everything else in between there are at least a hundred-plus supplements you could take. And that's without getting into any crazy esoteric-based supplements and combinations

I can confidently say that 95% of the supplements available to buy in shops and online don't do anything except burn a hole in your wallet and give you expensive urine. The idea of supplementing with nutritional extracts can be incredibly exciting, especially when you consider the roles and functions particular nutrients play within the body.

I was thrilled when I bought my first tubs of protein and creatine. In fact, with the fancy labelling and the concept of scooping out servings of dry powder that claimed to pack on 'serious mass', I felt a new edge to my training.

Researching these supplements was just as fun as buying them. On reflection, my research and understanding of supplement claims wasn't the best.

- I wasn't sure how to tell the difference between credible scientific research and polished marketing claims.

- I didn't know supplement companies could fund and publish research behind their products.

- I didn't understand nitrogen balance, and how it can easily be made positive by adding more protein and this didn't necessary equate to more muscle mass.

- I didn't know that studies done in rats weren't truly applicable to humans.

- I didn't know the shredded guy or beautiful girl on the supplement packaging was pumped full of additional chemical support or, better yet, Photoshop.

- I didn't know many supplements don't actually contain the amount of active ingredients that their label claims.

- I didn't know some supplements contained unsafe, illegal or banned substances.

Fast forward a few years, and a few thousand pounds lighter I've come to learn there are only a select few supplements worth buying.

More of one nutrient doesn't always mean better health, better performance and a better body. In fact too much of one nutrient can prove detrimental to health and leave you deficient in others.

As a person with diabetes you may require more nutrients than your healthy counterparts, especially if you lack self-control or consume an energy-restricted diet.

However, it's important to be mindful that some supplements need to be approached with caution because of their impact on certain organs and blood sugar control.

CALORIE RESTRICTION = MACRO + MICRO NUTRIENT RESTRICTION = POTENTIAL FOR DEFICIENCY

In fact, the traditional approach to dieting of eating clean foods and avoiding dirty foods in addition to doing exercises popularised by many bodybuilders and diet gurus can restrict the micro density of the diet and result in micronutrient deficiencies (47, 48, 49, 50, 51).

Deficiencies can lead to all sorts of problems with health, body composition and performance. Key problems include: immune dysfunction, down regulation of the thyroid, bone density problems, reduction in metabolic rate and many others.

I am always hesitant to write about supplements, because too many people prioritise them above proper diet, training and lifestyle. Also, some people may simply get more than enough nutrients from their diet and have zero need to buy supplements.

I can't stress enough if you're not eating, training or resting correctly no supplement on the planet will help you.

I've comprised a list of fundamental evidence-based supplements that I feel are a worthwhile investment to any person with diabetes looking to improve their health, muscle building and fat loss efforts. I've also outlined the evidence-based recommend doses for each supplement.

NEVER STOP TAKING YOUR PRESCRIBED MEDICATION AND RESORTING TO ANY SUPPLEMENT WITHOUT CONSULTATION AND MONITORING FROM A QUALIFIED AND REGISTERED MEDICAL PRACTITIONER.

GENERAL HEALTH SUPPLEMENTS

DO I NEED A MULTIVITAMIN?

No. Given the limited dose of nutrients in a single multivitamin tablet you should be getting more than enough baseline nutrients from your diet. Also, not all nutrients are always present in a multivitamin and, in some cases it may be more important to supplement isolated vitamins and minerals to eliminate deficiencies and take advantage of their nutraceutical and performance benefits. By all means feel free to use a multi vitamin to 'cover your bases', but not as an essential investment.

VITAMIN D

Vitamin D is a fat-soluble nutrient essential for human survival.

Vitamin D is synthesised in the skin from cholesterol upon exposure to sunlight containing sufficient ultraviolet B (UVB) radiation. This is the main source for most people. However, it can also be obtained from foods, such as fish, eggs and certain dairy products and dietary supplements.

Dietary sources are essential when sunlight-containing UVB radiation is limited (e.g. during the winter months) or exposure to it is restricted (e.g. due to lack of time spent outdoors or too little skin exposure).

There are a host of benefits associated with supplementing vitamin D, especially if deficient. They include improvements in:

- Musculoskeletal health [52] (calcium and phosphorus metabolism).
- Immune health [53].
- Insulin secretion and sensitivity [54,55].
- Testosterone production [56] (in men, not women).
- Reduced risk of falls in the elderly [57] (due to better strength).
- Reduced risk of cancer[58,59], cardiovascular[60] disease, diabetes [61, 62] and mortality[63].

DOSING

1,000-2,000 IU (25–50 mcg) per day is more than adequate [64].
If deficient, a higher dose may be required. Research suggests the safe upper limit is 10,000IU/day. (250mcg/day)

Vitamin D3 (cholecalciferol), is recommended over its counterpart D2 (ergocalciferol) because of its enhanced absorbability and use in the body.

Vitamin D is best supplemented alongside a fat-based meal or supplement like fish oil.

TESTING VITAMIN D STATUS

Testing vitamin D status is a worthwhile investment if you're serious about your training and recovery.

The 25(OH)D blood test is widely used as a biomarker of vitamin D status because it reflects vitamin D production from the skin and diet. Vitamin D has a long half-life in the circulation (about 2-3 weeks) and is not under tight homeostatic control.

VITAMIN K

Vitamin K is another of the four essential fat-soluble vitamins. It is typically found in plants and can also be produced by the gut micro biome (bacteria) found in our digestive tracts.

Vitamin K is available in a number of different forms, known as vitamers. These are phylloquinones (vitamin K1) and menaquinones (vitamin K2). Further vitamers exist within the vitamin K2 class, known as MK-'X', all of which have different absorption properties. The RDI of vitamin K is deemed enough to support healthy blood coagulation. However, research has shown intakes above this to be beneficial in promoting cardiovascular, bone health [65] and reducing cancer [66]. These levels can be reached by supplementing with vitamin K.

VITAMIN K AND DIABETES

An interesting study found that a relative deficiency of vitamin K resulted in a higher than normal insulin spike following a standard oral glucose tolerance test. After a single week of supplementing 90mg of vitamin K2 (MK-4) the response was remedied [67].

Another study showed an improvement of insulin sensitivity after supplementing 30mg of vitamin K2 (MK-4) over four weeks in healthy individuals [68]. Further studies are warranted surrounding vitamin K's potential role in diabetes management.

DOSING

The doses for each form of vitamin K differ. A daily dose of 500mcg vitamin K1 (phylloquinone) and Vitamin K2 (MK-7) seems reasonable [69]. Since vitamin K is a fat-soluble vitamin it is best supplemented alongside a fatty meal or fish oil.

SIDE EFFECTS

Vitamin K is best avoided if you're on blood clotting medication, such as warfarin.

FISH OIL

Fish oil is the richest source of the omega-3 essential fatty acids DHA & EPA. The research on fish oil supplementation on various aspects of health, including mortality, mental health, skin health, pregnancy, and cognitive function is somewhat mixed, with some studies showing significant benefits and others showing no change.

Interestingly, many studies show an inverse relationship between fish consumption and heart disease and mortality, so while fish oil may not guarantee you better health, eating fish seems to. This may be due to the fact fish oil is devoid of other nutrients typically found in real fish, including zinc, iron, selenium and highly absorbable protein rich in essential amino acids.

When it comes to getting enough EPA/DHA the best strategy would be to consume between 340-453g (12–16 oz) of cold-water, fatty fish each week, if personal taste allows for it.

WHAT IF YOU DON'T LIKE FISH?

Supplementing with EPA/DHA and cod liver oil may be a valid strategy.

A good starting point would be one teaspoon of high quality cod liver oil and an additional 1g of EPA + DHA supplemental fish oil per day.

Cod liver oil is rich in the active form of vitamin A and vitamin D, both of which are difficult to obtain elsewhere in the diet. Fish oil is purely EPA/DHA based. People living in hotter climates mightn't need additional vitamin D, however. It's fair to say the minuscule amount obtained from one teaspoon serving will pose little to no risk of toxicity.

Research shows no harm in supplementing with 1 gram or less of fish oil per day, even in those who eat fish regularly. I don't see the need to consume high doses of fish oil (i.e. >3 g/d) over the long term.

MAGNESIUM

Magnesium is an essential dietary mineral, and the second most prevalent electrolyte in the body besides sodium.

Magnesium has a strong relationship with insulin (70, 71) and thus plays an important role in carbohydrate metabolism. Low magnesium levels are common in people with T1D and T2D for a number of reasons.

- Low dietary intake of magnesium-rich foods, such as nuts and leafy vegetables.
- Increased excretion of magnesium due to chronic fluctuations in blood glucose control.
- Insensitivity to insulin affects the ability to transport magnesium in and out of cells.
- Use of diuretics in certain individuals to combat excess fluid retention and blood pressure issues.

This presents an array of implications for people with T2D, notably insulin resistance, impaired glucose tolerance and decreased insulin secretion (72, 73, 74, 75). Increased blood pressure and neural excitation are other negative traits.

This isn't an ideal scenario for a hard training individual with an increased demand for magnesium caused by sweating and the increased physical demands of exercise.

If magnesium is supplemented to treat a deficiency, it may also act as a sedative to improve sleep quality (76) and help reduce blood pressure and improve insulin sensitivity (77).

An interesting study from the Taiwan water industry even reported an inverse relationship between the amount of magnesium in the country's drinking water and death from diabetes mellitus (78). These findings were based on 6,781 controls (deaths) and the correlating levels of magnesium in the drinking water over this death span (1990-1994). Although these findings demonstrate the importance of magnesium, even in drinking water, there is always scope for further research.

Magnesium hasn't been shown to boost exercise performance or reduce cramps in healthy individuals. However, more research is needed in respect of people with diabetes as their potential for deficiency may be greater, which would have obvious implications on performance and muscle tissue susceptibility to cramping.

The intestinal absorption of magnesium varies, depending on how much magnesium the body needs, so there are few side effects associated with supplementation.

The body regulates circulating levels of magnesium carefully, as much of the magnesium consumed is either stored in bone or eliminated in urine.

The body will only absorb as much as it needs. Large doses of magnesium (over 500mg) can be used as laxatives, so excessive intake can result in diarrhoea and related gastrointestinal symptoms. People with impaired kidney function may need to speak to their doctor prior to supplementing with magnesium.

DOSING

Magnesium supplements come in several different forms, including magnesium citrate, magnesium oxide and magnesium bound to various amino acids.

Magnesium oxide is abundant and cheap, but is not absorbed well by the body.

Magnesium citrate is more readily absorbed and used by the body. Magnesium L-threonate can be used for cognitive enhancement.

Magnesium should be taken daily with food in line with the following:

The standard dose for magnesium supplementation is 200-400mg [79].

If a deficiency does exist, individuals have been known to super load to treat the deficiency using magnesium diglycinate or magnesium gluconate. This is only advised under the professional guidance of a doctor [80].

I'm also a big fan of applying transdermal magnesium post-training, especially to freshly trained muscle groups. This allows me to bypass the digestive system and rapidly replete magnesium to fatigued and potentially depleted muscle cells.

Transdermal magnesium is applied topically, using either magnesium oil, magnesium gel, magnesium lotion or magnesium bath (Epsom) salts. Dose as instructed.

Q.GUT HEALTH SUPPLEMENTS - DO I NEED A BIOTIC SUPPLEMENT?

The gut is crucial to human health. It plays a number of important roles, including digesting food, absorption of nutrients, production of vitamins and hormones and the ability to fight infections and regulate the immune system.

Bacteria are generally found throughout the entire gastrointestinal tract, but in various amounts. The small bowel has a lower level of bacteria (less than 10,000 bacteria per millilitre of fluid) compared to the large bowel, or colon (which has at least 1,000,000,000 bacteria per millilitre of fluid). Also, the kinds of bacteria typically found in the small bowel differ from those in the large bowel, or colon.

Regardless, the role of these bacteria is important.

There are an exponential number of studies connecting imbalances or disturbances of gut microbiota to a wide range of diseases, including obesity, metabolic disease, inflammatory bowel diseases, depression, fatigue and anxiety (81, 82, 83, 84, 85).

Gut health can be negatively affected by a host of factors including:

- Stress.
- Overuse of certain medications, such as contraception, pain killers, chemo therapy and antibiotics.
- IBS, Crohn's disease, Coeliac and other bowel diseases.
- Food borne bacteria (food poisoning).
- Auto-immune diseases.
- Bowel surgery.

Biotic supplements can be taken to influence the growth and development of specific strains of bacteria living within the large intestine (colon). The actions of these bacteria are intended to be symbiotic (work in harmony) with the host and provide benefit through their actions.

Biotic supplements can be divided into three categories:

1. **Prebiotic supplements are indigestible carbohydrates, or at least indigestible to us, that reach the colon intact and selectively feed many strains of beneficial bacteria within the large intestine. Think of them as bacteria food.**

As far as prebiotics go, aim to consume as wide a variety of plant foods as you can. Top sources of soluble fibre include carrots, winter squash, starchy tubers, turnips, rutabagas, parsnips, beets, plantains, taro and yuca.

Supplementing with resistant starch or another prebiotic formula is also a valid strategy.

Resistant starch is a type of starch that resists digestion in the stomach or small intestine, reaching the colon intact. It has minimal-to-no impact on blood glucose or insulin levels nor is it a significant source of calories. Green bananas and unripe plantains (which you can dehydrate to make chips) are good whole-food sources of resistant starch. Bob's Red Mill unmodified potato starch is another great source.

Several studies have shown that resistant starch may improve insulin sensitivity, and decrease blood glucose levels in response to meals (86, 87, 88). In one study, consumption of 15 and 30g per day of resistant starch showed improved insulin sensitivity in overweight and obese men, equivalent to the improvement that would be expected with weight loss equal to approximately 10% of body weight (89).

Be mindful that certain prebiotics can aggravate digestive issues, such as IBS. As such, speak to your gastroenterologist prior to consuming.

2. **Probiotic supplements are isolated or mixed strains of bacteria that change the overall bacteria population of the colon. Most bacteria sold as dietary supplements are probiotics and are measured in CFU.**

PROBIOTIC VS ANTIBIOTICS – WHAT'S THE DEAL?

The term antibiotics means 'anti-life'.

While taking them is never ideal, in many cases it's essential.

They have a negative effect on the microbiome living in your gut and increase the potential for dysbiosis (impaired microbial imbalance). Restoring a symbiotic microbiome takes time and effort but there are many things you can do both during and after a course of antibiotics to minimise the damage and encourage regrowth and diversification of your gut flora.

Supplementing with probiotics is a valid first step. There are a number of randomised and placebo-controlled trials that demonstrate the effectiveness of probiotic use during a course of antibiotics for lessening side effects and preventing gut infection (90, 91, 92, 93, 94, 95, 96).

3. **Synbiotic supplements have both prebiotic and probiotic properties.**

DOSING

Given the benefits of biotic supplements, you want them to develop a diverse symbiotic microbiome on their own.

FERMENTED FOODS

One of the most cost-effective and natural ways to build a diverse ecosystem of beneficial bacteria is by consuming fermented foods.

Fermented foods, including kefir, sauerkraut and kimchi are very much in their infancy with regards to clinical evidence. However, they have been shown to promote the growth of healthy symbiotic microflora and possess other anti-fungal, antibacterial and anti-carcinogenic roles (97, 98).

Based on survey data from 710 university students, a recent study found that consumption of fermented food likely to contain active probiotic cultures was inversely associated with predicted levels of social anxiety (99). However, due to many limitations and confounding variables, further research is needed before any assertions can be made.

Although highly unlikely, some people may be unable to tolerate probiotics and fermented foods due to a histamine allergy.

Ginger can be extremely helpful for reducing inflammation and calming the digestive system (100, 101).

BERBERINE

Berberine may be of great interest to people living with T2D.

Berberine is a plant extract commonly used in traditional Chinese medicine that can be supplemented for anti-inflammatory, glucose-lowering and intestinal health benefits.

The strong evidence surrounding berberine's use establishes it to be just as effective as pharmaceuticals.

DOSING

Human and animal research demonstrates that 1,500mg of berberine, taken in three split doses of 500mg each, is just as effective as taking 1500mg of metformin or 4mg glibenclamide, two pharmaceutical drugs used for treating T2D. Its effectiveness was measured by how well the drugs reduced specific biomarkers of T2D.

EXERCISING CAUTION

Berberine has a high potential to interact with medications, sometimes seriously [102]. Never stop taking prescribed medication and resort to taking Berberine, or indeed any other supplement, without consultation and monitoring from a medical practitioner.

SIDE EFFECTS

Too much berberine at once can result in stomach upset, cramping, and diarrhoea.

PERFORMANCE SUPPLEMENTS

WHEY PROTEIN

Whey is one of two proteins found in milk, the other being casein. Whey is the water-soluble fraction of milk that is left when the curds and solids have been removed. Casein protein is the curds and has gel-forming properties.

Whey is used as a protein supplement and comes in powders, bars and ready to drink mixes. There are various forms:

- Whey Concentrate
- Whey Isolate
- Whey Hydrolysate
- Hydrolyzed Whey

Supplementing with whey protein is a great way to hit your daily protein targets. It is absorbed much quicker than any other form of dietary protein, including casein and provides a plentiful supply of amino acids, making it highly bio available (usable by the body).

IS WHEY PROTEIN SAFE?

Whey does not harm the liver or kidneys but may accelerate existing damage if over-consumed. People with damaged livers and kidneys should always consult their doctor prior to supplementing with whey.

People with lactose intolerances should avoid regular whey protein and instead opt for lactose-free varieties including isolate, colostrum or plant protein.

DIABETES AND WHEY PROTEIN

You can use whey protein if you have diabetes.

Whey proteins (along with a number of other forms of protein) have insulinotropic effects, meaning they have the ability to stimulate insulin, which has the capacity to lower blood glucose in healthy individuals. The mechanism is not known, but insulinogenic amino acids and the incretin hormones seem to be involved.

One interesting study [103] involving 14 diet treated subjects with T2D set out to investigate whether supplementing meals with a high glycemic index (GI) with whey proteins might increase insulin secretion and improve blood glucose control.

- Fourteen diet-treated subjects with T2D were served a high-GI breakfast (white bread) and subsequent high-GI lunch (mashed potatoes with meatballs).

- Both breakfast and lunch meals were supplemented with whey protein one day and not the next. Lean ham and lactose were provided on the days where whey wasn't supplemented.

- Blood samples were taken before, during and after breakfast and lunch to assess blood glucose, serum insulin, and two stomach hormones called glucose-dependent insulinotropic polypeptide (GIP), and glucagon-like peptide 1 (GLP-1).

The study concluded that adding whey protein to meals, alongside rapid digesting and absorbed carbohydrates, stimulates insulin release and helps reduce post-meal blood glucose in people with T2D after they consumed a meal of mashed potatoes and meatballs.

Therefore supplementing with whey protein may have fewer adverse effects than commonly used therapeutic agents.

Other interesting observations from a study conducted by the American Journal of Clinical Nutrition showed the insulin-releasing effects of whey protein were greater than reconstituted milk, cheese, cod, and wheat gluten that contained the equivalent amounts of lactose. It was also greater than an equivalent carbohydrate load of white-wheat bread, which was consumed as a reference meal. (see fig)

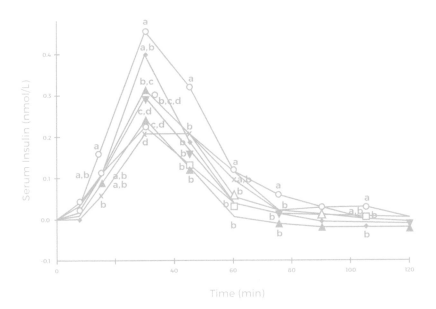

Mean (±SEM) Incremental changes (Δ) in serum insulin in response to equal amounts of carbohydrate from a white-wheat-breadreference meal (X) and test meals of whey (O), milk (♦) cheese (▲), code (□), gluten-low (▲), and gluten-high (▼) meals

Mikael Nillsson et al, Am J Clin Nutr 2004;80:1246-1253

2004 By American Society for Nutrition

Research in T1D is lacking, but it is fair to say that whey proteins have the capacity to increase blood glucose levels, as insulin secretion is lost, therefore negating the insulinotropic effects of whey.

I've found this to be true. Faster acting whey, such as concentrate and isolate will increase blood glucose levels the quickest even though they may be low carb. Be mindful of this and administer the appropriate medication for healthy glycemic control if you have T1D.

HOW TO TAKE?

The amount of whey protein to supplement with will depend on your daily protein goals.

Athletes or highly active individuals looking to build muscle and lose body fat could opt for a daily intake of (1.0-2.2g/kg bodyweight/0.68-1g/lb bodyweight [104, 105])

Sedentary people and those looking to maintain body composition should aim for a daily target of (0.8g/kg bodyweight/0.36g/lb bodyweight[104, 105]) and upwards.

If you meet your daily protein needs through food alone, there is no need to supplement.

As a general rule of thumb, I don't like to consume more than 25% of my daily protein goal from protein supplements. Along with many others, I have been guilty of over-consuming high-priced protein bars at the expense of high quality food. Try to get away from eating supplements by consuming as much natural food sources as possible.

A NOTE ON 'HIGH PROTEIN' FOODS

Just because a food says 'high protein' doesn't mean it's healthy or worth buying.

I've seen high protein bars, ice cream, bread, crisps, sauces, dips – you name it!

First of all, let's put things into perspective.

I've never come across a fitness enthusiast who is deficient in protein.

Secondly, why pay above the odds for a nutrient you have no need for?

Let's take a popular example - protein bars. They're made out to be a guilt-free option – they look and taste like normal chocolate bars but just pack more protein, usually in the form of whey.

The reality is they cost nearly four times as much, contain the same, or in some cases more calories, than non-protein chocolate bars and usually don't taste as good. They also include fillers, like sugar alcohols that often leave us feeling bloated, dizzy and smelling like a horse.

Provided I've met my minimum protein requirements and feel the need for some chocolate I'll just buy a normal chocolate bar. The only time I'll eat a protein bar is when I'm speaking at exhibitions or busy with business and don't have the time to eat properly.

CREATINE

WHAT IS CREATINE?

Creatine is a molecule made from amino acids that is produced naturally within the human body. It plays a role in energy production.

Scientifically speaking, creatine stores high-energy phosphate groups in the form of phosphocreatine (creatine phosphate). During periods of stress, phosphocreatine releases energy to aid cellular function by making a substance called adenosine triphosphate (ATP). ATP provides the energy for muscle contractions. This is the reason creatine increases strength after supplementation. It can also aid the development of the brain, bones, muscle and liver.

The body can produce some of its own creatine. It also comes from protein rich foods, such as eggs, meat or fish.

IS CREATINE SAFE?

Creatine is often touted as a dangerous drug and in many cases the gateway to steroids. However, it is one of the most thoroughly researched compounds in sports nutrition, and no adverse side effects have been noted through supplementation in healthy individuals [106, 107, 108, 109, 110, 111] since the 1960s when it was first studied. In fact, it's been suggested that it could be beneficial for older people who suffer from muscle weakness and loss.

WHAT ABOUT PEOPLE LIVING WITH DIABETES?

The research to support creatine consumption in people living with T2D is relatively large. Unfortunately there is zero research investigating the effects of creatine consumption in people living with T1D.

People living with T2D can safely consume creatine [112]. The so-called dangerous drug has been shown to be safe for them. It has also demonstrated significant benefits on glucose metabolism when used alongside exercise [112], raising its potential as a possible nutritional therapy in this population [112].

There is some confusion about the role of the kidneys and the waste product of creatine, 'creatinine', which is also used as a diagnostic marker for kidney problems. The supplement's ability to elevate this marker is a false marker and is in no way harmful. In fact, there isn't one single peer-reviewed study or case report suggesting creatine as the causative factor behind kidney damage, which is a marked complication of poorly controlled diabetes.

MECHANISM OVERVIEW

We already know weight training increases the translocation of GLUT-4 in muscle tissue, allowing for non-insulin dependent transport of glucose into and out of cells.

Creatine's ability to improve glycemic control is based on its ability to increase performance, which consequently leads to further increases in translocation of GLUT-4, and greater uptake of glucose [112].

DOSING

Creatine is usually dosed at 5 to 10g per day.

There is no need to do a special loading phase of creatine. Just take it.

Nor is there a need to cycle it; just take it everyday

SIDE EFFECTS

The side effects of creatine are highly variable between individuals and can include:

- Improved performance.
- Increased potential for hypoglycemia post-exercise (as a result of performance/work load increase).
- Weight gain, due to water retention. This may have implications for those with elevated blood pressure, oedema or those competing in weight restricted sports.
- Stomach cramping can occur if consumed with inadequate water.
- Diarrhoea and nausea are possible if too much is consumed at once.
- Potential allergic reaction – best avoided in this case.

CARNOSINE/BETA ALANINE

Carnosine is a dipeptide formed from the two amino acids β-alanine and histidine. It is found in large amounts in the brain and muscle, especially fast twitch skeletal muscle.

Carnosine has an antioxidant role and accounts for about 10% of the muscle's ability to buffer the metabolic stress that are associated with lactic acid, a by-product of high intensity exercise, which is believed to be one of the primary mechanisms responsible for the development of muscular fatigue.

There are a number of clinical studies highlighting the benefits of carnosine supplementation. They include: improvements in high intensity anaerobic exercise performance [113], anti-aging effects [114] on the skin, glucose metabolism, including the prevention of T2D and even enhanced quality of life in people with heart problems [115].

The popular sports supplement β-alanine is a precursor to carnosine. This means when beta-alanine is ingested, it turns into the molecule carnosine.

The rate-limiting factor of carnosine synthesis is beta-alanine availability.

Supplementing with beta-alanine will increase muscle carnosine content and increase the muscle's ability to buffer H+, (Hydrogen ions) increasing the potential to elicit improvements in physical performance during high-intensity exercise.

Carnosine and beta-alanine haven't been compared to each of their potential benefits, so it isn't currently known if carnosine supplementation has unique benefits in humans.

CARNOSINE OR BETA ALANINE?

Beta alanine has been shown to be more effective than carnosine at increasing muscle carnosine [116] levels and therefore might be a better option for training performance.

The research surrounding its benefits aren't game changing, but nevertheless it may serve as the icing on the cake to a finely-tuned diet and training programme.

DOSING

2–5 g at any time of the day.

SIDE EFFECTS

Large doses of beta-alanine can result in a tingling sensation in the body called paresthesia.

This is a harmless side effect, which can be avoided by using smaller doses (0.8–1 g) several times a day.

Beta-alanine or carnosine supplementation may be a good idea for vegetarians and vegans as carnosine is typically found in red meat.

USE OF STIMULANTS

The use of pre-workout supplementation has exploded in the last few years. One of the most notable ingredients, caffeine anhydrous, is the pharmaceutical form of naturally occurring caffeine that is typically found in everyday drinks like tea and coffee.

Caffeine has been shown to elevate the stress hormones cortisol and epinephrine [117, 118]. As previously discussed, these hormones are known for their role in increasing blood glucose levels.

IN TYPE 1s

Ingestion of caffeine prior to weight training may amplify the affects of glucose-raising hormones that are usually increased by this mode of training. This increases the potential for hyperglycemia, which in the grand scheme of things may reduce training performance and defeat the much sought after ergogenic 'performance boosting' properties of caffeine.

IN TYPE 2s

There is a similar concern with research showing exaggerations in blood glucose and insulin response when caffeine is ingested alongside carbohydrates, and also when fasted.

TAKE HOME MESSAGE

Be mindful that caffeine can increase blood glucose levels.

Supplemental caffeine, termed caffeine anhydrous, is more potent than the naturally occurring caffeine found in coffee, tea and dark chocolate and therefore may have a greater effect.

Be mindful of timing caffeine in and around training. A lot of people make the mistake of consuming their pre-workout caffeine fix 5-10 minutes before the gym.

Caffeine peaks in the blood stream 30-45 minutes after consuming it and can last for up to six hours. Consuming caffeine too close to training will allow for peak activation at the end of training. Although this may be useful, once fatigue hits in, it would be more beneficial to time your peak from the start of training. Also, too much caffeine in the evening can jeopardise the quality of sleep, due to its stimulant properties.

DO I HAVE TO DROP MY PRE-WORKOUT OR COFFEE PICK ME UP?

Certainly not. Just be aware you may need to inject extra insulin or take extra medication to accommodate the increase in blood sugar from caffeinated foods and drink. Exercise caution with pre-workout supplements, which tend to contain super high doses of caffeine or other popular bodybuilding stimulant-based supplements, such as yohimbine and ephedrine. These products should be supplemented with extreme caution and under the guidance of a physician, if at all.

It's also worth noting that as with any stimulant, the body develops a tolerance to caffeine so you may need to increase the dose. This could affect your day if you crash later on due or can't sleep due to high caffeine levels. You may find it beneficial to wean yourself off it or stop to detox to ensure that you benefit from moderate levels.

SLEEP

Melatonin is a neuro-hormone secreted by the pineal gland in the brain. Its primary job is to decrease the time it takes to fall asleep by regulating our natural body clock (circadian rhythm). Supplementation has been shown to effectively induce sleep and improve the quality of sleep, particularly in those suffering from insomnia [119, 120]. It also serves as a powerful antioxidant and possesses anti-carcinogenic properties, and is currently being researched for its role in fighting breast cancer [121].

DOSING

Melatonin in doses between 500mcg (0.5mg) and 5mg has been shown to work effectively. Start small, with 500mcg and if it doesn't work, increase up to 3-5mg. Ideally take it 30 minutes before bed. The benefits of melatonin are not dose-dependent. In other words, taking more doesn't mean you will fall asleep faster [122].

Anyone taking any neurally active agent (pharmacotherapy such as antidepressants or ADHD medication) should consult with their doctor prior to taking melatonin, as it is highly involved in many body systems and drug interactions are very likely.

Valerian is a plant used to treat insomnia and anxiety. A recent meta-analysis suggested valerian could be of benefit in improving insomnia and sleep quality. However, there may be more promising treatments [123].

DOSING

Valerian can be supplemented at a standard dose of 450mg one hour before bedtime [124].

L-Theanine, a unique amino acid present in tea has been reported to promote feelings of calmness and take the edge of stimulants such as caffeine [125, 126, 127], which may prove useful for the coffee enthusiast.

DOSING

L-Theanine tends to be taken in the dosage of 100-200mg (128).

SUPPLEMENT FAQS

Q. Do I really need to buy a protein powder?

No. Whole food is perfectly fine. If digestion is an issue post-training, a good quality Greek yoghurt loaded with probiotic strains is an awesome alternative. Alternatively, milk is another great option.

For those that are lactose intolerant, simply opt for a whole food protein source.

Q. What about Branched-Chain Amino Acids (BCAA)?

There is no strong evidence to support BCAAs being any more effective for stimulating muscle growth than high quality protein derived from solid food.

Save your money and eat your food although most, if not all, BCAAs contain high doses of leucine, the benefits of which have been described in the section in this chapter on protein.

Q. Do I need to detox?

You see plenty of claims about certain detox diets and supplements, despite a lack of scientific evidence to support their use. Marketing and anecdotal reports support their effectiveness for weight loss and overall health.

Calling a compound toxic is naïve and doesn't take into account other key factors, like dose and frequency of exposure. The reality is there are a wide variety of natural and non-natural substances that are toxic and non-toxic.

The body can accumulate toxic compounds and elements like heavy metals and fat-soluble substances. However, it is built for this and has the necessary mechanisms in place to eliminate them over time.

Even heavy metal poisoning is rare and can be treated with chelating agents rather than detox diets or products.

In a nutshell, there is no need for fancy detox supplements or diets provided you eat a healthy, balanced diet in line with your calorie needs and keep blood glucose levels in check. You and your wallet will be far better off and it will allow your body to do what it's built to do by using its own natural detoxification system to deal with so-called evil toxins.

Q.   Do I need to supplement with antioxidants?

Various vitamins and chemical compounds with antioxidant properties and effects on mitochondria have been used in attempts to prevent, control or reduce the complications of diabetes.

These include coenzyme Q, vitamin E, α-lipoic acid, N-acetylcysteine (NAC), vitamin C and other more complex compounds. The therapeutic use of these antioxidants, particularly in human studies directed at combating cardiovascular disease, a major complication of diabetes, has been disappointing [129, 130].

The ever-popular water-soluble ascorbic acid (vitamin C) is widely marketed for its antioxidant properties [131], yet there is no evidence to support its role in the management of diabetes [132]. In fact, it is suggested that antioxidant supplementation should be avoided in and around periods of strength training.

Why is this?

The reactive oxygen species (ROS) and reactive nitrogen species (RNS) produced during exercise by the mitochondria and other subcellular compartments cause skeletal muscle damage and fatigue. This signalling process is a stimulus for the remodelling of skeletal muscle following resistance and high intensity exercise.

Supplementing with antioxidants in and around training has been shown to blunt this process, which jeopardises muscular adaptions [133]. Imagine paying for a supplement that blunted your gains. A well-balanced diet that includes a diverse range of fruits and vegetables should provide more than enough antioxidants for health and human development. There is no need to supplement.

TAKE HOME MESSAGE

Supplements can serve a purpose in promoting wellness, muscle building and fat loss. However, I suggest dedicating the majority of your energy and spare cash into consuming a diverse diet of fresh, minimally processed food.

FURTHER READING

If you wish to read more about this topic, or see if a supplement dealer has conned you, head over to Examine.com, an evidence-based supplement information website with a mission to empower consumers with the knowledge they need to make worthwhile supplement purchases.

In fact, for just a few bucks, you can grab their Supplement Goals Reference Guide. This book will save you wasting a ton of money on useless supplements. Copy this into your address bar **http://bit.ly/1VySEC1**

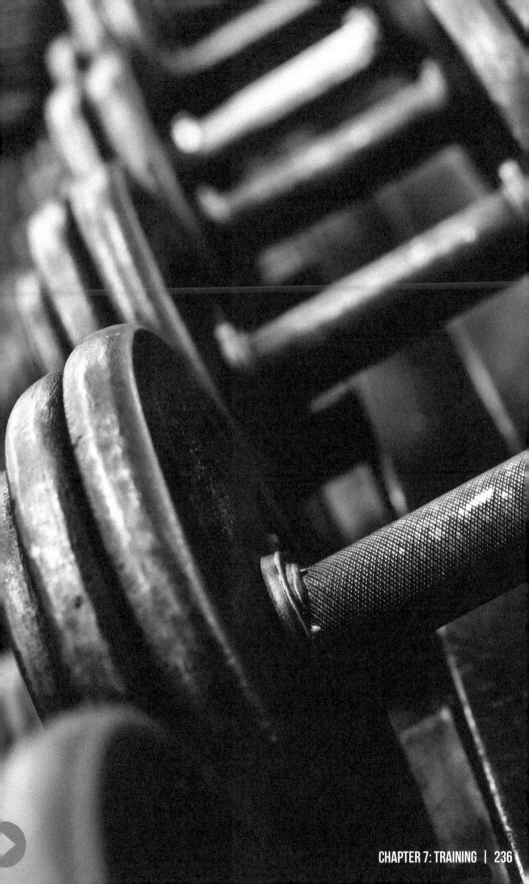

CHAPTER 7: TRAINING

After reading this chapter you should be able to:

- Understand the difference between commonly confused terms; health and fitness + physical activity and exercise.

- Gain a fundamental understanding of exercise physiology in someone living with diabetes.

- Understand why blood glucose levels behave differently with different forms of exercise.

- Training principles needed to build a fitter, stronger, better-looking body.

- The effects of strength training and cardio exercise on people living with diabetes.

I also dig deep into the practical aspects of strength training and provide a fully actionable training plan for you to get stuck into.

Now you understand the basics of nutrition and have a clear strategy to build a personalised diet, let's shift your attention to training.

Although exercise has long been considered a cornerstone of diabetes management, many people living with the condition don't have adequate knowledge or experience of training to get the most out of it.

In addition to this:

- Some diabetes healthcare professionals do not understand the underlying physiology of exercise.

- Many fitness professionals aren't aware of the complexities people living with diabetes face when it comes to exercise.

ALWAYS SEEK ADVICE FROM A HEALTHCARE PROFESSIONAL WHO UNDERSTANDS BOTH EXERCISE AND DIABETES.

Provided blood glucose levels are kept in check, exercise is a worthwhile investment for people with T1D and T2D who are looking to improve their health, body shape and overall quality of life.

PLEASE APPRECIATE…

The underlying physiology of diabetes and exercise is extremely complex, with many aspects beyond the scope of this text. I've done my best to simplify the information, along with referencing the most up-to-date and credible research to support my findings.

If you want to learn more about the very complex science, feel free to follow-up on the resources and references at the end of the chapter. If the science seems too much, or you already understand it, feel free to skip ahead to the practical elements of training found later in the text.

Either way, I hope this chapter settles your curiosity about why blood glucose levels behave in the way they do in response to exercise, and it helps you make an undying commitment towards achieving robust glycemic control.

THE BETTER YOUR CONTROL, THE BETTER THE RESULTS!

THE BIG CONFUSION: PART 1 - HEALTH VS FITNESS

Before we get into the benefits of weights and cardio, let's first define the difference between two wrongly interchanged terms: 'health' and 'fitness'.

WHAT IS HEALTH?

According to the World Health Organization (WHO), 'health' is a state of complete physical, mental and social wellbeing and not merely the absence of disease or infirmity [1]. In layman's terms, health relates to the harmony and interplay between all the body's systems and organs.

Can someone living with diabetes be healthy?

In my opinion, yes.

Are they normal?

No, not completely but health is a continuum and people living with diabetes have a choice to achieve wellness. Globally, there are plenty of people living with diabetes who are healthy, fit and accomplishing amazing things.

I pride myself on being one of them. Let's discuss some of the challenges facing people with T1D and T2D.

TYPE 1 DIABETES

The ever-changing dynamics of day-to-day life make perfect blood glucose control a never-ending challenge for T1D. On top of that, you have to contend with insulin pens breaking, pumps malfunctioning and unexpected illnesses.
Do your best to maintain control by treating blood glucose issues with lightning speed. This is the best way to limit complications and be the healthiest version of yourself.

TYPE 2 DIABETES

This condition is often accompanied by a host of other metabolic abnormalities, which have the potential to reduce life expectancy and quality of life. Individuals living with T2D have the opportunity to drive their diabetes into remission and protect themselves, provided they still have some functional beta cells and they make a conscious effort to change their lifestyle.

DIABETIC EXERCISE CHECK LIST

- Keep a clear head.
- Know what you're eating.
- Know when you last took your medication.
- Know how your body reacts to exercise.
- Know the best options to regain control.

WHAT IS FITNESS?

Fitness is simply the ability to do a task, nothing more, nothing less. The context and nature of the task will require different attributes.

Never confuse health with fitness; they are completely different.

Table 1.0 provides a generalised overview of how fitness can be categorized.

CATEGORY	INCLUDES
Health Related	<ul><li>Physiology</li><li>Psychology</li><li>Body composition</li><li>Cardiovascular fitness</li><li>Strength and endurance</li><li>Mobility (Movement quality)</li></ul>
Skill Specific	<ul><li>Motor skills (Co-ordination)</li><li>Power</li><li>Speed</li><li>Reaction times</li><li>Eyesight</li></ul>
Sport Specific	<ul><li>Sport specific fitness (Skill Development)</li></ul>

HEALTH-RELATED FITNESS

This includes well-known fitness-related attributes that are recognised for their direct relationship to promoting good health.

Physiology relates to how an individual performs a specific task or activity. It takes into consideration the interplay between organs, hormones and cells.

Exercise Physiology governs the human body's response to exercise. This includes a host of processes ranging from fuel utilization right through to the growth of new muscle tissue. Diabetes has a profound effect on the body's physiology, especially if poorly controlled.

Psychology relates to your state of mind and includes everything from your ability to get motivated to overcoming adversity. There is a very close relationship between your psychology and physiology. In fact, you could argue your psychology becomes your physiology.

Diabetes and its complications can be stressful to live with. This makes safeguarding psychological (mental) health a priority.

Body composition is about how much of your body is and isn't fat. The non-fat part of your body is called lean body mass. It includes muscle, water, bone and organs. Fat mass is purely body fat, and there are various types. The primary source of body fat is adipose tissue, the fat located under the skin and around the organs.

Lean body mass is metabolically active and burns significantly more energy than fat mass. This is one of the main reasons why increasing muscle mass helps increase resting metabolic rate, the amount of calories you burn at rest.

A myriad of evidence demonstrates a direct relationship between improvements in body composition and key markers of health.

Diabetes and high levels of body fat are not a good combination, which is why obesity is considered one of the major contributor's in the development of T2D.

Cardiovascular fitness (aerobic fitness) is defined as the ability of your circulatory and respiratory systems to supply oxygen during exercise or strenuous activity [2].

Poor cardiovascular fitness is typically associated with obesity and low levels of physical activity and exercise. Whether you live with Type 1 or 2 Diabetes, a healthy cardiovascular system is a worthwhile asset.

Musculoskeletal fitness consists of three components: muscular strength, endurance and flexibility [3].

- Strength is the ability to express force through the production of joint movements [4].

- Endurance is the ability to maintain or repeat a given force or power output over a given period of time [5].

- Flexibility is the ability to move through a specific joint range of motion [6].

Low levels of musculoskeletal fitness are another by-product of low levels of physical activity and exercise.

How you train determines the end result. If you train like a marathon runner, you can expect your body to develop the necessary physiological adaptions needed for marathon running. If you train like a strength athlete or bodybuilder, you can expect your body to develop different adaptions.

This is known as training specificity and is an essential aspect of exercise programme design.

MOBILITY

There is a lot of confusion and controversy about mobility. Often it is used interchangeably with flexibility and some say it's the same thing but others say it isn't. You could consider mobility an undefined term in fitness.

I personally define mobility as movement potential.

Ask yourself the following

- Can you exercise pain-free?
- Can you feel the intended muscles working during exercise?
- Can you move well outside the gym in day-to-day life?

If you answered no to any of these, you may have an underlying mobility issue.

It has been suggested that those living with diabetes may be at increased risk of limited joint mobility due to glycation-based cross-linking of the connective tissue structures, including in and around the joints, as a result of poor glycemic control. This gives the exercising diabetic even more reason to obsess over their blood glucose control. Nothing ruins a training session more than crappy mobility.

I've outlined a number of mobility strategies tailored to the modern day man and woman within the practical training section of the text. These focus on overcoming the many common nags, niggles and muscle weakness that play a big role in hindering movement quality.

If you've suffered from an injury you may need to seek specific advice from a professional physiotherapist.

SKILL-SPECIFIC FITNESS

This refers to the ability to complete a specific task using particular skills. It could involve anything from the motor skills needed to juggle balls to the hand-to-eye coordination necessary for sewing a needle.

Certain skills are required more than others during specific tasks. The degree to which they are developed depends on how frequently they are trained.

When it comes to exercise, you must gain the necessary balance and coordination to perform all five basic human movements.

Are you fit to squat, deadlift, press, pull and carry?

SPORT SPECIFIC FITNESS

The skills required for certain sports are highly dependent on the nature of the activity and movements involved.

For example, the fitness skills of a rugby player are different to those of a golfer.

If you play sport your training must complement the unique skills required for your sport, otherwise your training is going to go to waste.

The primary goal of this resource is to encourage individuals to engage in appropriate lifestyle, nutrition and exercise behaviours that promote positive health and fitness outcomes.

There are many different forms of exercise available. This book focuses exclusively on weights resistance training and supplementary cardiovascular exercise, for those wishing to get lean(er).

THE BIG CONFUSION: PART 2 – PHYSICAL ACTIVITY VS. EXERCISE – THE DIFFERENCE

Many people are confused by the difference between physical activity and exercise. This is unsurprising as the two terms are used interchangeably by medical and fitness professionals, as well as in most mainstream health promotional material.

WHAT'S THE DIFFERENCE?

Physical activity is defined as any bodily movement produced by skeletal muscles that require energy expenditure (7).

Exercise Training refers to planned, structured and repetitive bodily movements performed with the intent of developing (or maintaining) physical fitness. This includes cardiovascular, strength and flexibility training options (8).

BEFORE YOU BEGIN - PRE EXERCISE CONSIDERATIONS

For most people with diabetes, low-level physical activity can be pursued without the need for medical examination. However, those looking to participate in planned vigorous exercise are strongly recommended to consult with their health professional team and undertake all the necessary medical evaluations beforehand.

This is especially true for individuals who struggle with their control and have underlying health complications including:

- Obesity (and everything that comes with).
- Cardiovascular complications associated with the heart, blood vessels, eyes, kidneys, feet and nervous system.
- Nerve damage and other neurological disorders, such as epilepsy.
- Orthopaedic limitations (e.g. previous joint surgery, unhealed ulcerations or wounds on the feet).
- Other underlying medical conditions that may hinder exercise performance.
- History of smoking.

A fitness professional must be aware of these complications before prescribing exercise plans. An orthopaedic limitation, such as unhealed ulcerations or amputation will significantly affect exercise programme design and possibly worsen the condition.

In any case, where complications do exist, an individual's response to exercise must be measured and progressed accordingly.

EXERCISE AND HUMAN HEALTH

I don't need to elaborate on the fact that exercise has been proven time and time again to be good for us. There is a substantial amount of evidence to support the role of regular weight training and cardiovascular exercise in protecting against many major health problems [9] and that more sedentary individuals are associated with a worse metabolic profile [10].

Key examples include:

* Obesity
* Diabetes
* Cardiovascular disease
* Cancer
* Mental health Issues
* Osteoporosis
* Sarcopenia and other muscle-wasting diseases resulting in frailty

EPIDEMIOLOGICAL EVIDENCE IS EMERGING THAT BEING PHYSICALY ACTIVE, RATHER THAN SEDENTARY, CAN LOWER MORTALITY AND MORBIDITY FOR ANY GIVEN LEVEL OF HBA1C. [11]

EXERCISE AND DIABETES

It is well established that exercise and daily physical activity are important for all individuals with any type of diabetes [12].

However, many people living with T1D and T2D avoid exercise for various reasons, including lack of knowledge, fear of injury, low self-confidence or fear of blood glucose issues like hypoglycemia.

TO GET THE MOST OUT OF EXERCISE, PEOPLE LIVING WITH DIABETES MUST MAKE STRATEGIC ADJUSTMENTS TO THEIR DIET, LIFESTYLE AND MEDICATION.

TYPE 1 DIABETES

Physical exercise is highly recommended for people living with T1D.

Combined weights resistance training and aerobic exercise has been shown to improve key health markers, blood glucose management and increase life expectancy [13, 14].

However, exercise for people with T1D can prove challenging. There are a number of reasons for this, including:

Hypoglyceima

1. Firstly, the use of injectable insulin can dramatically increase the chances of hypoglycemia if mis-dosed or mistimed. Frequent episodes of hypoglyceima can result in 'Hypoglyceima Unawareness'. A metabolic condition that impairs the body's production of counter regulatory hormones.

2. This condition reduces the body's ability to recognise the warning signs of hypos – increasing the risk of experiencing severe hypoglycaemia (and injury). The body's natural stress response to exercise is also impaired.

3. The good news is the condition can be reversed fairly quickly, with research showing improvements within 3 weeks of sound blood glucose control and hypo avoidance.

Hyperglyceima

1. Lack of insulin production can promote hyperglycemia which, when uncontrolled can cause a host of problems that result in fatigue and reduce performance.

Prolonged hyperglycemia can cause a number of problems for the exercising individual, including:

- Muscle Loss via increased protein breakdown and reduced protein synthesis.
- Complications with electrolyte metabolism.
- Abnormal secretion of inflammatory/oxidative factors, (which, in healthy amounts are considered a key component of exercise-associated cardio-protection.)

These issues can make exercise seem to be more hassle than it's worth. However, they don't render exercise harmful.

People living with T1D must be aware of complications and work tirelessly to find an optimal strategy for sound blood glucose control, which in turn will allow them to reap the full beneficial health effects of exercise.

TYPE 1 DIABETES - KEY EXERCISE CONSIDERATIONS

- Must have hypoglycemia and hyperglycemia prevention/treatment strategies in place when following an exercise programme.

- May experience an increase in blood glucose levels from high intensity exercise due to glucose-raising hormones.

- Must make appropriate adjustments to their insulin medication both pre- and post-exercise.

MORE RESEARCH IS NEEDED

Surprisingly, research about T1D and exercise is somewhat limited in comparison to T2D and thus warrants further investigation.

TYPE 2 DIABETES

Many people living with T2D have never exercised and remain inactive post-diagnosis due to lack of confidence, knowledge and fear of injury.

Yet there is a substantial amount of evidence to support the value of combined resistance training and cardiovascular exercise in the treatment of T2D.

The research has largely shown the effects of resistance training are more efficacious than aerobic [15] exercise or diet [16] alone at improving rate of fat loss, body composition change and a decrease in the likelihood of peripheral neuropathic amputations [17] (i.e. the feet).

The risk of hypoglycemia is much lower in people with T2D, with the exception of those using insulin medication.

TYPE 2 DIABETES - KEY EXERCISE CONSIDERATIONS

- Calorie restriction in conjunction with exercise and increased physical activity-based lifestyle interventions are critical to obesity and T2D diabetes management.

- Appropriate adjustments must be made to medication when pursuing exercise.

Individuals with no exercise experience may need to build a foundational level of fitness before progressing to more advanced exercise options like weight training.

Simple increases in physical activity, such as trying to stand more during the day or using a pedometer to track daily step count are incredibly simple lifestyle changes that can have a profound effect on preventing obesity.

UNDERSTANDING DIABETES AND EXERCISE

I want to highlight the key processes that occur in the body during exercise and how they differ between people living with T1D and T2D.

To fully understand this it is important to refer back to the physiology of someone without diabetes and highlight the differences.

UNDERSTANDING GLUCOSE UPTAKE

Glycemic balance is achieved through a variety of important metabolic and hormonal processes that stimulate the uptake and production [18] of glucose.

Glucose uptake is governed by:

- The rate at which glucose enters the blood stream from diet and internal production via the liver.

- The amount of glucose transported into cells for use, via insulin and the physiological response to exercise.

Insulin Mediated Glucose Uptake involves the secretion of insulin, stimulated via food intake or increased concentrations of glucose in the blood.

In healthy individuals increased levels of insulin stimulate the translocation of intracellular glucose transporters GLUT 4 onto the surface of fat and muscle cells, which increase glucose uptake for use as fuel or to be stored as energy (in the form of muscle glycogen or fatty acids). The fate of glucose generally depends on the quantity consumed in relation to the energy demands at the time.

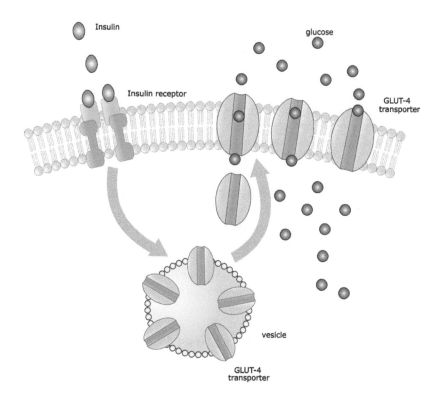

Additionally, insulin suppresses the output of glucose from the liver. The effect is a lowering of blood glucose.

In people living with T1D, insulin production is non-existent. In cases of T2D, insulin action is impaired. In both instances the body becomes ineffective at processing nutrients; such derangements in insulin action have widespread and devastating effects on many organs and tissues, if uncontrolled.

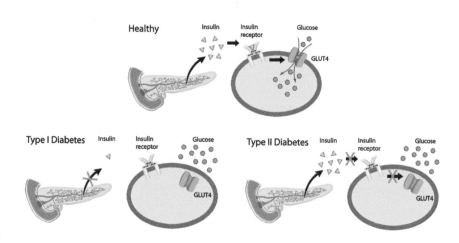

Exercise Induced Glucose Uptake involves muscular contraction, which increases the translocation of glucose transporter GLUT 4 to the surface of skeletal muscle tissue specifically, the primary tissue responsible for glucose disposal [19, 20].

Figure: Simplified representation of exercise mediated translocation of GLUT4

CAPILLARY

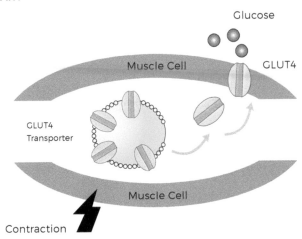

Whilst an insulin mediated response is impaired in people living with Diabetes the exercise induced glut4 translocation is maintained. Therefore, people with diabetes, especially T2D, can increase the clearance of glucose through exercise as effectively as non-diabetics.

While this mechanism of glucose transport can be beneficial to people with complete deficiency of insulin production. It's important to be aware that the liver's production of glucose will inevitably outweigh what can be transported from blood and into the muscle. Consequently, hyperglyceima will result.

People with T1D or advanced T2D cannot rely on exercise mediated transport of glucose 24 hours a day for practical reasons. Therefore, the need for injectable insulin is still required.

THE LIVER AND BLOOD GLUCOSE REGULATION

GLUCOSE PRODUCTION

The liver plays a key role in the maintenance of blood glucose levels during exercise by producing and releasing glucose into the blood stream. It does this via two processes:

Glycogenolysis: Stored glycogen in the liver is broken down and released into the blood stream as glucose. This is the main source of internally produced glucose during exercise of varying intensity.

Gluconeogenesis: The liver produces its own glucose from non-carbohydrate sources, such as glycerol, lactate and amino acids. This is the main source of glucose used during fasting and certain exercise conditions.

These processes act as a counter regulatory response to provide an immediate source of fuel for the system when it needs it most, or to prevent and correct substantial decreases in blood glucose levels that may lead to hypoglycemia.

COUNTER REGULATORY HORMONES

Increased concentrations of counter regulatory hormones, such as glucagon, growth hormone, cortisol and other stress-related hormones known as catecholamines, are responsible for glucose production in the liver.

Glucose produced from the liver must be in balance with the glucose utilised by the muscle cells otherwise problems with blood glucose levels can occur.

Hypoglycemia occurs when the liver's production of glucose fails to match the elevated uptake of glucose by muscle cells. This is usually the result of prolonged exercise, when liver glycogen stores become depleted, and the process of gluconeogenesis doesn't produce enough glucose to keep up. A very rare circumstance in healthy individuals.

Hypoglycemia can reduce exercise performance and impair concentration, which may increase the risk of injury. In rare cases, it can also lead to increased consumption of excess calories, which may hinder fat loss efforts, which is a particular concern for those competing in bodybuilding, powerlifting or weight-restricted combat sports.

Hyperglycemia occurs when glucose production exceeds utilization by the working muscles.

Depending on the severity of hyperglycemia, unfavourable changes in body chemistry result, which if left uncontrolled can jeopardize health, exercise performance and recovery.

THE EFFECTS OF DIFFERENT TYPES OF EXERCISE ON BLOOD GLUCOSE CONTROL

Different forms of exercise rely on different energy systems within the body. This translates into different blood glucose responses for each form of exercise.

So the blood glucose response you have from a hard weight training session will differ over the course of 24 hours from that of a leisurely walk around the park with your dog.

In order to understand which fuels are being used, you must learn the difference between aerobic and anaerobic exercise, and how they affect the blood glucose levels of a diabetic.

Aerobic Exercise is an activity that uses large muscle groups at relatively low rates of muscular contraction that can be maintained continuously for prolonged periods of time (minutes to hours).

During aerobic work, the heart pumps out oxygenated blood to deliver oxygen to the working muscles. As exercise demand increases, the heart and lungs work harder to supply more oxygen to the working muscles.

Aerobic exercise includes both low intensity steady state exercise, such as walking and also more vigorous aerobic exercise, such as high intensity interval training, which combines low intensity work with periods of high intensity.

To promote adherence (and benefit), the type and duration of aerobic exercise you choose needs to be tailored specifically to personal preference and fitness levels.

THE EFFECT OF AEROBIC EXERCISE ON BLOOD GLUCOSE LEVELS

Generally speaking, aerobic exercise has been shown to reduce blood glucose levels in T1D and T2D for 2-72 hours after the last bout of activity (21, 22).

Obviously, the effect depends on aerobic exercise choice and duration. More vigorous aerobic exercise may cause a transient increase in blood glucose levels due to the release of glucose raising hormones (discussed soon).

Anaerobic Exercise is characterised by high rates of intense muscular contraction performed over a relatively short period of time. During anaerobic exercise, the body's demand for oxygen exceeds the oxygen supply available. Anaerobic exercise is not dependent on oxygen but relies on stored energy sources in the muscles.

Weights resistance training and high intensity cardiovascular training are examples of anaerobic that are particularly relevant to this book.

THE EFFECT OF ANAEROBIC EXERCISE ON BLOOD GLUCOSE LEVELS

Resistance training is known to be a potent stimulator of the counter-regulatory hormones catecholamines, cortisol and growth hormone. These hormones serve a number of purposes, including the ability to increase blood glucose.

High intensity aerobic exercise also generates a lot of lactate, which is a precursor to gluconeogenesis, one of the body's glucose-producing processes.

Lactate produced during exercise is processed in the liver via a metabolic pathway called the Cori cycle and is then converted into glucose and recycled back to the muscles to be metabolised back into lactate. Some of this recycled lactate may lead to an increase in blood glucose levels.

In healthy individuals, the temporary rise in blood glucose levels is compensated at the end of training, keeping blood glucose levels in range.

But people with T1D fail to produce enough insulin to bring blood glucose levels back down to normal levels, which can lead to hyperglycemia if insulin medication isn't administered.

There are currently no guidelines in place to suggest how much insulin someone with T1D should administer to treat post-exercise hyperglycemia.

SMALLER ADJUSTMENTS IN INSULIN DOSE CLOSER TO EXERCISE MAY HELP PROMOTE BETTER BLOOD GLUCOSE CONTROL.

People with T2D respond differently to exercise depending on their degree of insulin resistance. The threat of hyperglycemia is not as high compared to those suffering from T1D.

BLOOD GLUCOSE LEVELS POST-ANAEROBIC EXERCISE

In the first few hours of exercising, blood glucose levels may initially rise.

However, anaerobic exercise generally depletes glycogen stores and can result in a blood glucose lowering effect 1-2 hours after exercise when the associated counter-regulatory hormones wear off.

The extent of glycogen depletion will depend on training volume and pre-existing glycogen stores, which are largely influenced by overall calorie and carbohydrate intake. Could eating a lower calorie - low carb diet increase the chances of a hypoglycemia post-exercise? Quite possibly. This is something that must be considered if fat loss is the end goal.

NOCTURNAL HYPOGLYCAEMIA FOLLOWING EXERCISE

The delayed blood glucose lowering effect of anaerobic exercise increases the potential for night time hypoglycaemia. The only way to prevent such episodes from occurring is to closely monitor night time blood glucose levels over time, identify reoccurring patterns and respond with appropriate adjustments to your diet and medication.

WEIGHTS RESISTANCE TRAINING AND ITS EFFECT ON GLUCOSE METABOLISM

Picture this: two cars, same model.

One car has a 1.0 litre engine; the other has a 3.0 litre engine

The 1.0 litre represents the non-training diabetic; the 3.0 litre represents the highly trained diabetic.

Which burns more fuel during rest and movement?

You guessed it – the 3.0 litre.

Weight training increases your engine size (metabolism) in a number of ways:

- Muscle is a relatively energetic tissue and burns significantly more energy than fat tissue. The end result is an increase in fuel consumption during rest and training.
- Increased fuel storage capacity – a bigger muscle creates a larger collection point for fuel, notably protein, carbohydrate and fat.
- Increased performance – you have the potential to burn increasingly more calories during and after exercise as a result of increased training performance (exercise thermogenesis).

PHYSIOLOGICALLY SPEAKING

Key adaptions to weight training in healthy individuals include an increase in muscle mass along with increased levels of GLUT 4 (glucose transporter) and a restoration of insulin signalling activity [23,24].

All of these adaptions assist carbohydrate metabolism by providing a better environment for insulin action and they also have the potential to facilitate greater glucose uptake, independent of insulin.

Since one of the major hallmarks of diabetes is impaired insulin action and glucose metabolism, surely these adaptions would be beneficial?

WITH INCREASED WORK LOAD, MUSCLE CELLS BECOME MUCH MORE SENSITIVE TO THE EFFECTS OF INSULIN (BOTH NATURAL AND ARTIFICIAL). THE MORE INTENSE AND PROLONGED THE WORK THE GREATER THE SENSITIVITY.

IN TYPE 1 DIABETES

Due to a lack of research and zero randomised controlled trials in testing the efficacy of high-intensity physical activity on glycemic control (A1C) or post-exercise hypoglycemia it remains unclear whether weights resistance exercise is highly beneficial for glycemic control in people living with T1D.

Based on the limited amount of research so far, the benefits of resistance exercise haven't been recognised as part of a strategy to improve T1D management. Some studies show improved A1C [25]; others show no significant improvement [26].

WHY SO?

The liver's counter-regulatory effect can increase blood glucose levels during training conditions. T1D'ss lack the compensatory insulin production to normalise levels post-training. Therefore high intensity weights resistance training has the potential to increase blood glucose and possibly conflict with T1D control.

In fact, research has suggested that performing weights resistance training prior to cardiovascular exercise may be a valid strategy to protect against the blood glucose lowering effect (and increased risk of hypoglycemia) that is commonly associated with aerobic exercise [27]. It has even been suggested that conducting a 10 second maximal sprint before or after engaging in low to moderate intensity exercise acts as a valid hypoglycemic prevention strategy [28].

For those living with T1D, rigorous glucose testing and daily insulin therapy in conjunction with an appropriate diet are crucial for optimal performance and recovery from training. Additionally, an individualised approach to pre- and post-exercise glycemic management must be employed. This can only be achieved through rigorous testing and the trialling of a number of control strategies

TYPE 2 DIABETES

The research clearly highlights the effectiveness of weights resistance training in the management of T2D over aerobic exercise [29] or diet alone [30].

A well structured randomised control trial led by Carlos Castaneda in 2002 [31] found that after 16 weeks of resistance training, subjects made marked improvements to their glycemic control (A1C), increased muscle glycogen stores and 72% of participants were able to reduce their prescribed medication dose.

CIRCULATING INSULIN LEVELS

People with T1D can't reduce the effect of the insulin they administer manually.

Too much circulating insulin limits the effect of the counter-regulatory hormones that stimulate the liver to produce glucose, meaning further decreases in blood glucose as exercise continues.

Therefore, appropriate medication and dietary modifications in T1D are crucial in the prevention of hypoglycemia.

Consider the dose, frequency and timing of both food and insulin in and around training.

Key questions to ask yourself include:

- Have you injected the correct amount of insulin for the source and quantity of food consumed, specifically carbs and protein?

- Have you adjusted your basal/bolus insulin dose correctly to account for the potential decrease in blood glucose levels associated with aerobic exercise?

- Have you adjusted your basal/bolus insulin dose correctly to account for the potential increase in blood glucose levels associated with anaerobic high intensity exercise?

- Have you consumed the meal too close to training, and risk indigestion or, worse, hyperglycemia?

- When was the last time you ate? Where you highly active during this period? Have you gone too long without food, and risk going hypoglycemic?

Hypogycemia in non-diabetic individuals is a rare occurrence. Individuals administering insulin exogenously as a performance enhancement aid are exceptions to this.

Episodes of hypoglycemia are generally less of a problem in those suffering from T2D as hepatic glucose production ramps up in response to any decrease in circulating insulin levels [32].

The success of an exercise regime or physical activity should never be gauged solely by how much blood glucose levels decrease during participation. Hypo prevention strategies should always be in place to maximise performance and reduce risk of injury.

CHECK BLOOD GLUCOSE LEVELS AND USE THEM TO GUIDE YOUR STRATEGY – IF THEY'RE TOO LOW THEN EAT, IF THEY'RE TOO HIGH THEN MAYBE SUSPEND INSULIN. IF THEY CROSS A THRESHOLD CONSIDER SUSPENDING EXERCISE FOR A DAY.

HYPOGLYCEMIA (INTRA-WORKOUT)

If you experience a hypoglycemic episode mid-workout you may want to consume additional carbohydrates to restore blood glucose to a tolerable level.

People with T1D who train in a low carb state should be mindful of this risk and always have carbohydrate to hand just in case hypoglycemia strikes mid-workout. Be mindful when treating a hypo that overconsumption of carbohydrate can lead to hyperglycemia later in the session and thus require additional administration of insulin to restore balance. Bouncing blood glucose levels during training session is highly irritating and can lead to drops in performance.

I prefer to use liquid carbs in this situation because overconsuming whole foods close to or in the middle of training can stress the gut, resulting in bloating, nausea and poor performance.

Sports drink yes; bowl of oats or cereal no, unless it's the only option, in which case you may need to take adequate time out from training to accommodate digestion.

It's also important to identify how the hypo occurred? Did you take too much insulin with your pre-training meal? Did you go too long without food?

WHAT ADJUSTMENTS WOULD YOU MAKE NEXT TIME?

If the hypo was severe and resulted in a lack of consciousness or the use of glucagon, it is essential that you report the issue to your healthcare team to come up with an effective plan to prevent future episodes.

HOW MUCH GLUCOSE SHOULD I CONSUME?

How low blood glucose levels fall and the degree of circulating insulin (caused maybe by a miscalculated dose or delay in eating a meal) should dictate how much glucose you need to consume.

Personally I treat hypos with 20g of glucose at a time. I wait about 5-10 minutes, check how I feel and only consume more glucose if I feel the need to.

SITE INJECTIONS

Remember that injecting insulin into a trained, fully pumped muscle group can increase the speed at which insulin works due to increased blood flow around the area.

There is a similar problem with people wearing pumps. Increased blood flow to the skin can increase insulin delivery from the insulin pump during exercise, which consequently has a quicker effect on blood glucose levels.

STRATEGIES TO PREVENT HYPOGLYCAEMIA ASSOCIATED WITH EXERCISE.

STRATEGY	AIMS	DISADVANTAGES
Pre-exercise insulin bolus. (Especially if 1.5-3 hours pre exercise).	Reduce risk of hypoglycemia. This requires no need to treat with Carbohydrate (calories). Highly beneficial for those chasing fat loss.	Hyperglycemia at the start of exercise, which can prove uncomfortable. Requires close monitoring and 'fine tuning'.
Adjust Basal Insulin Dose. (especially if using a pump)	Reduce risk of hypoglycemia. This requires no need to treat with Carbohydrate (calories). Highly beneficial for those chasing fat loss.	Requires close monitoring and 'fine tuning'. Basal rates generally need to be adjusted ahead of time. Typically 1-4 hours depending on type of insulin used. Always be conservative with dose corrections.

↓ Basal insulin Post Training	Reduces the chances of experiencing night time hypoglycaemia	If miscalculated, may result in elevated fasted Blood glucose. Requires close monitoring and 'fine tuning'.
↓ Insulin outside of training as muscle mass increases	As per above	As muscle mass increases ad fat mass decreases, sensitivity to insulin will increase. Be mindful of monitoring and 'fine tuning' insulin dose in response to changes in body composition.
Consuming carbs 'intra' training	To fuel high volume or lengthy training sessions. Provides faster digesting fuel compared to whole foods. This may be ideal at certain times of the day, such as first thing in the morning when getting up to prepare food will result in less sleep. or, when preventing a hypo before eating out after training.	Can lead to digestive upset. Source of highly palatable calories. This will be probleamtic for fat loss if overconsumed.

Pre Workout Caffeine Consumption (stimulant)	Increases blood glucose (dose dependant) and may reduce potential of hypoglycemia.	If sensitive, caffeine may cause agitation and nausea, which can't reduce exercise performance. If consumed too late in the evening (within 6 hours of bed time) caffeine may reduce quality of sleep.
High Intensity Sprint pre/post weight training or cardio.	Weight Training: Can be used to quickly bring blood glucose up. Not as useful post training as weight training will elevate glucose due to stress response. Can be used to bring blood glucose up pre and post training.	Time consuming. May generate fatigue. Little to no effect when performed intra workout.

HYPERGLYCEMIA AND KETOACIDOSIS PRE EXERCISE

It's worth avoiding exercising whilst hyperglycemic or in a state of ketonaemia (abnormally high concentrations of ketone bodies in the blood) as they have the potential to generate fatigue quicker and decrease strength [33].

Reasons for this include:

- Increases the reliance on muscle glycogen as a fuel source and limits the capacity to switch from carbohydrate to lipid as an energy source.
- Depletes muscle glycogen quicker than normal.
  Promote dehydration and problems with electrolyte metabolism.
- Increases muscle protein breakdown and reduces levels of protein synthesis (muscle loss).
- Exacerbates further deteriorations in blood glucose levels.

EXERCISING WITH HIGH BLOOD GLUCOSE CAN JEOPARDISE PERFORMANCE AND BURN VALUABLE MUSCLE TISSUE FOR FUEL.

I hate the idea that my muscles aren't receiving the muscle-building nutrients they should be. Research suggests delaying exercise if blood glucose is higher than 14mmol/L or 252 mg/dl and if blood/urine ketones are present [34].

If you're tight for time and blood glucose is slow to respond skip the session and train another time. If you're serious about making strength and body composition goals, high performance in the weight room is essential – not just training for the sake of it so don't be afraid to call off a session if your glycemic control isn't spot on.

TRAINING ENVIRONMENT

The impact of the training environment extends beyond the obvious increase in perspiration and hydration needs.

TEMPERATURE

It has been shown that increased room temperature increases subcutaneous blood flow, which in turn can accelerate insulin absorption [35]. Consequently, this may increase the risk of hypoglycemia and reduce exercise performance, especially in T1D.

Interestingly it has been demonstrated that the body's ability to generate heat in colder environments (18-19 Centigrade) during episodes of hypoglycemia may be compromised [36].

ALTITUDE

Altitude has been shown to pose challenges to blood glucose control in an exercising individual with diabetes.

Reduced oxygen availability at higher altitudes increases reliance on anaerobic energy metabolism, which increases carbohydrate use for fuel.

AN OVERVIEW: BLOOD GLUCOSE RESPONSE DURING EXERCISE

A number of key factors can affect blood glucose control during exercise. They include:

↓ BLOOD GLUCOSE	STABLE BLOOD GLUCOSE	BLOOD GLUCOSE ↑
Too much circulating insulin medication pre exercise.	Appropriate meal timing.	Not enough insulin medication to cover pre-training meal.
Aerobic-based activity.	Insulin medication dosed and timed correctly for set meal and planned activity.	Ketoacidosis pre exercise.
Increased. Insulin absorption (such as into a muscle tissue being trained).	Insulin Medication adjusted appropriately for counter regulatory response during anaerobic or high intensity exercise.	Insulin pump Disconnected for a prolonged period of time.
Being unfamiliar with exercise type, duration or volume.		High intensity/anaerobic training (HIIT, weight training).
Hypoglycemia unawareness.		Excessive carb intake.
Training environment (altitude and temperature).		Stimulant use.
		Anxiety/Stress
		Illness

PRE-EXERCISE DIABETES BLOOD GLUCOSE CHECK

The impact of the training environment extends beyond the obvious increase in perspiration and hydration needs.

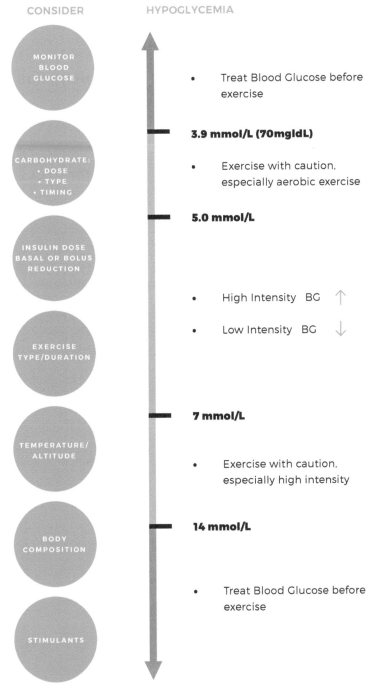

CONSIDER

- MONITOR BLOOD GLUCOSE
- CARBOHYDRATE:
  - DOSE
  - TYPE
  - TIMING
- INSULIN DOSE BASAL OR BOLUS REDUCTION
- EXERCISE TYPE/DURATION
- TEMPERATURE/ ALTITUDE
- BODY COMPOSITION
- STIMULANTS

HYPOGLYCEMIA

- Treat Blood Glucose before exercise

3.9 mmol/L (70mgldL)

- Exercise with caution, especially aerobic exercise

5.0 mmol/L

- High Intensity BG ↑
- Low Intensity BG ↓

7 mmol/L

- Exercise with caution, especially high intensity

14 mmol/L

- Treat Blood Glucose before exercise

HYPERGLYCEMIA

BLOOD GLUCOSE GOALS DURING PHYSICAL ACTIVITY (37)

If using oral diabetes medications 90mg/dl (>5mmol/l)

If using insulin 110mg/dl (>6.1mmol/l)

DIABETES, DEEP SQUATS AND INSULIN SHOTS – IS IT WORTH THE EFFORT?

Generally speaking, Yes.

Taking up the iron is worth it! Especially for people with Type 2 Diabetes. The research for Type 1 Diabetes is weak and desperately needs further investigation.

The benefits of weight training won't come overnight.

Successful body composition change, fitness and improved glycemic control require long term adherence to a training plan in conjunction with rigorous self assessment, and appropriate changes to lifestyle, diet and medication.

EVEN IF HBA1C LEVELS AREN'T IMPROVED THERE ARE STILL MANY HEALTH BENEFITS TO REGULAR EXERCISE.

TRAINING PRINCIPLES

Now you've come to terms with exercise and diabetes, let's review your training goals and discuss the underlying principles needed to build a stronger, better-looking body.

If you want to skip the theory (which I don't recommend) and get straight into the gym, head over to the resources section at **www.diabeticmuscleandfitness.com** and download the set training programmes.

STARTING WITH THE END IN MIND

Maybe you want to lose fat and reveal your first set of abs?

Maybe you want to increase body mass and avoid feeling undersized?

Regardless, the end goal is the same. You want to look better naked. And, of course, out-lift everyone else.

FAT LOSS OR MASS GAIN?

In order to get the most out of your diet and training, you must know your end goal.

Fat loss is a popular goal amongst people living with diabetes, especially those living with T2D. If you feel you're carrying too much body fat or you've been told by your doctor to lose weight your goal is set. Fat loss is also a necessity for those competing in bodybuilding and other weight-restricted sports.

Highly effective fat loss should be sustainable over the long-term and where possible preserve and promote both muscle mass and training performance.

Mass gain is suited to individuals who feel weak and undersized or who want to participate in sports like rugby that require a high level of muscle mass. It's also a suitable goal for individuals who've just finished a fat loss phase and want to gain further muscle mass and size.

Highly effective mass gain involves maximum muscle gain and increases in performance. Fat gain, although inevitable should be kept to an absolute minimum.

Maintenance of current levels of body fat and muscle mass is also a goal, often during periods of stress, such as prolonged periods of travel or high volume of work.

PICK YOUR GOAL AND STICK TO IT

A big issue I see with many bodybuilding and fitness fanatics with diabetes is hopping between mass gain and fat loss. This is especially true in males.

This yo-yo approach results from ignorance and paranoia about losing valuable muscle mass and size when weight begins to fall during fat loss.

If your approach is set up properly and glycemic control in check, muscle loss will never be an issue.

TRAINING PRINCIPLES

The principles I'm about to share with you are grounded on years and years of knowledge and experience. They stem from endless hours of coaching and training and everything I have learned from some of the best minds in the world of physical strength and fitness.

Many of these principles get overlooked, often even by trainers. I've always been a firm believer that if you look the part, you must be able to perform the part also.

Would you want a Ferrari or Lamborghini with a 1.0 litre engine?

No.

Would you be surprised if I told you many of the well-polished physiques you see on the front of muscle magazines are riddled with injury?

What if I told you a good majority of these physiques lack the basic mobility needed to bend over and tie their shoelaces? Or that a great number of people who appear physically fit are actually far from it, with many lacking the cardiovascular fitness to climb up a few flights of stairs without blowing smoke out their back ends.

Don't get me wrong – this isn't the case for everyone. However, I'd say 9/10 of the most important aspects of fitness are overlooked when chasing an aesthetic-orientated goal.

SURFACE DETAILS DON'T COUNT

To build the best version of you, you must be willing to work under the hood just as much as on the surface. A great body looks and feels great, both inside and out.

PRINCIPLE 1: EXERCISE = INFORMATION

Just like nutrition, exercise provides information to the body. How the body responds depends on:

- Exercise type
- Exercise duration
- Exercise frequency
- Exercise quality

Collectively this is known as training specificity.

YOUR PHYSIQUE AND PERFORMANCE ARE THE RESULT OF THE TYPE OF EXERCISE YOU DO ON AVERAGE.

STRENGTH TRAINING FOR A STRONGER, BETTER LOOKING BODY

Strength training has been established as the best form of exercise known to man for improving overall body strength and shape.

The Diabetic Muscle and Fitness Guide promotes a buffet of strength training options that deliver a number of key benefits, including:

- Overall body strength and power.
- Hypertrophy (muscle size).
- Improved mobility.
- Fat loss.
- Corrective exercises that target commonly underdeveloped muscles.

Other exercise methods, including cardiovascular exercise, stretching and specific mobility work can complement but not replace the benefits of a well-structured strength-training regime.

TRAINING DIFFERENCES: FAT LOSS VS. MASS GAIN

Both fat loss and mass gain are grounded on strength training.

The main difference between the two is energy balance; one requires a calorific surplus whilst the other requires a calorific deficit.

Calorie intake is determined by food intake, whilst calorie expenditure is determined by how active you are both in the gym as well as during your normal daily routine, along with other important body processes.

Exercise and physical activity play the biggest role in influencing energy expenditure. Weight training serves the purpose of stimulating muscle gain, whilst cardio serves the purpose of increasing energy expenditure. When cardio is added tactfully to a weight-training regime, it can help promote an energy deficit, which is essential for fat loss.

Performing cardio whilst striving for weight gain will make it harder to achieve an energy surplus. Depending on the type and duration of cardio it may contribute towards unwanted fatigue, which can hinder your performance and ability to stimulate growth in the weights room. This is the exact reason why endurance training conflicts with strength training.

I'm not saying you can't do cardio when trying to gain weight. You can – just be mindful you'll need to eat more calories to compensate what you burned off. You'll also have increased recovery demands depending on the type of cardio you do.

PRINCIPLE 2: STRENGTH FIRST

The stronger you are, the more effective you are at everything.

Strength is the most important aspect of physical existence. A lack of strength compromises performance and quality of life as we age.

Strength can be generally classified into physical and mental strength. As a person with diabetes, you must possess a great deal of strength in both paradigms in order to get the most out of life and exercise. Let's discuss the quality of physical strength – what it is, why it's important and how to build it.

WHAT IS STRENGTH?

Strength is simply the production of force with your muscles. It can be easily measured by the amount of weight you lift.

WHY IS IT IMPORTANT?

We produce force every day in our living environment. This includes everything from brushing your teeth to lifting the groceries right to carrying our children to bed or forcing open a door in an emergency. Everything we do involves the application of force.

A healthy heart and lungs are important but if you're not strong enough to effectively function in your physical environment, your quality of life will suffer.

The loss of strength is a consequence of ageing, lack of physical activity, poor diet and illness.

If you haven't prioritised strength, you're missing the boat. Don't build your house on sand. Strength is the platform for more muscle mass.

Get strong on a regular, trackable basis!

HOW TO INCREASE STRENGTH?

The best way to increase strength is to train it.

Not all exercise regimes train strength. They must be specific.

Strength training is about skill acquisition, neurological adaptation and muscle mass. In other words, using specific movements and exercises to apply force/load to the body. Training with barbells, kettlebells, machines and of course bodyweight is the best way to develop it.

For the majority of people reading this who use their bodies and physical strength on a day-to-day basis, you must become strong and proficient across five basic human movements. Rarely, if ever, does the body function in isolation; the body functions as a whole.

The bulk of your training will, therefore, focus on loading and strengthening the entire human system across the following basic human movements.

- Squat
- Hip hinge
- Push
- Press
- Carry or Lift

I also throw in some isolation and finishing exercises for good measure to ensure maximum stimulation.

THE PROCESS FROM IRON TO MUSCLE:

1. **Lift and Load**: Training serves as a controlled stress. Exercises are conducted over the greatest range of motion and loaded progressively. This disrupts the body's natural state and provides the necessary stimulus for change.

2. **Eat, Rest and Recover**: To take advantage of this stimulus the correct resources must be in place. With the right diet and rest, the body kick-starts numerous growth and repair processes to accommodate the stress initiated through training.

3. **Adaption**: During the recovery process key physical and mental changes occur to accommodate the specific stress applied. Think stronger muscles and better quality movement in response to the set exercises or movements.

For those starting out, adaptions take place very quickly; the process eventually slows as your training age increases. You simply become more efficient at adapting over time.

IT IS IMPORTANT TO APPRECIATE THE PROCESS TAKES TIME, AND ANY INTERRUPTION (POOR BLOOD GLUCOSE CONTROL, STRESS, LACK OF SLEEP, POOR NUTRITION, ETC.) WILL SLOW PROGRESS.

The training programmes are designed to get you stronger over time. They're not not just a random collection of exercises that leave you hot, sweaty and sore.

PRINCIPLE 3: PERIODIZATION - PLAN YOUR TRAINING

To get the most out of your training, it must be planned.

Periodization is a concept, not a defined training model or regime. It's simply a way to manipulate training variables, most notably training volume.

TRAINING VOLUME IS BEST DESCRIBED AS:

Load X Sets X Reps

Irrespective of load, volume can also be summarised as the total amount of reps performed per muscle group, per workout, and per week. The frequency of training sessions and or exercises will play a big role here.

Volume is extremely important because it dictates the amount of work and practice we get. The more practice you get moving loads with specific exercises, the stronger you get at those specific movements using that load and rep range.

To progress, you must increase training volume over time. (38) This doesn't mean you need to increase the load, number of sets and reps every time you step into the gym. This simply wouldn't be possible. Too much volume can be counterproductive as it can accumulate too much fatigue.

Don't get me wrong: you can build an impressive physique with a low-volume lifting routine. However, you can build an even better physique with a higher volume routine. Make no mistake, there is a dose-response relationship between volume and muscle growth.

"Try to progress with as little work as possible. Increase volume only when you plateau, provided the necessary recovery resources are in check."

ONLY COUNT THE HARD WORKING SETS AS PART OF YOUR TRAINING VOLUME. NOT LIGHT WARM-UP SETS.

Besides volume, we also need to consider other training elements that can be periodized. They include:

- Rest Periods – The amount of rest between sets.
- Exercise Choice – Revolving exercises that provide fresh stimulus and attack weak points.
- Exercise Techniques – Methods and tactics to provide a progressive stimulus.
- Cardio – Cardiovascular exercise may be added progressively over time to generate a calorie deficit and promote fat loss.

These training variables can be adjusted over time to optimise a given fitness outcome and can also:

- Reduce the potential for plateaus.
- Reduce the possibility of burnout (overreaching/overtraining).
- Keep things fresh and reduce boredom.
- Prevent injury.

There are endless ways to periodize a training routine to achieve individual goals.

The training programmes included have been carefully periodized over 16 weeks, meaning the volume for each week and training block is different and builds on the previous block. The programmes also include periods of lower volume training, which serve as recovery or de-training weeks.

YOUR TRAINING PROGRAMME IS A ROUGH GUIDE – PREPARE TO TAKE A DETOUR

Occasionally set your programme aside... you must be flexible with your training approach.

Your training programme doesn't take into account the spontaneous and ever-changing circumstances life throws at us.

This includes everything from personal and work-related stress to illness.

Don't panic.

It's OK to skip a workout and move it by a day if you don't feel like training; it's OK to stay away from the gym until your cold gets better; it's OK to finish your workout early and deal with a personal emergency; it's OK to use another piece of equipment if one of the machines you want to use isn't available.

Don't let the thought of any of these get you down. Stressing will do more harm than good. Get over it!

THINK LONG GAME

Remember you're in this for the long haul!

If you're labouring under the assumption that extreme suffering is part and parcel of getting in shape, you're wrong. Don't get me wrong, there will be times when you will feel uncomfortable and tired, especially when gunning for ultra low levels of body fat. However, there is a big difference between laziness and full blown fatigue.

When you're in a state of fatigue, you must do your very best to recover instead of building fatigue on top of fatigue. No one will congratulate you on training through a period of burnout or injury.

Training smart is everything – you must know when to back off. I discuss how to approach this in the practical element of this chapter.

CHASING OPTIMAL IS NOT NECESSARILY THE SAME THING AS BEING REALISTIC.

Always think about fitting your training programme around what is sustainable and realistic in your life first, before assessing anything else. Always focus on the time and resources you have available in the present moment.

Is this really the right time to start the programme, or do you just not want it badly enough?

Avoid mistakes by planning and understanding your day-to-day routine. Do your best to stick to the plan.

Consistency is what makes progress rather than perfection. Realise building a strong, healthy physique is a journey of stops, starts and detours.

PRINCIPLE 3: ASPIRE TO MOVE WELL

To get the most from your training, it's essential to aspire and learn to move with integrity both inside and outside the gym.

Fitness should revolve around movement because movement is a big part of everyday life. You'd be surprised by how many people appear to be in great shape but struggle to tie their shoelaces or pick up their underwear without discomfort.

I used to be like this until I realised and respected the benefits of movement training.

WHAT'S THE POINT IN LOOKING GREAT IF YOU STRUGGLE TO MOVE?

Natural movement is the very essence of life.

Your training should be grounded on principles that help you look and move well.

TRAIN MOVEMENT NOT MUSCLE

As discussed, don't assemble workouts solely according to individual body parts. Think and programme primarily in terms of movement.

Don't think legs; think squat. Don't think chest; think push. Don't think back; think pull.

We want exercises that when done in a programme produce total body adaptation towards better strength and movement quality.

I have also included a limited number of extra isolation training options for those looking to bring up specific body parts.

Ensure full range of motion with each movement.

There is no such thing as half-assed training. When it comes to movement-based training, quality comes before quantity – always.

Quality movement is about training movements or exercises through their full range of motion.

Take a body weight squat, for example.

A poor quality squat would include a half or quarter squat whereas a quality squat is ass to grass, all the way down. And – before you ask – no it's not bad for your knees provided there is no underlying tissue problems or injury.

Quality range of motion promotes:

- Optimal stimulation of all the muscle fibres within a given movement.

- Better efficiency and motor control (co-ordination) in conducting the specific movement, provided technique is correct.

- Reduced chance of injury.

MOTOR SKILLS

Think of motor control/skills like a car journey.

If you don't know where you're going you'll stop, start and take plenty of wrong turns. Overall you'll be pretty inefficient at getting there.

Over time, as you repeat the journey you get better at remembering the route and arrive at your location quicker and more efficiently.

Each journey represents a specific exercise. Longer, more complicated journeys resemble the big bang whole body movements that require a lot of skill.

At first, you may not be familiar with the technique. You stop, start, jerk and do all sorts – it can get pretty ugly.

Over time as you practice with the right teaching cues you get better. Just like you would if you repeated the journey over and over again. However, it's important to be aware your practice must be perfect in order to get perfect.

It's easy to develop bad habits. Just think of the drivers who text when driving, curb their wheels, get fixed penalty notices or cut people off along the way. These are prime examples of bad habits, which eventually can cause damage (or injury, as far as our exercise analogy is concerned).

It's, therefore, important important to iron out bad habits as soon as possible to get the most out of the exercise. They are very hard to undo. Repetitive behaviours become patterns and these patterns require re-programming of technique (brain to muscle) when they become problematic – don't go there! Try re-learning your driving test and see what I mean.

GOOD MOTOR CONTROL

QUALITY MOVEMENT & SOLID TECHNIQUE

REDUCED CHANCE OF INJURY

BETTER STRENGTH AND HEALTH OUTCOMES.

PERFECT FORM – DOES IT EXIST?

There is no textbook definition for perfect form, simply general guidelines. Everyone is unique and may require specific adjustments to their form to get the most out of particular movements.

Keep it simple and assess:
If it looks like shit – it is shit!
If it feels like shit – it is shit!

Basically, if a movement feels good, hits the intended muscle groups and doesn't cause pain you're good to go.

PRINCIPLE 4: TRAIN PAIN AND INJURY FREE

Why do most people fail to move well?

In a nutshell:

- Injury/pain/illness.
- Modern day posture,

INJURY

Being injured isn't nice.

Safety and speed of progress go hand-in-hand; nothing will jeopardise your progress faster than injury.

Always weigh up cost and benefit.

There are two things to consider when training with an injury.

1.   Biomechanical changes

If you've torn a muscle, broken a bone or lost a limb, there will be obvious implications to your natural biomechanics and range of movement. As such, it's important to find specific exercises that allow you to illicit a safe and effective training effect. This requires professional guidance from a qualified physiotherapist, injury rehab specialist and/or chiropractor.

2.   Fear

Fear of re-injuring yourself can hold you back from getting the most out of your training, especially if you've experienced an injury in the gym. I tore my left pectoral muscle five years ago on the second rep of a 180 kg bench press. It was sore before lifting, but I ignored what my body was telling me and paid the price (eight weeks off training). To this day I haven't dared placed that amount of weight back on the bar. I've compromised and utilised different methods to achieve my goal

OVERCOMING FEAR...

There's nothing wrong with fear. It's a natural protective mechanism. I say to my clients and myself that if you don't fear some of your workouts you're not training hard enough.

Fear doesn't have to relate to a single all-out max rep. It could stem from the thought of a particular tough workout. For example, most people fear the thought of training legs due to the amount of work involved. The body knows what's coming.

Dwelling on fear can be the difference between hitting a new personal best, progressing your physique and, at worst, hitting a very long plateau.

The next time you experience fear, embrace it! I always visualise the weights or workout laughing at me. Sounds crazy right? Just try it next time your under pressure and see who has the last laugh.

The last thing you want to do is freak out and walk away unless you're injured, suffering from severe fatigue or lifting a weight that is unrealistically heavy in relation to your current strength. Be realistic, not stupid. Ambitious, not lazy.

Fear is good in the right circumstances.

PAIN

Pain inhibits quality movement.
If you experience pain when you exercise it is important to identify the root cause, report it to a professional and modify exercise activity.

THE SAYING 'NO PAIN, NO GAIN' IS WITHOUT DOUBT, ONE OF THE MOST FOOLISH MINDSETS TO HAVE WHEN IT COMES TO TRAINING THE BODY.

If you want a catalyst for injury and burnout – these four words would be it.

Don't be DAFT!

If you decide to train on, you'll encourage the body to find alternative ways and means of moving. Think of this as compensatory movement. The body shifts stress/load from the intended area and onto other tissues. If repeated it is likely to aggravate the problem and cause secondary movement problems if left unaddressed.

Don't go there – if it's sore, stop, rest and do something else.

Train smart.

ILLNESS

Poor health can seriously impair your ability to recover and perform. Some illnesses have a greater impact than others.

In respect to diabetes, exercising whilst in ketosis or with a blood glucose level above 14 mmol/L or 252mg/dl is not advisable and will impair performance and recovery. Dehydration, joint/muscle stiffness/weakness and reduced concentration are of no benefit to a hard training individual.

Exercising whilst suffering from common ailments like the flu or food poisoning will have obvious implications on performance and recovery. It doesn't take a rocket scientist to work out the gym is one of the most unhygienic environments known to man.

Knowing that your ability to perform in the gym and recover is directly linked to your diabetes control should provide you with an unstoppable drive to control your condition and be increasingly mindful of further stresses.

You must learn to mange stress and listen to your body's internal cues to avoid stressing the system even further.

We will touch on this later on in the book under the subject of auto-regulating training.

MODERN DAY POSTURE

Modern day movement patterns are toxic to a hard-training individual.

We sit too much. We spend too much time on computers, phones and tablets.

How many times have you held your hands above your head today? Have you sat more than you've stood?

Many of the important muscles involved in strength and total body conditioning become weaker, tighter and inhibited with our modern day lifestyle.

Take sitting for example.

We all sit. It's inevitable in almost everyone's daily routine. The problem arises when we sit more than we stand. Spending eight hours in a chair at work then another three-to-five hours on the sofa at home is not uncommon.

Sitting for prolonged periods of time can decease lung capacity, which leads to fatigue, encourage lordosis (when the spine curves inwards on the lower back) and tighten the hip flexors, calves and connective tissue.

All of these reactions can hinder movement quality – when coaching I refer to this as 'gummed-up' mobility. It's exactly how I feel after sitting all day.

A standing desk can be a great way to prevent this and keep the system fresh for training later in the day.

Another issue I see that contributes to poor mobility is excessive use of smartphones.

How many times have you checked your phone today?

Relentlessly checking your smartphone every 10 minutes could be the root cause of your neck and shoulder pain as well as impaired performance in the gym.

According to a recent study by marketing agency Tecmark, a person looks at their smartphone on average 221 times a day for a total of 3 hours 16 minutes.

Over a year that's 1,200 hours spent moving your neck up and down 80,000 times to stare at your phone. This can only get worse as apps and technology evolve.

How many times did you move your neck up and down 10-15 years ago? Nowhere near as much.

And, smartphones were supposed to make life easier?

DON'T TRY TO BE A HERO

The bulk of your mental energy must be focused on ensuring you achieve quality-loaded movements rather than fear of being crushed.

If you put more weight on the bar than you can handle, you're simply straining your system, encouraging bad habits, limiting range of motion and increasing your risk of injury.

Looking impressive in the gym may be important to you but the reality is your best shot at making a good impression with your body is outside the gym.

Load appropriately – train your body not your ego.

PRINCIPLE 6: MAXIMISING RECOVERY

STRESS MANAGEMENT

Stress can be both harmful and useful to the body, depending on the form, dose and frequency.

Generally speaking, the body is susceptible to a wide range of stressors on a daily basis. Key examples include sleep deprivation, emotions, work, financial concerns, poor diabetic control, other illnesses and even training stress.

Rare and extreme doses of stress are also possible, and include everything from getting hit by a car to getting shot.

Generally speaking, short-term stress is your friend. Long-term and extreme stress is not.

Taking advantage of stress, whether it's learning a new skill or training in the gym, must be done in a controlled manner you can adapt to.

TRAINING IS STRESSFUL

Training is a prime example of a controlled short-term stress. Just think a one-hour workout is only 4% of your day. During this hour you train hard and stress the body – the remainder of the day is spent resting, nourishing and recovering. The end result (if repeated over time) is a fitter body.

MAXIMISE RECOVERY

Your ability to adapt to stress depends on the recovery resources you have available. You must ensure you have a grip on the following variables:

- **Blood sugar management**

You must keep your sugars in check if you want to get the most out of your training sessions. Poor glycemic control will wreak havoc with your mood and body's ability to recover. This includes both hypo and hyperglycemia.

Hypos will ruin your mental and physical performance whilst at the same time increasing your intake of unwanted calories, which may encourage fat gain if you go above your set calorific level.

Running high, especially for prolonged periods of time, such as overnight, will starve your tissues of fuel, hinder muscle repair, increase the risk of dehydration and leave you feeling exhausted. Focus extra attention on controlling sugar at night because this is one of the key times for recovery. Running high throughout the night is one sure way to screw-up body chemistry and ruin early morning training sessions.

- **Appropriate nutritional intake**

Calorie intake and essential nutrients are crucial for maximising performance and recovery, provided blood sugar levels are in check.

Protein is required for the growth and repair of muscle tissue. Fat is required for healthy hormone production and carbohydrate is required for the refuelling of muscle glycogen (the primary fuel source for weight training) and maintenance of blood sugars.

- **Hydration**

Exercise, building muscle and losing fat is thirsty work.

Higher protein intakes, episodes of hyperglycemia, training in a hot climate, and use of certain supplements, particularly creatine, also influence hydration needs.

There is strong evidence to support dehydration having a detrimental effect on mental and physical performance [39]. Other research links dehydration to false signs of hunger [40].

Dehydration gives me a false sense of hyperglycemia, which if left unchecked could increase the likelihood of me mistakenly administering insulin or avoiding food, which in turn increases my risk of hypoglycemia.

Ensure you keep hydration in check pre, intra and post exercise. The recommended amount of fluid to consume each day is highly specific to the individual in question. Key factors, such as body weight, training type/frequency/duration and health status all influence intake.

I recommend using a water container to reference your intake across the day instead of going by the glass.

- **Sleep**

We all know what it feels like to lose out on sleep - you wake up the next morning feeling like you've had a night on the town. Your mind is slow, your body stiff and motivation at an all-time low. No matter how many coffees, you still feel lethargic. As for food? Stuff that, grab me the nearest ready meal, takeaway or sandwich.

There's no doubt about it, sleep is good for you - whether its in promoting good health, feeling great, helping you burn body fat or recovering from training - sleep is good and in fact essential for life.

However, the problem is many of us don't get enough. It's either too short or interrupted. Smart phones, social media, over consumption of stimulants and stress are all to blame. Either way, you're shooting yourself in the foot (big time) if you're missing out on your zzz's.

- **Environment**

You are a product of your environment.

The company you keep inside and outside the gym will have a huge impact on your health, mindset and progress in the gym.

If you're around nine negative, jealous, lazy people you will become the 10th. If you're around nine positive, successful and proactive people, you'll become the 10th.

A toxic friendship or a poor work and gym environment will drain your mental and physical energy, leaving little room for personal development and the people closest to you.

Research supports this by showing that people who experience more negative life occurrences (stress) are less likely to recover from and adapt to their training programmes [41].

Your psychology (mental) becomes your physiology (physical).

Eradicate relationships and environments that hold you back. Your health and future are worth it.

- **Illness**

If you experience a bout of illness or sickness during a training phase, you must respect the fact your body has more stress to contend with. As a result you may have to take time out from training, consume the appropriate medication and pay closer attention to your blood sugars.

Pushing through this in the hope of 'sucking it up' or 'no pain no gain' is ludicrous and only adds further stress to the system, which may open the floodgates to something worse.

From a diabetic perspective, illness, particularly infections, can wreak havoc with the body's internal chemistry and lead to worsened glycemic control. This compounds the original stress and may potentially make things worse, especially if left untreated.

TAKE HOME MESSAGE

You must respect how you recover on a day-to-day basis and learn to balance your training stress with outside stress.

Not every day will be perfect therefore you must adjust your training based on how you feel.

If you can't bring high quality effort to the gym, it's important to step back, identify the problem and do something about it.

No one is going to thank you for pushing through pain, and neither will your most prized possession – your body.

PRINCIPLE 7: MEASURE

Keeping a close tab on your performance is a great way to highlight the effectiveness of your recovery and plan in general. Know that training progress will never be linear for long; there will be times when it progresses, plateaus and regresses.

Pay special attention to plateaus and regressions.

Plateaus may simply indicate you've adapted to your training routine and need to change things up. Don't worry the plans in this book take this into account.

Regressions highlight under recovery and the need to back off or revaluate your recovery variables.

Ask yourself:

- Have you missed out on sleep?
- Have you added in any extra exercises unnecessarily? This includes those one-off activities like marathons or walks with friends and family.
- Have you missed meals or forgotten to drink fluid?
- Have you been subject to a sudden physical or emotional trauma?

All of these factors can hinder your progress – it's simply a matter of identifying them and doing your best to work round them.

I highly recommend buying a personal jotter/dairy and logging your performance from session to session.

'If you aren't assessing your diet or training don't expect your physique or performance to reach its full potential...'

DO I NEED TO GO HEAVIER FROM WORKOUT TO WORKOUT?

It's not necessary to lift heavier from workout to workout. It's incredibly difficult, no matter how good your recovery strategies are.

But long-term (across the year) you should strive to get stronger on a regular, trackable basis. Progressive resistance is the name of the game

To lift more weight, learn to overload intelligently as time goes on.

KNOW THAT INFINITE PATIENCE BRINGS IMMEDIATE RESULTS.

ADJUST YOUR TRAINING BASED ON HOW YOU FEEL

Sometimes you'll feel like training; other times not.

Training, just like nutrition, provides information to the body. Under no circumstances do we want to provide crappy information in the form of a half-assed or pathetic training session.

I'm not a huge fan of the whole 'just show up' mind-set.

It's much better to show up, train smart and provide the best possible information for maximum growth and development.

You can do this by adjusting your training based on how you feel. Simply score yourself according to the chart below and take the appropriate action with your training. The best time to score would be first thing in the morning. However, appreciate things may change across the course of the day (due to missed meals, emotional trauma etc.).

This allows you to be flexible with your training programme and get the most out of your workouts and recovery – meaning better adherence, better progress and less chance of suffering burnout or a nasty injury.

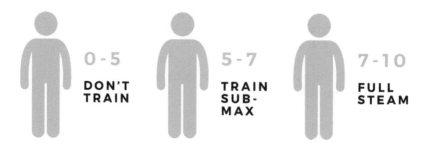

0 - 5
DON'T
TRAIN

5 - 7
TRAIN
SUB-
MAX

7 - 10
FULL
STEAM

WHEN TRAINING SUB-MAXIMALLY CUT DOWN ON TRAINING VOLUME (SETS) OR EXERCISE SELECTION. CUT THE WORKOUT SHORT IF NEEDS BE.

NEVER BE AFRAID TO REST. IF YOUR BODY'S TIRED, LISTEN AND ALLOW RECOVERY.

PRINCIPLE 8: CARDIO

Cardiovascular exercise should form a smaller proportion of your training. Three types of cardio exist: two are beneficial to your goal; the value of the third is debatable. They can be identified by activity or their effect on heart rate.

USEFUL CARDIO

Low Intensity Steady State includes slow, lazy activities like a stroll in the park, gentle swim or cycling along the toe path. It doesn't have any impact and is the kind of activity you can do while still holding a conversation.

The calorie burning effect is lower so you have to do more for it to add up. It places minimal stress on the body, doesn't interfere with muscle growth and can work extremely well for fat loss.

This form of cardio promotes fat loss via increased energy expenditure. It doesn't stress the system and can also be used for relaxation and regeneration.

High Intensity Interval Training is an extremely taxing form of cardio and unlike low/moderate intensity cardio cannot be performed over prolonged periods of time without rest.

It is usually performed in bursts of 30 seconds of all-out effort followed by one minute of rest or light, active recovery intervals for a set time, usually no more than 20-30 minutes. Hill sprints, battle ropes, prowler pushes and Tabata are good examples. Individuals starting this form of cardio are advised to work in shorter intervals of 10 seconds and work up to longer 30-second intervals over time as fitness levels improve.

There are a number of key benefits to HIIT. Firstly, it can lead to similar, if not better metabolic adaptions than lower intensity cardio but over less time [42]. Secondly, it has been shown to provide a short-term, small, but significant elevation in metabolic rate that other forms of cardio do not [43]. This is a huge advantage to anyone looking to maximise fat loss.

On the flipside, the recovery demands of HIIT and the risk of injury are higher than all forms other cardio. In fact, sprinters (mainly HIIT) are much more likely to suffer injuries than long distance runners, despite the fact they run for less distance and time [44].

Generally speaking, I don't recommend any more than 180 mins HIIT per week if chasing a body composition and strength ordinated goal. It's important to build up to this level over time, and not all at once for adherence issues.

HIIT HYPERGLYCEMIA KEY NOTE:

As noted in the previous chapter, high intensity exercise like HIIT can cause acute hyperglycemia in people with T1D. This is due to a number of factors, including:

- The increase in glucose-raising hormones that are produced under stress to increase physical alertness and mobilise fuel.
- Increased production of lactate, another by-product, which can be recycled into glucose by the liver, therefore increasing blood glucose.

To compound the situation, high intensity exercise also has the potential to lower blood glucose levels much later on after exercise, such as during sleep.

A person with T1D certainly has a lot to think about. It is important to be aware of these fluctuations and react appropriately with specific diet and insulin therapy to regain control. I talk about this in more detail later on in the book.

THE OUTLIER – APPROACH WITH CAUTION

Moderate Intensity Cardio is essentially endurance training. A good example is road running. The adaptions and work required with this type of cardio can interfere with muscle growth and recovery especially if overused. The depletion of muscle and liver glycogen as well as the molecular signalling that derive from endurance training are thought to play key roles (45) in this. Also take into account the potentially damaging impact of this type of cardio, particularly if performed on a hard surface. It can result in muscle and joint stiffness/soreness, which can have obvious implications for performance in the weight room.

Try training legs the day after a 10-mile run and you'll catch my drift.

HOW MUCH CARDIO DO I NEED TO DO?

The amount of cardio to do depends entirely on how much body fat you have to lose and in what period.

A big problem with many people's fat loss progress is a drop in their physical activity levels as calories are reduced from the diet and increased from exercise in the hope of losing more fat.

As a result, many people become more fatigued and change their behaviours. This includes the likes of napping more often and taking the lift instead of the stairs.

What they fail to realise is lowering their physical activity preserves energy, rendering any calorie drops and increased exercise less effective at creating a negative energy balance. This negatively affects fat loss progress.

Low-intensity cardio is technically physical activity. It doesn't have to be on a treadmill and can include many different types of daily activities parking as far away as possible from the front of the supermarket to doing laps around the office.

Use a Pedometer

I am a massive fan of using a pedometer to track physical activity levels outside of training.

Step counts give an accurate gauge of how active you are. As mentioned earlier physical activity levels (outside of exercise) play a huge role in energy expenditure which helps control body weight. This data is particularly useful if fat loss is your goal.

Closely tracking your physical activity via a step count is a great way to build the habit of being more active while also setting a benchmark to work from when your fat loss progress plateaus.

As you plateau, you can increase your step count progressively over time. This is an excellent way to increase energy expenditure and burn more fat.

In fact, using a step count allows you to be much more efficient with your time. Instead of dedicating set periods of time to go to the gym and walk on boring 'get you nowhere' treadmill. You can simply walk around more, build your steps and confidently know your burning calories.

Pedometers aren't sufficient for tracking certain activities like bike exercise. In this case, I attach the pedometer to my ankle and get a rough step count for set time. I then tailor this reading for future activity. Sometimes you might have to guesstimate.

Pedometers are useful but not 100% accurate. However, they do give you a constant gauge to work from. And, therefore prove useful at building the habit of moving more often.

A great place to start with any fat loss is 10, 000 steps per day.

I use an Apple Watch. However, there are many other great pedometers available from Garmin and Fit Bit, etc.

THE TRAINING PROGRAMMES

Now you understand the main principles behind training, let's put it all together into a solid plan of action.

TRAINING OVERVIEW

I've created two full training programmes, one for fat loss and one for mass gain. The programmes are tailored according to skill level, from beginners to intermediate/advanced trainees.

You can access the training plans and other valuable resources over at **www.diabeticmuscleandfitness.com**

Each programme is based on a 16-week journey of strength and conditioning and includes everything from exercise choice to sets and reps. Workouts are broken up into blocks of training time, with one week of de-training in between to maximise recovery.

For those looking to go the extra mile…

There are a ton of training resources available on The Diabetic Muscle & Fitness members' site. They include workout plans, video tips, live webinars and much more. Visit www.diabeticmuscleandfitness.com for more details.

TRAINING STRUCTURE

The workout programme trains all three energy systems.

1.   **The creatine phosphate system**, which deals with high-intensity, short duration activity (generally lasting up to 10 seconds).

2.   **The glycolytic system**, which deals with moderate-intensity, moderate duration activity (up to a minute or so).

3.   **The Aerobic System**, which deals with lower-intensity, long duration activity.

Training all three energy systems stimulates every muscle fibre type, strengthens the cardiovascular system, fortifies connective tissues and improves bone density.

In layman's terms, your training plan will be grounded on:

1. Heavy compound exercises (1-5 rep range).
2. Some higher-rep pump work (6-20 rep range).
3. Finishing moves that generate a lot of blood and get your heart pounding. This includes everything from drop sets to supersets to giant sets. Individuals looking to lose fat may need to perform increasingly more cardiovascular exercise than those looking to gain mass.

WORKOUT FREQUENCY

Workouts will be segmented into a mix of upper, lower and whole body training days. This style of training is incredibly time effective, allowing you to hit different muscle groups and movements with increased frequency. It is brutally effective if training volume and fatigue are managed correctly.

Beginners will initially work on a four-day training split and progress to five days as they become more adapt.

Intermediates will train five days per week.

Professional athletes or trainees need to contact me personally at **hello@diabeticmuscleandfitness.com**

GETTING STARTED

Before you get started take some time to run through the following checklist.

STEP 1. ESTABLISH WHICH TRAINING PROGRAMME SUITS YOU BEST.

CHOOSE YOUR SKILL LEVEL

Are You A Beginner?

- Minimal-to-no training experience.
- Can dedicate four days per week to training.
- May need the assistance of a qualified trainer to take you through the first few workouts.

Coaching Point:

- Beginners need less variation in the lifts in order to master the movements.
- Beginners initially get incredible results from a minimal amount of work. This plateaus as training age increases.

Are You Intermediate/Advanced?

- At least 3-5+ years training experience.
- Can demonstrate sound technique in all the key compound lifts.
- Can lift at least double their body weight in all key compound lifts.
- Respect and conduct regular mobility work.

Coaching Point:

- Intermediates need to work harder to get results than beginners.

STEP 2. CHOOSE A GYM

Your training environment is extremely important and plays a huge role in your ability to adhere to your training programme over the long haul.

I've designed the programmes in such a way to include all the basic machinery and tools most gyms should have. But in reality remember you will get so much more out of free and bodyweight training over fancy machines anyway.

Other questions you need to ask yourself:

Q. What are the staff like – are they helpful and engaging or do they just take your money?

Building relationships and relatedness is a huge factor when it comes to acquiring and keeping motivation. Friendly and helpful gym staff are a great asset to your fitness efforts. They can provide positive criticism and a helping hand on big lifts when you most need it.

Q. What are the members like? Do you feel intimidated?

Sometimes an intimidating environment can work in your favour and motivate you to work harder. Other times it can hold you back. It all depends on the type of people around you.

I recall the first time I went to my local bodybuilding gym. The sounds made by a few of the guys who were training made me fear for my life. I didn't quite know how to take it; part of me was trying not to laugh; part of me was shitting myself! The last thing I wanted was being shouted at for being weak, fat and diabetic.

For the first few weeks, I stuck to the recumbent bike in the cardio room. It was boring. Deep down I knew I was pedalling nowhere (literally).

Eventually, I said 'f**k!' it and plucked up the courage to go in.

I put on my best pigeon chest, spread my arms, and marched in like a TV deliveryman. I wasn't long until I tired out and got a reality check that I wasn't in shape.

A few weeks later I began to thoroughly enjoy training. Being in an environment with people stronger than me, drove me to do better.

Hand on heart, I would not have been as driven if I had trained in a commercial gym loaded with fanny packs and selfie-obsessed posers who spend more time in the changing room mirror than in the weights room lifting.

Never judge a book by its cover. You'll be surprised just how many experienced trainers are willing to help you out or give you a spot.

Of course, there was always the odd idiot but needless to say, once I got a taste of the alpha male environment I wasn't going to go back to the recumbent bike any time soon. The good guys outweighed the bad.

There will be gyms you'll train in where the crowd just isn't right. The best piece of advice I can give is, give it a chance and if it doesn't work - move!

The gym is your escape from the real world – you need strong positive people around you.

Q. Is the gym tidy?

Who wants to train in a dirty untidy and unmaintained gym? No one. If you train in a dirty gym then tell the manager. That's what you pay your membership for.

Q.   Is the gym easy to get to?

If the gym takes an hour or more to get to everyday you may need to weigh up your options and see if there is anywhere closer. Dedicating a lot of time to travel to and from the gym can soon wreak havoc with work and your personal life.

PRE-EXERCISE WARM-UP STRATEGY

Warming up is preparing your body to train. Think of it like taking a test drive. It is the transition from everyday job to gym. It is the best time to work on areas that are inhibiting movement and also prime your brain on the technicalities of certain exercises.

Sometimes you'll need more; sometimes you'll need less. It all depends on what you've been doing that day and what you plan to do over the next hour or so.

I've outlined below a very generalised warm-up protocol for the everyday working person who sits too much and spends hours in front of a screen hunched over. This warm-up strategy applies to all skills of trainee.

WARM-UP PROTOCOL

An effective pre-training warm up routine should ramp up your heart rate, free up tight, pesky tissue and prime the muscles for action.

STEP 1 – PREP THE ENTIRE SYSTEM

The first stage of any warm-up is to prime the entire system. We want to increase blood flow, raise body temperature and activate your fight or flight mechanisms to increase mental focus.

There are a host of different exercises and manoeuvres you can perform. The ones I've found most beneficial include:

- Med ball slams.
- Jumping jacks.
- High knee walks.
- Lunge with press.

Perform 3-5 sets for 10-20 reps of each with around 1-2 minutes rest in between sets.

STEP 2 – FOCUSED MOBILITY

Focused mobility aims to address tightness and limited range of motion in specific areas. You will need the following tools to get the job done.
- A good foam roller.
- Lacrosse ball.
- Red resistance band (lightest version).

These tools aren't expensive and can be picked up at any good sports store or online retailer.

The most common areas that tend to be jacked-up include:
- T-spine (upper–middle back)
- Hips
- Ankle
- Shoulders
- Pectorals
- IT Band (outer thigh)
- Glutes

As with Step 1, there are 101 different moves for each body part. It's simply a matter of finding out what works best for you through trial and error. Here is a list of my favourite go-to moves. Choose 1 or 2 moves and don't focus on reps; instead look to improve your range of motion until you're satisfied you've achieved this.

Area	Exercise
T- Spine	• T-Spine rotations • Back extensions on the foam roller
Hip	• Lying hip rotations
Ankle	• Knee-to-wall touches • Ankle rocks and circles • Foam roll both calves individually
Shoulders	• Scapula wall slides • Band pull aparts • Banded dislocations • Lying single-arm windmills
Pectorals	• Pec smash with a spikey mobility ball
Glutes	• Roll tight spots on lacrosse ball.
Iliotibial Band (IT Band)	• Foam rolling

WHY AM I SO SORE?

If it's your first time doing mobility work, it is inevitable you will be subject to some discomfort with tight muscle groups. There could be a number of reasons behind your tightness, but in most cases it's down to overuse.

When you start incorporating mobility work into your training, this pain and tightness has a much better chance of subsiding than if you just leave it alone. Tender spots and underlying tightness in certain muscles will prevent you from moving freely, hinder your exercise experience and possibly increase your risk of injury.

STEP 3 – DYNAMIC MOVES

I incorporate these to activate inhibited muscle groups, most notably the core and glutes, two extremely important muscle groups that play a major role in force production. My go-to moves include:

- Glute bridges.
- Banded X walks.
- Planks.
- Bird Dogs.
- Standing walkout.

Perform 3 sets of 1 or 2 moves for 10-15 reps each.

WHAT ABOUT STRETCHING?

I'm not a big fan of performing too many stretches prior to training. In my opinion they are best used outside of training to reduce tension in over-facilitated muscles. I've outlined the key areas I like to stretch along with my favourite go to moves.

Area	Stretch
Pecs	• Basic door frame stretch
Lats	• Banded lat stretch
Calves	• Step stretch • Basic wall stretch
Hip Flexor	• Banded hip flexor stretch
Adductors	• Butterfly stretch
Glutes	• Pretzel stretch

Perform 3 sets of 30-45 seconds per stretch. Perform 3-5 sets for 10-20 reps of each with around 1-2 minutes rest in between sets.

OTHER RECOVERY STRATEGIES

I've found the following strategies and treatments highly effective in recovery and regeneration.

- Deep tissue massage.
- ART (Active Release Therapy).
- Acupuncture.
- Epsom salts bath.

More Is Better, Right?

When it comes to mobility work, enough is enough; you can overdo it and waste precious training time.

As already discussed in this chapter, mobility is of paramount importance. It not only encourages us to move with integrity, but also allows us to load the muscles safely through a full range of motion – meaning greater stimulation and better muscle and strength gains.

UNDERSTANDING THE WORKOUTS

In order to get the most out of your training you must understand the structure and layouts of the workouts.

I've highlighted some of the key elements below.

EXERCISE GROUPING

Your exercises are listed in groups. Each specific group of exercises is labelled with a letter, for example A.

The number of exercises in a specific group will be listed after the group letter.

For example, A1, B1, C1 would denote 1 exercise for each group.

Whereas A1, A2, A3 would symbolise three exercises in Group A. These exercises are performed in this exact order with designated rest times between each.

Multiple exercises within one group are often termed supersets or giant sets due to the fact they are combined together.

EXERCISE SELECTION AND DISTRIBUTION

Generally speaking, exercise selection depends on skill level, individual anatomy, previous injury and the equipment you have available.

I've tailored each programme specifically to skill level, with simplified and more advanced exercise variations for the five basic human movements we discussed previously: squat, push, pull, hip hinge and carry/lift.

TEMPO

Tempo defines the speed of the rep. If you're a beginner, feel free to ignore this and simply focus on training the movement in a controlled fashion.

Tempo is typically written like this 2/1/X/1, which means:

2 – 2 seconds on the lowering phase.
1- 1 second pause at the midpoint of the rep.
X- Perform the positive part of the rep as quickly as possible.
1 – 1 second rest at the end of the movement.

Then repeat.

This example rep should take four seconds to complete.

REST PERIODS

The rest periods for each exercise are outlined in your programme. Rest periods are longer for compound exercises compared to smaller isolation exercises because they are more stressful on the system.

Rest times between grouped exercises like supersets are shorter for both a desired training effect and efficiency.

FAQS

Q.   How many sets do I need to do?

The number of working sets is outlined in the set training programmes. Note these are full effort work sets. Feel free to perform a number of lighter warm-up sets prior to the work sets to prime your brain and body with the movement.

Q. How much weight do I need to lift?

How much you lift will be depend on your current level of physical strength and fitness. There are no set weights to life, simply ensure you are lifting as heavy as possible for in and around the prescribed number of reps.

If you fall short, it's too heavy. If you complete the set with ease, you've gone too light. Find the sweet spot.

Q. Do I need to go to failure on every set?

Not always, especially on the days when you feel tired and drained. Remember, progressive overload is the name of the game. Do your best to shift more weight from workout-to-workout – not just on one lift but across the whole session.

Exercise Volume = Sets x Reps x Load

Extra volume could be in the form of an extra rep, or even an extra 1 kg (2.2 lbs) on the bar.

If you find yourself lifting less, you may be under-recovered and need to back off training effort. Resort to the auto-regulation scale I talked about in the training principles section.

You could also be under-fed, dehydrated or stressed out. Make sure diet, sleep and glycemic control are kept in check

Q. Do I have to warm up before every training session?

No, if you feel ready to rock the minute you walk into the gym – go for it!

However, if you skip mobility and warm-up work just to save time, you may not be training at your full potential.

THE MODERN FITNESS PROFESSIONAL - TRAINING CLIENTS WITH DIABETES

Personal trainers can play a massive role in promoting health. They can also play a considerable role in the management and prevention of certain lifestyle-controlled health issues, especially obesity and T2.

A fitness professional should be capable of the following health promotion roles:

- Educating and empowering the client on the benefits of exercise.
- Coaching safe exercise technique.
- Prescribing well-structured exercise and physical activity regimes.
- Promoting healthy lifestyle change relating to diet, sleep, and stress management.
- Working collectively with other healthcare professionals, especially if there is an underlying health concern or pre-existing injury.
- Being conscious of their abilities, knowledge and scope of practice and not giving advice beyond this, and using the expertise of others where needed.

This particular section of the text will discuss the role of modern fitness professionals, or personal trainers. I want to tackle this from two angles. Firstly, from the perspective of someone living with diabetes, what makes a great trainer? Secondly, from the perspective of a coach, how do you safely and effectively coach someone living with diabetes?

HIGHLY ACTIVE PEOPLE LIVING WITH DIABETES ARE FAR LESS LIKELY TO SUFFER A CARDIOVASCULAR EVENT, WHICH IS THE MOST COMMON CAUSE OF MORTALITY IN DIABETES, COMPARED TO SEDENTARY INDIVIDUALS. (46,47)

FIRST THINGS FIRST,

WHAT MAKES A GREAT PERSONAL TRAINER?

Today's fitness industry is saturated with uneducated, over-confident, non self-aware and irresponsible trainers who have little passion for evidence-based practice, the science behind it and helping others. Their passions rarely extend beyond lining their own pockets.

When looking to hire a personal trainer, it's important to separate the wheat from the chaff. A true fitness professional will possess the following qualities, which are a rarity nowadays.

- Respect their scope of practice - refer out and ask what to do when they lack knowledge or experience in a particular area.
- Be dedicated to lifelong mastery of their trade. They'll regularly attend seminars, workshops and undergo mentorships etc.
- Talk with evidence, and in context. Never in absolutes. Typically, this involves responding to most questions with, 'It depends...'
- Measure data and adjust accordingly.
- Listen attentively.
- Educate and empower the client – give them the 'why' to everything they do.
- Motivate and encourage.
- Demonstrate they are capable of getting results – look for proof, including prior testimonials and case studies etc.
- Be willing to work as part of a team (especially a clinical health team).

PERSONAL TRAINING A CLIENT WITH DIABETES

When it comes to coaching people with diabetes, a personal trainer's role is limited. The only exception to this would be trainers who have undergone the necessary education and qualifications specific to the condition they are dealing with.

The majority of trainers nowadays possess a basic level of knowledge regarding exercise and human physiology. This excludes elements of clinical nutrition, diabetes medication, endocrinology, interpretation of diabetes diagnostic measures and psychology, all of which are important in diabetes management.

Not every trainer will be a walking encyclopaedia. This is also the same for most experts working in diabetes, However, each and every personal trainer has a responsibility to ground their coaching on solid principles that prioritise the health and wellbeing of their clients, especially those suffering from diabetes.

GENERAL COACHING PRINCIPLES FOR PEOPLE LIVING WITH DIABETES

As previously discussed, lifestyle improvements, paying particularly attention to diet and physical activity are important in the control of blood glucose for all types of diabetes. They also reduce the risk of short and longer-term diabetes-related health complications.

However, poorly controlled diabetes, its complications and lack of understanding of how to exercise properly, are huge barriers to exercise participation for many people.

A personal trainer can play a key role in the promotion of exercise through guided instruction and a basic understanding/awareness of how the diabetic body responds to different forms of exercise. Depending on their level of qualification, they may also be solicited to offer dietary advice, however this should always be approved by the client's health professional team. In no circumstances should a personal trainer make suggestions about a client's medication unless they are fully qualified and insured to do so.

GYM ETIQUETTE

Be mindful of how you communicate to clients suffering from diabetes.

Bearing in mind diabetes is one of the most patronised diseases you will come across. Your client won't appreciate jokes about eating sweets and sugar, which are often cracked by family members and friends. The last thing they need is a mentor joking and making fun of their condition.

Also, the term 'diabetic' is not widely regarded as appropriate, especially in the United States. Refer to your clients as people living with diabetes. This is a much more subtle way of communicating their identity, rather than branding them as a diseased 'diabetic'. I personally hate being called diabetic.

When working with the younger generation, choose language appropriately. Critically, avoid language that implies 'overweight' or in any way discusses unacceptable body shape or size. Emphasise getting health, managing blood glucose, fuelling performance and training appropriately.

THE ADVICE YOU GIVE AS A PERSONAL TRAINER BOILS DOWN TO THE LEVEL AND EXTENT OF YOUR QUALIFICATIONS.

In order to provide the safest and most effective coaching to clients with diabetes, a fitness professional must understand and respect the following issues. Some of the physiological aspects have already been discussed in depth, so please refer back to the respected chapters for more detail.

1.   **Energy Systems and Fuel Metabolism During Physical Activity/Exercise**

People living with diabetes have a reduced ability to match glucose production with glucose utilisation and, as such, may need to adjust medication to accommodate. Blood glucose levels can change during and after physical activity or exercise. These changes are largely dependent on the type of exercise conducted.

Low-level physical activities, such as arm chair aerobics or slow lazy walking will burn energy. However, its effect on blood glucose will be minimal. Moderate level activity such as brisk walking and light jogging and cycling has a greater potential to lower blood glucose and cause hypoglycaemia (depending on how diabetes is treated).

High Intensity exercise, such as weight training or interval training, may result in transient hyperglycaemia because the liver (hepatic) glucose output tends to exceed muscular glucose uptake, particularly post-exercise.

Consequently, the two main problems with exercise and diabetes are hypoglycaemia (low blood glucose) and hyperglycaemia (high blood glucose). However, specific alterations to medication and diet can be made to offset these problems.

2.   Blood Glucose Monitoring

Use of self or continuous blood glucose monitoring is essential, especially for clients using insulin. This allows the client to accurately adjust their diet, insulin dose and other medications in response to training sessions.

Blood glucose management can also be reviewed by asking to see a client's blood glucose test results. After starting an exercise programme, you'll be able to see if their control has been on average good or bad. Simply take the meter and look at the average results over the last few days or set time period since starting.

If low blood glucose or hypoglycaemia is reported frequently there is a high probability that the client may be overeating calories to treat their condition. This may have implications for fat loss and body weight management, which may be of concern in weight-restricted sport.

If hyperglycaemia is reported frequently, it could suggest impairments in the client's recovery and performance. Recall hyperglycaemia is a catabolic condition that increases muscle protein breakdown and promotes dehydration, a key limiting factor in exercise performance.

Long-term hyperglycaemia has been linked to joint stiffness, foot problems, amputation and muscular weakness, all of which will affect individual exercise prescriptions.

3.   Acknowledge different elements of the client's health care team.

Firstly, obtain a client's permission to contact members of his or her team. Introduce yourself and relay feedback relevant to their diabetes control, body composition change and other factors, such as illness and injury rehab.

4. Respect Your Scope of Practice.

There is a clear line that separates a personal trainer from others working outside their scope of practice. Unfortunately, many personal trainers are naïve and take on more than they can chew. This can be due to ignorance or in many cases a passion to self-experiment and help others.

Refrain from advising clients on topics you are not qualified to work with, including (but not limited to) diet, medication, depression and other underlying health complications/injuries.

5. Question Everything.

The quality of your coaching service boils down to the quality of questions you ask before, during and after your client begins works with you. Here's an example of key questions worth asking:

PRE-COACHING ASSESSMENT

The first consultation with your client is extremely important. It gives you a background check of who they are and what they've been doing on average with their lifestyle before coming to work with you.

Ask about the following factors:

DIABETES HISTORY

Q. What type of diabetes do you have?
Q. Do you have the contact details of your diabetes team, and would you grant me permission to speak to them (outline your intentions and approach then ask for a critique and key pointers)?
Q. How well have you managed your condition? (HbA1C is a good reflection of the last 3-4 months' control)
Q. Have you had any complications with your diabetes? (If so refer out).

Consider the following factors before training someone with diabetes:

- People living with poorly controlled diabetes are at risk of muscle atrophy, impaired muscle mass development and reductions in muscular strength (48).

Be cautious with people with advanced disease complications, including:

- Blood pressure: Avoid isometric muscle contractions (loaded exercises where the muscle fibres don't change in length).

- Neuropathy: Be mindful of loading the feet, especially if there are reports of nerve damage or ulcerations.

- Retinal Disease: Complex exercises like squatting and clean and jerk may be problematic. Also be mindful of equipment lying on the gym floor that can be easily tripped over. As fatigue builds, concentration can decline, increasing injury risk.

Take care to properly medically screen these individuals before recommending any exercise programme. Consider graded exercise stress testing before initiating any new vigorous exercise programme.

- People living with diabetes are far more susceptible to overuse injures and impaired mobility because of structural changes that occur in their joints as a result of long term hyperglycemia, abnormal glycation and oxidative stress. These problems can be alleviated by improving blood glucose control and by auto-regulating/periodising training with easy, hard and rest days.

- Ask for a client's permission to test their blood glucose if they collapse and go unconscious. If you don't know how to take a reading, ask them to show you it. Depending on this result, this may sanction this use of glucagon during episodes of severe hypoglycemia. You should also be aware of how to use this prescription drug in times of emergency.

HEALTH

Q. How is your sleep?
Q. Are you taking any other medications?
Q. Other illnesses or injuries that I need to be aware of?
Q. Are you currently going through a period of emotional stress?

NUTRITION

Q. What has your diet been like over the last six months on average?
Q. Have you ever tracked calories or macronutrients? (if so, what?).
Q. Food intolerance, allergies?
Q. Food dislikes?

BODY COMPOSITION

Q. How has your body weight changed over the last six months or has it remained constant?

Q. How active are you during the day (job details)?

GENERAL COACHING

Q. Have you worked with a coach before. If so, how did it work? If not, why not? What didn't you like?

DURING COACHING ASSESSMENTS

The coaching period is a key time to assess the effectiveness of your exercise programme and whether the client has been able to stick to it.

Ask the following:

Q. Did you stick to the programme? If not, why not?

Q. Are you in pain?

Q. Did you enjoy it?

Before you make any adjustments to a client's programme, you must first score their adherence. If they haven't stuck to the programme, what's the point in changing anything? The variables you originally prescribed need time to take effect.

If they are constantly failing to adhere, you might need to readdress your approach or question their level of motivation.

Look for the following symptoms when training people with diabetes. Cease exercise if symptoms worsen or remain unresolved.

- Typical symptoms of hypo and hyperglycaemia.
- Lack of energy.
- Pins and needles in the hands and feet.
- Dizziness or light headiness.
- Pain or discomfort in the chest, neck, jaw, arms or other areas linked to cardiovascular problems.
- Heart palpitations (learn to differentiate from stimulant-induced anxiety).
- Severe muscle cramps.
- Extreme thirst.

All of these symptoms will jeopardise a client's exercise experience and increase the potential for injury. Try your best to identify the problem by assessing the following general factors

- Blood glucose behaviour across the day and during training.
- Biomechanical issues that arise from previous injuries, muscular imbalances, poor foot wear and poor exercise technique (maybe self-taught or taught by a previous coach).
- Physical activity levels across the day.
- Stress – are they anxious about something and not present during the training session.
- Food and fluid intake prior to training – have they missed meals or fluid?
- Sleep – are they sleep deprived?
- Caffeine intake - in the form of coffee, tea, or pre-workout sports supplements.

If you can't pinpoint a problem based on the above, refer to a health professional for additional tests.

HYPOGLYCAEMIA UNAWARENESS

One of the best risk indicators for hypoglycemia is personal experience. However, if an individual has a history of frequent hypoglycaemia then hypoglycemia-associated autonomic unawareness may be an issue, especially in those suffering from T1. The more frequent occurrences of hypoglycaemia, the greater the chance hypoglycemia may go unnoticed until blood glucose reaches dangerously low levels. This is a result of defects in glucose counter-regulation that reduces the production of key stress hormones (epinephrine and norepinephrine) in response to falling blood glucose levels.

Fortunately, asking the client to check their blood glucose levels during an exercise session is made easy with a self-monitoring blood glucose test or use of a continuous blood glucose monitor. Hypoglycemia can be prevented with adjustments to insulin dose and food intake during and following intake.

Test the client's blood glucose levels more frequently when engaging in new activities or exercise modalities.

OTHER KEY NOTES

- It takes at least two hours for most fast-acting insulin analogs to clear the bloodstream. If a client has injected to treat high blood glucose (14mmol/L or 250mg/dL) pre-exercise, they must wait until the insulin takes effect before taking more.

- Encourage the client to monitor their blood glucose levels for several hours post-training. This will help detect delayed-onset hypoglycemia from exercise, especially during the night.

- Depending on the client's dietary goals, consuming a carbohydrate-based meal or snack within one hour post-training can help prevent hypoglycemia, restore muscle glycogen and kick-start muscle protein synthesis.

TREATING SEVERE HYPOGLYCEMIA

You must treat severe low blood glucose differently from how you would treat normal low blood glucose. There is a high probability the individual will be unconscious, and unable to concisely swallow food or drink. Trying to treat the problem by jamming food or drink into the mouth is not advised and may result in you suffocating the individual or having your fingers bitten off.

First of all, you must ascertain what the client's blood glucose level is and determine whether or not it is actually a true case of severe hypoglycemia. Blood glucose can easily be tested by looking at a client's CGM or by taking a finger prick sample. It's good practice to obtain a client's permission to do this if such conditions arise. This should be discussed in your pre-training consultation.

If the client's blood glucose reading denotes a severe hypo you have two options: administer an injection of glucagon or ring the emergency services.

Glucagon, as discussed in the diabetes medication section is a prescription drug people using insulin should carry as a safety precaution. Glucagon is usually kept in a bag, or the car, rather than carried in a pocket like an insulin pen since it's used only in extreme circumstances. I highly recommend you ask your clients who use insulin to bring it with them to training sessions and carry it afterwards just in case. Also make sure they carry a medical identification tag, especially if they have a busy day of work post-exercise.

Most glucagon kits contain pre-filled syringes, a small vial of glucagon in powder form and set instructions. The instructions are usually in pictographs and are fairly self-explanatory.

However, administering glucagon may be difficult especially if it's in a stressful gym environment or your first time.

The general procedure for administering glucagon is as follows:

1. Call an ambulance.
2. Pull the plastic cap of the glucagon vial.
3. Inject all the fluid (water) into the vial.
4. Remove syringe from the vial whilst ensuring no air escapes from the vial.
5. Swirl and dissolve the powder entirely.
6. Hold the vial upside down then reinsert the tip of the needle into the vial via the rubber stopper.
7. Don't put the needle the whole way in and draw in air.
8. Draw the fluid back into the syringe based on the instructions. A smaller amount may be needed for children aged 6 to 12 years old.
9. Use an alcohol swab or sterile wipe on the skin (if possible)
10. Insert the needle as per the instructions into the thigh, glutes or shoulder.
11. Inject the entire contents of the syringe.
12. Put the client into the recovery position and wait for the emergency services.

The client should regain consciousness 10-25 minutes after the injected dose of glucagon. After things have returned to normal, ask to speak to the client's healthcare team and identify what went wrong to prevent it from happening again.

AFTER COACHING

After finishing with a client it's common courtesy, and the sign of a great coach to evaluate your service.

Ask for feedback.

Q. Was the client happy with the result? Did it meet or exceed their expectations?

Q. Are there any areas of your coaching that need to be improved?

On the last training session ask your client to score the following elements of your service out of ten:

- Level of accountability (was it enough?).
- Ability to motivate.
- Punctuality.
- Understanding – were the various approaches clearly explained?

Set a reminder to follow up on the client's progress after they finish their coaching period. I've found the three and six month marks to be ideal. Ask them how they've been, and whether or not they've sustained the lifestyle, diet and training principles you taught them. Progress photos will tell you a lot. Clients always appreciate a follow-up. It shows you care and brings more trust and value to your relationship, which increases the potential for recurring business.

CAN WE TRUST PROFESSIONAL EXERCISE GUIDANCE?

The harsh reality is not many medical professionals know how to prescribe exercise. I'm not saying medical professionals are useless when it comes to diabetic fitness management. Their role is essential, especially when it comes to diagnosis, evaluation of blood work during treatment and prescription of necessary medication. However, they are unlikely to have had the required training to make effective exercise prescriptions and therefore, as we discuss below, it may be a good idea to start an exercise programme with the assistance of an exercise professional alongside the backing of your diabetes management team.

Appropriate exercise remains significantly under-prescribed for people living with diabetes. Prescription of exercise is highly specific and requires expert advice. This is especially true given the sheer amount of exercise options available today.

The same goes for nutrition. Dietary requirements should be adjusted for individuals pursing different exercise goals, and volume. This requires the advice of a qualified clinical and sports nutritionist.

THE FITNESS TRAINER

The common fitness professional may be extremely versed on 'how to' exercise but be ignorant about the management of diabetes around exercise.

Synergy Between Fitness and Medical Professionals. The fitness trainer and medical professional must work in unison to promote the most effective exercise strategy for their diabetic clients.

Each person's exercise regime should be modified according to his/her habitual physical activity, physical function, health status, exercise responses and stated goals (49). This requires the expertise of both parties.

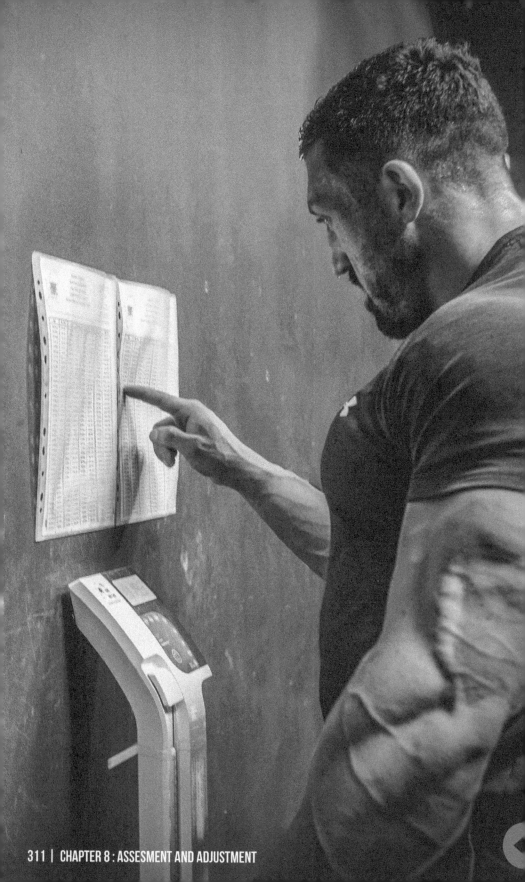

CHAPTER 8: ASSESMENT AND ADJUSTMENT

"If you don't know where you are headed, you'll probably end up someplace else." -
Douglas J. Eder, Ph.D

1. **DIETARY AND TRAINING ADJUSTMENTS ARE NECESSARY BECAUSE ENERGY NEEDS CHANGE AS WE PROGRESS.**

2. **TRAINING ADJUSTMENTS ARE NECESSARY, AS YOU CAN GET TIRED.**

3. **LOGGING THE RIGHT DATA CAN PROVE INVALUABLE TO YOUR ONGOING PROGRESS. LOG OBJECTIVE MEASURES, SUCH AS BODY WEIGHT, ADHERENCE TO DIET, WHICH CAN BE INTER-CONNECTED WITH SUBJECTIVE MEASURES, SUCH AS BLOOD SUGAR CONTROL, MOOD, HUNGER AND ENERGY.**

4. **YOU MUST BE PATIENT BEFORE MAKING ANY DIET OR TRAINING CHANGES. THIS INVOLVES TAKING TIME TO COLLECT AND EVALUATE YOUR MEASURES.**

5. **WHETHER YOUR GOAL IS TO INCREASE MUSCLE MASS OR LOSE BODY FAT, IT IS IMPORTANT TO KEEP BLOOD GLUCOSE LEVELS IN CONTROL.**

Now that you have a solid plan of action to follow it's important to back this up with regular assessment and evaluation. This chapter will teach you everything you need to know about evaluating and adjusting your approach, whether your goal is to lose fat or pack on serious muscle mass.

WHY MEASURE?

The human body is an extremely smart and adaptive organism and consequently a training plateau is inevitable. In fact, it is just around the corner. The rate at which adaption or plateau occurs will vary from person to person.

Your fat loss, muscle gain and performance are all subject to plateau. If you want to get the most out of your time, effort and hard earned cash you must measure consistently and adjust things as needed.

The process of measurement and adjustment will either make or break your progress.

Tracking anything is better than nothing.

ALWAYS LOOK FOR THE DISCONNECT

ACCOUNTABILITY

Accountability from an experienced coach, close friend or family member can prove invaluable when it comes to tracking progress.

It's important that this feedback is honest and open. Being told you look great out of fear of causing offence serves no benefit and gives a false sense of progress that will eventually be shattered when you're told the truth.

Positive comments are evidence your approach is working – take note and keep going. Negative comments are evidence that work still has to be done or your approach isn't working well and needs to be changed. Don't take it personally; use it as feedback to fuel your efforts.

Other feedback from people you haven't seen in a while can also prove valuable – especially when you shock them with noticeable physical changes.

Set up some form of accountability measure. Ideally, every fortnight as this gives you a fair chance to test your approach.

Social media blogging is a great way to get accountable. You'll often find your efforts will inspire other people.

THE WRONG REASONS FOR ADJUSTING

Before I discuss the various measures you need to take, lets take a quick look at some of the biggest reasons most people screw up their adjustments.

How many can you relate to?

- They don't see progress quickly enough.
- The scales remain the same.
- They compare themselves to others (usually on social media).
- They adjust when they hear of someone else doing something.
- They adjust when they miss a workout or meal – usually throwing the head up and getting up.

The reality is most people adjust for the sake of it, with no clear reason why. This disorientated approach often leads to burnout and dietary failure. Furthermore, it makes it that bit harder to get started again.

Unless you're a competitive athlete looking to make a particular weight class you must be slow, diligent and tactful in your adjustments.

ASSESSMENTS PROVIDE US WITH A SERIES OF INTER CONNECTED TRUTHS.

The sum of these truths gives reason for adjusting. Resist the temptation to go by one measure alone.

WHAT TO TRACK?

Measurements can be divided into objective and subjective measures. I've outlined a list of the key measures you can take along with specific action points.

1.   Compliance

In order to assess the effectiveness of your approach, you must be able to honestly review your adherence to the diet and training plan.

If your measures show zero progress from the previous check, yet you've missed workouts and overeaten on a few occasions, do you think it's fair to say the variables didn't work or you didn't give them a chance?

The odd mishap isn't a problem, but regular reoccurring mistakes pose a problem and highlight your level of focus and commitment isn't where it needs to be.

If you do mess up, start afresh and wait until you've had a good two weeks to reassess.

2.   Bodyweight

1.   For fat loss, a loss of 0.5-1% body weight per week is a good aim.
2.   Daily weight fluctuations are normal.
3.   Look at average weight across the week instead of daily.

The health and fitness industry would have you believe the more weight you lose, the healthier and better looking you will become. This has led many people to have an unhealthy and somewhat obsessive relationship with the scales.

People looking to lose fat should focus on fat loss over weight loss. Weight loss is non-selective and includes everything from body fat, valuable muscle tissue right through to bone mineral content. This is the kind of scenario you want to avoid. The only exception to this is in the context of clinically obese individuals needing to drop weight fast for certain medical interventions.

On the contrary, individuals looking to gain body mass should focus their efforts on lean muscle gain. No one wants to add unsightly and unhealthy body fat.

The problem with relying on the scales is body weight tends to fluctuate day-to-day. This is perfectly normal yet it freaks people out. There are numerous reasons why body weight fluctuates. To name a few:

1. Bowel contents.
2. Fecal matter.
3. Gains in lean muscle mass.
4. Perspiration rate.
5. Water retention from injury, illness or certain medications.
6. Hormonal influence (female monthly cycle).

Daily fluctuations of 1-3 lbs are fairly common and place an obvious question mark above the validity of bodyweight as a single progress measure.

ACTION STEP: WEIGH DAILY AND AVERAGE YOUR BODYWEIGHT

Take your weight first thing every morning, naked, after the toilet and before eating.

To get the most accurate representation of how your body weight is changing, I get my clients to weigh daily, average their total body weights (across the week) and subtract from the week prior. This helps account for the daily fluctuations mentioned above and gives a valid representation of how their body has responded to their set calorie intake and level of physical exercise.

The difference in weight is then correlated with other measurements to determine a specific programme change or to carry on doing the same thing.

3.   The Mirror – Physical Appearance

1.   PHOTO IMAGES WORK BETTER THAN THE MIRROR.

2.   ENSURE PHOTOS ARE TAKEN IN THE SAME SPOT USING THE SAME LIGHTING.

3.   MIRRORS CAN BE DECEIVING AND AREN'T THE MOST RELIABLE WHEN USED ALONE.

Trust me when I say visual appearance trumps the credibility of any body composition measure tenfold. No one will come up and ask your body weight or skin fold stats. But they will look at you and make their mind up as to whether or not you're in shape.

Take time to assess yourself honestly before asking anyone else's opinion or subjecting yourself to the scales and other measures.

AM I LOOKING BETTER?

Look for progress. The signs could include anything from looser fitting clothes and more visible muscle definition to the emergence of new vascularity (veins) under the skin. Generally speaking, I've found first thing in the morning or post-training the best time to assess progress.

There will be times when you'll feel out of shape, bloated and uncomfortable. There are a huge number of factors that influence the way we look on a daily basis, including everything from dietary intake that day, sleep, travel, training, sweat rate right through to hydration. Anticipate some days you'll simply look better than others.

When you do capture yourself looking great, congratulate yourself, build self-esteem and even capture the moments on camera if you must – this is a great reference when you experience a bad mirror day.

You will only regress when you consciously go majorly off the diet for more than a few days, don't train, lack sleep and undergo poor blood sugar control. Simply don't expect to look your best during this time.

ACTION STEP: TAKE PHOTOS

I feel photos do a better job at showing progress than mirrors. Mirrors can be deceptive, depending on the glass they use or where they're located.

When taking photos, I keep to the following rules:

1. Photos are taken on the same day, every week/fortnight.
2. Photos are taken in the same location (usually marked with an x).
3. Photos are taken using the same camera setting, angle and backdrop.
4. Photos are unedited and raw (no Instagram filter).
5. Photo angles: front relaxed, side (hands on head, showing torso) and rear relaxed.
6. Males: wear shorts.
7. Females: wear shorts and sports bra.

You can also ask your coach or closest friends for their honest opinion on the photographs.

4. **Body Measurement**

GIRTH MEASURES ARE USEFUL FOR ASSESSING RATE OF BODY FAT CHANGE.

BODY COMPOSITION TESTING IS AN ESTIMATE, NOT A MEASURE.

DEXA OR RAW SKINFOLDS ARE THE MOST USEFUL.

The simplest, most convenient and cost-effective way to measure changes in body size over time is to measure the girth of certain body parts and assess how you feel in your everyday clothes.

To take measurements, you will require a high-quality body composition tape measure, which doesn't stretch. You can record measurements yourself or have someone take them for you. When recording, make sure the tape measure is not too tight or too loose, is lying flat on the skin, and is horizontal. In all circumstances, it is ideal if you can work off a landmark, like a freckle, tattoo or scar to allow for better accuracy.

ACTION STEP: MEASURE THE FOLLOWING

Waist Circumference – Take the measure two inches above the belly button. This is usually the narrowest part of the waist.

Most muscular individuals score as overweight/obese when assessed under the standard BMI chart and are therefore automatically considered higher risk even though they may be super lean and in a very good state of health.

If you are able to access a Dexa scan there is no need to assess girths.

if you want a cheaper, more convenient option than a Dexa scan opt for raw skinfold measures.

Skinfolds, although not as accurate as Dexa, are another convenient way to assess body composition. Always make sure someone experienced does the test. We are only interested in the actual mm measurement of the skinfold site – not the actual % body fat that can be calculated. The less processed the data the more accurate the findings.

It doesn't take a rocket scientist to work out, if you measure 30 mm on your umbilical site one week and 28 mm the next – you've lost body fat in that area.

"Measurement is the first step that leads to control and eventually to improvement. If you can't measure something, you can't understand it. If you can't understand it, you can't control it. If you can't control it, you can't improve it."
- H. James Harrington

5.   Performance

In an ideal world, your performance will improve from week to week, whether you're trying to lose fat or increase body mass. An increase in performance indicates that your recovery is on point.

All you need to track performance is a logbook and pen. Some people like to use their smartphone. However, this is more of a distraction given the temptation to dip into social media.

WHAT TO TRACK?

Track how the session went, note down your total volume shifted (weight x reps x sets) for each exercise and compare it to previous training sessions. You'll know if you have progressed or regressed.

You won't get stronger on a session–by-session basis. Plateaus are inevitable. Your main goal is to get stronger on a regular, trackable basis. A well-kept logbook allows you to identify plateaus and highlight the need to address specific issues that may be negatively affecting your recovery.

Hip - The hip girth should be measured naked or with minimal clothing at the level of the greatest protrusion of the buttocks. Stand upright,t with both feet evenly distributed on the floor and keep your glutes soft (unlocked).

Thigh – The measure is taken at the visually largest part of the upper thigh, which is usually high up on the leg. The measure is best taken in shorts. Note that the measuring tape will not be quite horizontal – it should be at 90 degrees to the line of the thigh.

CLOTHING

The feel of your clothes will tell you a great deal about your rate of body composition change. For those looking to lose fat, looser clothing is an obvious sign of fat loss, whereas for those looking to gain mass, clothing may appear tighter and more fitted, especially around the arms and chest.

ANTHROPOMETRIC MEASUREMENT

Anthropometry refers to the measurement of the human body. It typically involves measurement of body length, width, circumference (C), and skinfold thickness (SF) (50).

We've already touched on girths as one of the simplest methods.

WHAT ABOUT OTHER TECHNIQUES?

Numerous methods are currently being used by personal trainers, including Dexa scan, skin folds, Bod Pod and underwater weighing – but how useful are they?

That so many different types of assessments exist demonstrates none is entirely accurate. One important point to make about body composition analysis techniques is that there is no way of accurately measuring the quantity of body fat that any person is carrying other than by cutting their carcass up and weighing the tissue.

Of all the methods a Dexa scan is the most credible.

Most universities' sports science faculties have a Dexa Scan machine and charge anywhere between £20-£60 for an assessment. These scans can also prove useful when it comes to supporting diabetic life insurance in heavily muscled individuals.

Resist the temptation to adjust just because one measure is showing a lack of progress. You must correlate all the measures together and see the big picture.

I've put together two decision trees for fat loss and mass gain. These will highlight the need for you to adjust your approach. Once you've decided whether or not you need to make an adjustment from your original intake, follow the steps below on how to calculate the adjustment unique to each goal.

FOR FAT LOSS

1. IF WEIGHT ISN'T LOST QUICKLY ENOUGH, YOU NEED TO BURN OFF OR TAKE IN MORE FUEL.

2. IF WEIGHT IS LOST TOO QUICKLY, YOU'LL BE RISKING MUSCLE LOSS AND INCREASE THE CHANCES OF REBOUNDING.

3. SUGGESTED DEFICIT CHANGE VALUE: 200-300 KCAL/DAY, OR~5-10% OF TOTAL CALORIE INTAKE.

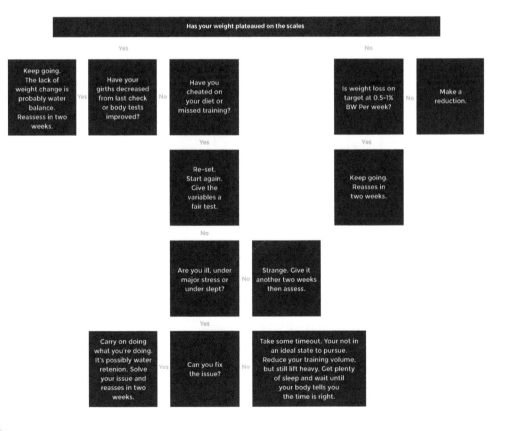

STEP-BY-STEP GUIDE

- Compare your average bodyweight from one week to the next.
- Note how much your weight changes on average across the weeks assessed.
- Beginners should initially take four weeks to assess their progress. The reason for this is simple: during the early stage of starting a diet there most likely will be a freak weight drop. Ignore this initial drop and use latter weeks for your assessment. If assessing over four weeks, you would rely initially on three weeks worth of data. After three weeks resort to every two weeks.
- More advanced dieters can assess every 1-2 weeks.
- Target weight loss is between 0.5-1.0% BW per week.

There are exceptions to the 0.5-1.0% BW drop, particularly in those competing in weight classed events.

Let's make this a little clearer with a practical example.

Take a beginner and advanced dieter who both weigh 220 lbs. The target weight drop of 0.5-1.0% BW/week would equate to 1.1-2.2 lbs per week.

If their diet and training are followed correctly their progress on the scales might look like this.

Fat Loss (Beginner) – 4-Week Overview				
DATE	WEEK 1	WEEK 2	WEEK 3	WEEK 4
Average Weight	220lbs	215lbs -5lbs	212lbs -3lbs	211lbs -1lbs

*Note the large weight drop between week 1 and week 2.

Q. Does this person need to make an adjustment?
A. No. If we ignore the first week and average the following three weeks of weight loss, the average drop is 1.3 lbs. This is perfectly in line with our target weight drop and justifies no need to change the approach.

Fat Loss (More Advanced) – 2-Week Overview				
DATE	WEEK 1	WEEK 2	WEEK 3	
Average Weight	220lbs	219lbs -1lbs	218lbs -1lbs	

*Note no extreme weight drop between first and second week, due to longer-term diet and training adherence.

Q. Does this person need to make an adjustment?

A. No. If we ignore the first week and average the following three weeks of weight loss the average drop is 1 lbs. This is perfectly in line with our target weight drop and justifies no need to change the approach.

WHAT KIND OF SCENARIO WOULD JUSTIFY A DIET ADJUSTMENT?

Provided you've gone through the process on the decision tree and failed to meet a weight drop target, you can justify a change. The severity of the adjustment will depend on how far off you are from the target, with minimal progress denoting a sharper adjustment.

HOW MUCH OF AN ADJUSTMENT DO I NEED TO MAKE?

As a general rule of thumb, I like I like to create a daily deficit of 5-10% from the total calorie intake. This can come from added exercise and/or a reduction in food intake; it is entirely up to you.

If you have spare time and love your food, added cardio may be the best option. If you aren't fussed about the cardio, take it from food. However, be mindful there is a fine balance between doing too much cardio and eating too little food.

Our 220 lbs example has stalled progress while consuming 2,800 kcals per day. A 5-10% deficit would equate to 2,660 kcal daily – 2,520 kcal or a 140-180 kcal reduction respectively. Applying the steeper deficit when further of from the target.

DEFICIT FROM DIET

1g of fat = 9 kcal, and 1g of carbohydrate = 4 kcal

I like to keep protein constant due to the fact it keeps hunger at bay. Therefore, I need to remove between 140-280 kcals from carbohydrate and fat. The proportion of which is entirely down to personal preference.

The quickest way to get this in motion is to adjust your calorie goal on the tracking software you use. Keeping animal protein portions the same whilst reducing fat or carbohydrate based foods

DEFICIT FROM CARDIO

I don't like spending any more than 50% of my time in the gym doing cardio. For example, if I were training for 5 hours per week in the gym – I wouldn't do more than 2.5 hours of cardio across the week.

You can also do a half and half mix of the two: it's entirely up to you. Conversely, if your rate of weight loss turns out higher than targeted, you would be wise to pull things back.

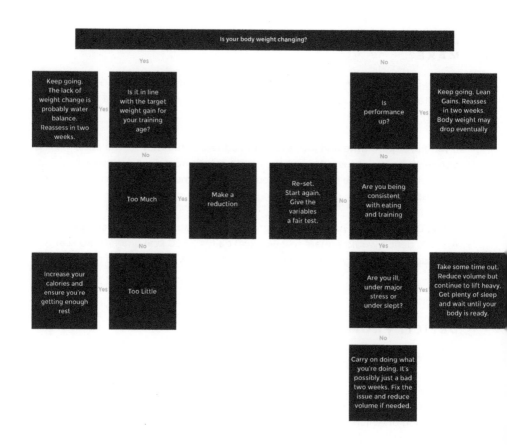

FOR HIGH QUALITY MASS GAIN

1. IF WEIGHT IS NOT GAINED QUICKLY ENOUGH, INCREASE CALORIE INTAKE.

2. IF WEIGHT IS GAINED TOO QUICKLY, YOU'LL HAVE PUT TOO MUCH FAT ON, SO DECREASE CALORIES.

3. SUGGESTED INCREMENTAL CHANGE VALUE: 100-200 KCAL/DAY, OR ~3-6% OF TOTAL CALORIE INTAKE.

I want to break this section into two different types of lifter, as each has their own unique targets in respect to mass gain.

BEGINNERS (NEWBIES)

- Zero training experience
- The first year of training is where you will get the greatest gains in body mass and strength.

INTERMEDIATE/ADVANCED TRAINERS

- 2.5+ years of training experience
- With every year of training, muscle growth will slow. You will need to work harder and longer to get results.

TARGETS

During a mass gain phase it's imperative that all gains are kept as lean as possible. From a diabetic perspective, excess body fat will prove unhealthy and unsightly.

Training Age	Weight Gain
Newbie	2-3 lbs
Intermediate	1-2 lbs
Advanced	0.25-0.5 lbs

KEY SIGNS YOU NEED TO ADJUST

There are a number of interconnected truths that will highlight the need for change.

An increase in performance, irrespective of changes in body weight signifies good recovery and muscle growth.

However, if you're not gaining weight according to the targets, you'll need to increase your calorie intake. On the contrary, if you're gaining too much weight above and beyond the targets, you may need to reduce your calorie intake.

HOW MUCH OF AN ADJUSTMENT DO I NEED TO MAKE?

As a general rule of thumb, I like I like to work an energy surplus up slowly at around 5-10% of total calorie intake daily

If we take an example client consuming 3,000 kcal daily, this would equate to 3,150-3,300 kcal daily. Aim for the higher value if you're well below the target.

WHERE DO THESE CALORIES COME FROM?

1g of fat = 9 kcal and 1g of carbohydrate = 4 kcal

Protein is most likely high enough and any further increase may fill you up too much and make it harder to eat other calories. In most cases, the extra calorie surplus could come from carbohydrate and/or fat. It really doesn't matter.

People with T1D should alter their medication strategy accordingly to accommodate the extra calories. The notion of weight gain is not applicable to those who are T2D, since their primary mode of treatment is usually weight loss.

A NOTE ON ALCOHOL

Alcohol does contain calories. However, they are useless from a body composition and performance perspective. However, if you wish to include a glass of wine or the odd beer as part of your calorie allowance, go ahead, just don't abuse it.

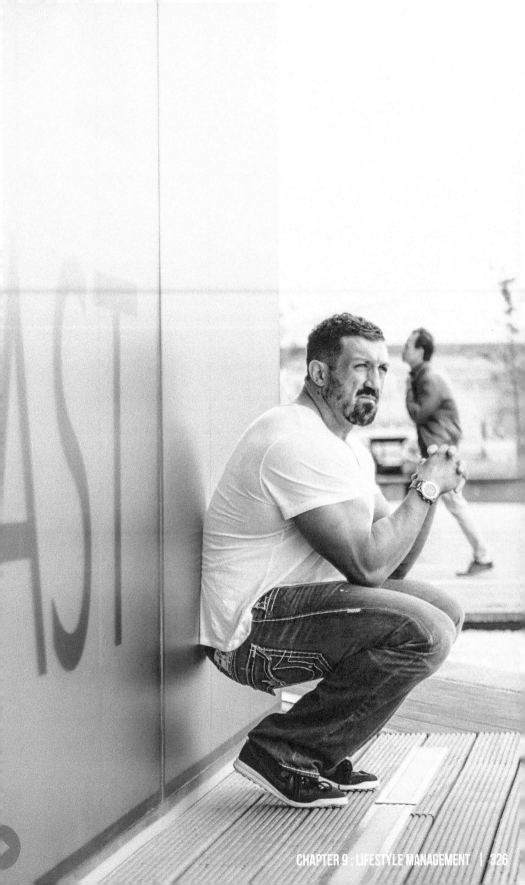

If you want to get the most out of your muscle building and fat loss efforts, you must be ultra-mindful of how you live your life.

Sleep and stress management are not only essential for health and wellness but also set the foundations for optimal physical performance and body composition change.

SLEEP

We all know what it feels like to lose out on sleep - you wake up the next morning feeling like you've had a night on the town. Your mind is slow, your body stiff and motivation at an all time low. No matter how many coffees, you just can't shake off that thick layer of fatigue that clouds your body and mind.

There's no doubt about it: sleep is essential.

However, many of us don't get enough. It's either too short or interrupted.

Research suggests that several nights of sleep restriction results in an increase in pain perception, decreased sociability, an increase in body discomfort and back/stomach pain.

Imagine the additional stress of weight training, day-to-day emotions and poorly controlled diabetes on top of all that.

Then take into account the increased use of smartphones, social media and drinking too much coffee and pre-workout just before bedtime and it becomes clear how sleep deprivation can become a real issue for many.

SLEEP DEPRIVATION WILL HAVE A SEVERE IMPACT ON YOUR HEALTH AND PROGRESS.

In this section, I want to provide some practical tips on how to optimise the quality of your sleep.

HOW MUCH SLEEP DO I NEED?

There is a myriad of evidence to support the value of a good night's sleep in promoting weight loss, mood state and sports performance.

Aim for 7-8 hours of deep, high-quality, uninterrupted sleep every night. If this isn't possible, try and accumulate any missing time through short naps.

ACTIVE AND STRESSED INDIVIDUALS NEED MORE SLEEP.

WHAT CAN I DO TO IMPROVE MY SLEEP?

Here are some of my favourite (anecdotal and evidence-based) tips to assist with sleep.

1. Research has shown greater REM sleep (deep sleep) occurs if you eat a high carbohydrate meal one hour before bedtime [51]. If trying this, ensure your medication is dosed accurately to avoid experiencing a hypoglycemia or hyperglycemia during the middle of the night. The meal must also be in line with overall calorie targets.

2. Limit stimulants before bedtime, most notably caffeine.

3. Avoid alcohol before bedtime. Research shows alcohol's fast metabolism leads to a decrease in REM sleep. Other possible consequences are tachycardia (rapid heart beat), headaches and a full bladder, which may increase nighttime toilet trips and interrupt sleep cycles. Limiting fluid consumption before bed might be a wise idea, unless you're thirsty.

4. Turn off all electrical devices (especially the ones with LED lights or displays) at least 1 hour before bedtime and try to sleep in a very dark room. Research has shown that over-exposure to artificial sources of light, especially at night-time can cause symptoms of depression and poor quality sleep [52].

5. Go to bed at the same time every night (or set an alarm).

6. Decrease body or room temperature before sleeping.

7. Invest in a high-quality mattress. It will do wonders for your mobiltiy.

8. Avoid watching horror or thriller movies; they can spike stress hormones such as adrenaline, which increase heart rate and mental alertness. Not an ideal situation before bed.

9. Some supplements have been shown to help induce sleep and improve sleep quality. Essential supplements for this purpose include L-Theanine, valerian, magnesium and melatonin. I talk more about this in the supplements section.

10. Use a hot water bottle – if you feel it helps.

STRESS MANAGEMENT

Nowadays we are under increasingly more stress. The bills keep pilling up and people can contact us whenever they want.

It can sometimes feel like there will never be enough hours in the day, and life is always going to be a demanding rush. The multiple demands on your time are extraordinary.

So I am here to tell you that you need to take extraordinary measures to meet your needs. Measures so far attached from the norm that others may question your sanity.

YOU HAVE MORE CONTROL OVER STRESS THAN YOU THINK.

Stress management is essential for health, blood sugar management and building a better body. No matter how stressful your life seems, there are a number of ways to relieve pressure and regain control.

Just thinking about it is a big step in the right direction. Awareness helps a lot!

Besides eating better, staying active and getting enough rest, I've outlined some highly effective ways you can manage your stress.

These tips are based on both my personal experience and from studying the behaviours of successful people.

GET AT LEAST 5 MINUTES OF QUIET TIME OR MEDIATION DAILY

Staying calm and acting cool doesn't come naturally to many of us, especially in today's hectic hustle and bustle world.

Ever notice how one bad event can shape your mood and interactions for the rest of the day?

Quiet time and meditation should come into your daily practice. At first, you'll laugh (I did). You'll conjure up all sorts of images and body shapes. I'm sure the first thing that comes to mind will be you doing a mantra pose on the shores of a beautiful lake or by a crystal blue tropical ocean on the other side of the world.

Of course, any activity outside our norm seems strange, and out of place. However, a week of mindfulness practice and quiet time to yourself will do you the world of good.

You will complain less, react less, and fill your life with what is most important and valuable to you. Investing in yourself first, pays huge dividends and sets you up in a far better position to help others.

WHERE TO START?

I don't suggest you go out and buy the biggest textbook on meditation or even look up the subject on the internet. You'll get overwhelmed and fail to start.

I am a big fan of guided meditations. It saves time and I'd rather have an experienced teacher talk me through the key essentials. It's far more efficient and gets you actively practising from the start.

If you don't fancy hiring a teacher, I recommend a great app called Headspace. I just put my headphones on and let myself become immersed in the calming sounds and guided story that follows. Check it out; it costs pennies to use, and they even offer a free trial.

At first, you'll find it hard to settle, but perfect-guided practice makes perfect. Ten minutes at the start of every day makes me calm, focused and ready to achieve.

I used to think sleep, quiet time and mediation were dead time. But as I've grown wiser I've come to realise they are pre-requisites to high-performance living.

Complain less, react less impulsively – do more!

KEEP A JOURNAL

Writing a journal is one of the simplest ways to improve wellbeing and happiness. It allows you to note down achievements, empty your brain of chatty thoughts and see things from a distance. I also use it for noting down random ideas and managing projects.

The key with any good journal is consistency. Every morning I have a full brain splurge – Whatever I'm thinking I empty onto the page, discuss it with myself and come to a conclusion.

Key elements include:

- 3 things I've learned in the past 24 hours about life, business, etc.
- 5 things I'm grateful for today.
- 3 big challenges I need to face today.

*I am fairly strict with the numbers to ensure qualitative writing.

The primary purpose of this journal is to teach me more about myself.

This leads me to the next point.

SPEND A MOMENT EVERY DAY THINKING OF SOMEONE TO THANK.

I always try and start my day by thinking of someone to thank. Gratitude and inner peace go hand-in-hand. Although I may have diabetes, I'm grateful for the gift of life, which always makes me feel at peace. You probably have many people in your life to be grateful for: friends, family, people from the past, mentors, teachers, as well as countless others. You may even want to thank a higher power for the gift of life itself, or for the beauty of nature.

When you're thinking of someone to thank, focus your attention on gratitude. Do this ideally first thing in the morning.

Starting the day with a sense of gratitude is a great way to distract you from slipping into various forms of negativity. As part of your journal, write down five things you're grateful for and shift your focus to all the good in your life. As you begin to jot things down, you'll find various people and circumstances will keep popping into your head. You'll surprise yourself.

If you wake up in the morning with gratitude on your mind, it's pretty difficult, in fact almost impossible, to feel anything but peace. You can then get the most out of your day and bring an incredibly positive attitude into the gym.

GET OUTSIDE MORE

Where do you spend most of your day?

For most people, it's indoors unless they're walking to the car or taking the bins out.

Few have the privilege of being outdoors regularly. Dog owners will tell you how rejuvenating being outdoors can be, especially when they go for walks at the end of a busy day or the weekend.

Just think about how many times you've been awestruck by nature, whether it's gazing in awe at a mountainous landscape, a beautiful lake or admiring the deep blue ocean and cliffs of your nearest coast. There is a lot to be said for being outdoors and experiencing nature's real beauty. Get distance and space to think; we spend too much of our lives trapped indoors.

Make a habit of getting outdoors at least once a day and, if possible, going to a local place of outstanding beauty once a month or so, weather permitting of course. Mind you, the sound, smell and look of rain hitting the trees is always better than an annoying email notification or alarm clock.

Another benefit to being outdoors is its ability to increase vitamin D production, a fat-soluble vitamin that plays a crucial role in both health and wellbeing and training performance.

The Best Way To End A Busy Day (and this chapter)

Pause and reflect.

You'll find a wealth of opportunity lies ahead, most of your paranoia is self-imposed (and usually somewhat laughable) and your biggest failing is inconsistency.

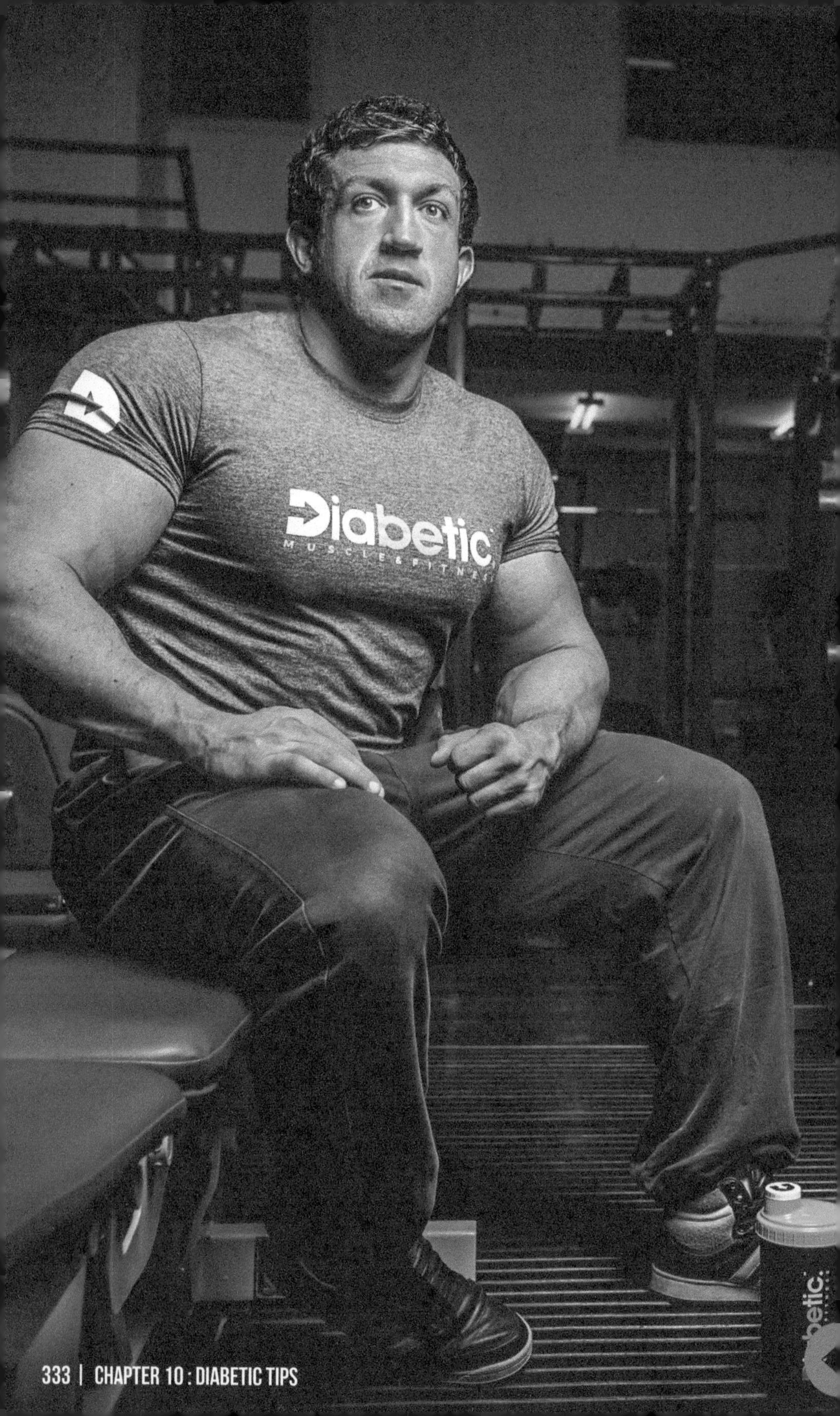
Diabetic

50 TIPS FOR PEOPLE LIVING WITH DIABETES

I've rustled together a list of 50 tips that have proven incredibly valuable in helping me manage and overcome diabetes. These tips cover a range of topics, form mind-set, diet, and training right through to living life as a diabetic.

TIP 1

Buy a set of high quality digital scales for weighing food. They are highly effective for counting calories, carbs and all the other macros. Ensure the scales have a tare function so you can weigh food accurately in Tupperware or other general kitchen crockery.

TIP 2

There's nothing worse than having a jammed needle on your insulin pen. Keep spare ones to hand and always check the needle is functioning first before injecting. I usually squirt out a few units of insulin to test.

TIP 3

Your blood sugar meter may fail to work in cold temperatures so do your best to keep it warm. If it does stop working, get some heat into it. I've found rubbing it against my leg or holding it against the hot air vent in the car to be the best and quickest ways of getting it functioning for a blood reading.

TIP 4

If in doubt about your blood sugar level, test.

TIP 5

A plastic bottle makes a great temporary sharps disposal.

TIP 6

Be mindful of wearing an insulin pump during exercise and sex. It might pull out.

TIP 7

If you ask for a diet soft drink, but think you've been served a non-diet version, don't jeopardise your control – check with the bar person and ask for a refill if needed. I always watch the bar staff like a hawk when they serve me.

TIP 8

I never inject in the same place. I rotate injection sites daily to avoid scar tissue build up. Be aware that where you inject may influence the rate at which insulin enters the blood. This is especially relevant when choosing whether to inject into muscle or body fat. Bear in mind a trained muscle group will allow insulin to enter into the blood stream more rapidly, which may increase the risk of hypoglycaemia.

TIP 9

Don't be afraid to say 'no' to a night out, a meal or a situation that you know will mess up your control.

TIP 10

Always carry a stash of fast-acting carbohydrates to treat a hypo. Key places to store them include: the car, a handbag or rucksack or your desk/locker at work.

TIP 11

When public speaking, always carry a liquid sports drink as a hypo prevention strategy. It works so much better than chewing sweets in front of an audience.

TIP 12

When travelling, take a copy of your prescription, just in case you run out of supplies. This saved my life in Mauritius when I dropped my insulin into the ocean on a fishing trip.

TIP 13

Don't confuse a hypo with anxiety. Test.

TIP 14

Look after your teeth and gums. A mouthful of rotting teeth and sore gums will jeopardize your nutrient intake and recovery from exercise.

TIP 15

Find a peer group. As hard as this may be, surrounding yourself with like minded people with diabetes who love health, building muscle and staying lean will do wonders for your motivation, knowledge and progress.

TIP 16

If you need a doctor's note for anything diabetes-related, don't be afraid to ask.

TIP 17

Don't let healthy people eat your hypo food, whether you store it in your house, car or workplace.

TIP 18

Sleep is paramount to your health and diabetic control. Respect it and do your best to get eight hours of quality shut eye every night. If you can't manage eight hours, try and have a nap at around midday.

TIP 19

Fluctuating blood sugars can affect your mood. Be mindful of this when you are around other people.

TIP 20

Never say 'f**k it!' when you go hyperglycaemic. If your sugars aren't in balance, fix them sooner rather than later.

TIP 21

Sugar-free sweets still contain calories.

TIP 30

Having a good A1c just because you go low all the time is not healthy and highlights the need for change.

TIP 31

Base your bolus dose of insulin for a set meal on how your blood glucose will sit three to four hours after the meal.

TIP 32

Injecting into muscle will bring your blood sugar down faster. There may be a time and place for this, especially if correcting a very high blood glucose reading.

TIP 33

Remember to change your lancets!

TIP 34

Reducing stress, increasing daily activity levels, adding muscle mass are valid ways to reduce basal insulin requirements.

TIP 35

Although slow to act, sugar alcohols can raise blood glucose levels. As a general rule, I count 50% of the sugar alcohol grams from total carbohydrate.

TIP 36

When drinking alcohol many people choose low calorie mixers like vodka and gin with diet soft drinks. Although low in calories, they can get you drunk quickly. When you're drunk, good food choice tends to go out the window along with common sense. Be mindful it's easy to mess up your diet and miscalculate medications the drunker you get.

TIP 37

Kinesiology tape or GrifGrips are useful for keeping technology like pumps and CGMs secure during extreme activities and training.

TIP 22

Always have your partner, wife or husband carry spare medication.

TIP 23

Dry your hands before testing. Too much water on your hands can dilute a blood sugar reading and give a false indication that you're going hypo.

TIP 24

Never leave insulin in the sun, especially on holiday.

TIP 25

Always clean your hands after using the gym and prior to testing post-exercise. The gym is an incredibly unhygienic environment. The last thing you need is an infected finger.

TIP 26

Never inject insulin or test your blood glucose whilst driving. It's not worth the risk.

TIP 27

Be careful wearing a powerlifting belt when wearing an insulin pump. It may snag during a lift and increase the risk of injury.

TIP 28

Sometimes on a night out bar staff mix up diet and non-diet soft drinks. When in doubt ask, and if you have your blood glucose monitor with you test a small sample. A diet soft drink will have no detectable glucose whereas a non-diet drink will be flagged as high.

TIP 29

Take note of why you experience hyperglycaemia. You might find the same circumstance reoccurring. This will help you predict and prevent future events.

TIP 38

Respect that what works for one person with diabetes may not work for you.

TIP 39

It is always best to fine tune your basal insulin dose before attempting to regulate mealtime insulin bolus.

TIP 40

Be mindful of other medications prescribed for diabetes-related health problems, including β Blockers, diuretics and statins, which can affect performance negatively.

TIP 41

Wear appropriate shoes and socks at all times, especially during exercise. Avoid exercising in shoes with an air bubble (unless you want a broken ankle and want to shear poundage off your major lifts). Also, check your feet regularly and keep them as clean as possible.

TIP 42

Be mindful of overtraining. It's easy to override fatigue and a dull system with willpower.

Symptoms include chronic tiredness, lethargy, lack of motivation to train, chronic stiffness and tightness in muscles/joints, poor performance and an element of depression.

This is typical after a show prep or photoshoot diet. Total recovery can take up to seven weeks, during which time proper nutrition, rest and down time from (full on) training are essential.

TIP 43

If you have been diagnosed with high blood pressure (hypertension), avoid near maximal aerobic work and heavy resistance training (especially forced reps and isometric holds, which often involve holding the breath).

TIP 44

Low blood sugars sometimes feel like high blood sugars, and vice versa. Take a few seconds to TEST.

TIP 45

If going for surgery, especially in a foreign country, tell the medical team you're diabetic and want your glucose closely monitored during surgery. They should frequently infuse insulin directly into your bloodstream to keep sugars in control.

TIP 46

Sitting or napping for prolonged periods of time can increase blood glucose due to decreased physical activity. Be prepared to dose insulin appropriately to keep glucose in check.

TIP 47

Your bolus insulin dose should be based on the following key factors:

1. Type of food.
2. Pre-meal blood glucose level.
3. Proximity of exercise or stressful events.
4. Proximity of substances that raise blood glucose.
5. Digestion issues.

TIP 48

If your blood glucose is high pre-exercise, consider taking half your usual correction dose and assess 25 minutes into training. A full correction dose might stimulate a hypo.

TIP 49

If you're a competitive physique athlete and need to wear artificial tan on competition day, injecting insulin can be difficult. Avoid injecting through tan, as this is extremely unhygienic. I apply a plaster to an unexposed area of my glutes then peel off and on, as and when needed to inject.

TIP 50

Avoid smoking or passive smoking at all costs. Be mindful nicotine patches can decrease blood glucose levels.

IN CLOSING

Having diabetes is a responsibility, almost like looking after a small child. Keep it in line, and life goes well, bar the odd curve ball outside of your control.

Neglect it, let it run rampant, and see what happens. Trouble.

One of the most important elements to building a healthier, better-looking body is accountability. I am a strong advocator of public accountability, especially on modern day tools like social media.

Holding yourself publically accountable gives you that much needed pressure to keep your diabetes, health and body in line.

I actively encourage you to blog, tweet, Facebook, YouTube and snapchat about your diabetes if you want to maximise your body composition and performance potential.

In addition to that, surrounding yourself with like-minded individuals is essential. Let's face it, those of us into fitness get a lot of negativity. From friends, colleagues and even family members.

Why are you eating like that? Why are you going to the gym again? Are You getting too big, too thin? Eat more! Don't be pushing yourself too hard! Let your hair down and come out with your friends (for once)!

Sound familiar? I've lived with it all my life! If you're new to fitness, don't worry – it's coming.

Living with diabetes and having a passion for fitness and building an incredibly strong, good looking body can be a lonely journey. It takes time, ruthless commitment and plenty of energy (physical and mental).

This is the exact reason why I created the online member's community. I want to build the world's strongest network of people living with diabetes who are highly passionate and committed to improving their mental and physical strength.

The community will primarily be geared towards those interested in strength training and bodybuilding (improving the look and feel of your body). However, the nutrition and diabetes related content will benefit anyone living with diabetes who takes part in other sports or who has a deep interest in staying healthy.

WHAT MAKES IT BETTER THAN ANY OTHER DIABETES SITE?

Let's face it, real world experience and knowledge on shredding fat and building muscle with diabetes is extremely rare.

As much as I value the work of healthcare professionals, they aren't the best source of advice when it comes to getting super strong and lean when living with diabetes.

Most of what you read on diabetes and fitness doesn't go into enough detail. Also, a good deal of what you read is written by people who don't know what it's like to suffer from diabetes.

There is a MASSIVE difference between theory (talking the talk) and practical application (walking the walk). Especially when you take into account emotions and the ever-changing dynamics of day-to-day life.

Having spoken to thousands of diabetic gym fanatics over the years. It kills me to see so many guys and girls working their asses off but ending up nowhere.

I'LL BE HONEST...

Not many are in shape.
Not many are strong.
Not many are fit.
Not many have good blood glucose control.

The majority of people living with diabetes don't get the results they deserve and end up feeling hopeless.

Something's not right.

I plan to fix that!

The members' site will be a no-holds barred information hub, focused on building a community of super healthy, ultra-strong diabetics who know how to train SMARTER THAN EVERYONE ELSE!

Currently, I'm in the midst of developing the content.

Here's what to expect:

- Regular article updates, inside tips, research reviews and other diabetes-related ramblings.

- Video modules covering everything you could want to know about diabetes muscle gain and fat loss.

- Monthly webinars [set topics - question & answer sessions].

- Workout plans.

- Muscle building and fat loss recipes.

- Rants.

- Interviews and case studies of incredible people living with diabetes.

- And much more.

I'll also be looking to develop a members' discussion board once the site matures.

The site only costs a few bucks a month, which is significantly less than the cost of a new training top, which will do very little other than get you through a few workouts.

WHEN IS IT BEING LAUNCHED?

The membership site is set to be launched on the 1st December 2016.

INVESTING IN YOURSELF, ESPECIALLY YOUR HEALTH AND WELLBEING WILL SAVE YOU A LOT OF TIME, MONEY AND HASSLE IN THE LONG RUN.

Ton find out more, visit **www.diabeticmuscleandfitness.com**

BEFORE I GO – ONE MORE THING!

Strive to surround yourself with like-minded people on the same mission as you!

REFERENCES

CHAPTER 3 – THE DIABETIC MONSTER

Defining Diabetes - Type 1

1. Babey M, Kopp P, Robertson GL. Familial forms of diabetes insipidus: clinical and molecular characteristics. Nat Rev Endocrinology. 2011 Jul 5. 7(12):701-14.

2. Ionescu-Tirgoviste, Constantin; Gagniuc, Paul A.; Gubceac, Elvira; Mardare, Liliana; Popescu, Irinel; Dima, Simona; Militaru, Manuella (2015-09-29). "A 3D map of the islet routes throughout the healthy human pancreas". Scientific Reports 5: 14634. doi:10.1038/srep14634. PMC 4586491. PMID 26417671.

3. BRS physiology 4th edition, page 255-256, Linda S. Constanzo, Lippincott publishing.

4. Sam AH, Sleeth ML, Thomas EL, Ismail NA, Mat Daud M, Chambers E, Shojaee-Moradie F, Umpleby M, Goldstone AP, Le Roux CW, Bech P, Busbridge M, Laurie R, Cuthbertson DJ, Buckley A, Ghatei MA, Bloom SR, Frost GS, Bell JD & Murphy KG (201) Circulating pancreatic polypeptide concentrations predict visceral and liver fat content. The Journal of Clinical Endocrinology and Metabolism 100(3): 1048-1052.

5. Suzuki K, Jayasena CN & Bloom SR (2011) The gut hormones in appetite regulation. Journal of Obesity 2011: 528401

6. British Liver Trust http://www.britishlivertrust.org.uk/liver-information/

7. Westman, Eric C et al. "The Effect of a Low-Carbohydrate, Ketogenic Diet versus a Low-Glycemic Index Diet on Glycemic Control in Type 2 Diabetes Mellitus." Nutrition & Metabolism 5 (2008): 36. PMC. Web. 15 June 2016.

8. Hemingway C, Freeman JM, Pillas DJ, Pyzik PL. The ketogenic diet: a 3- to 6-year follow-up of 150 children enrolled prospectively. Pediatrics. 2001 Oct;108(4):898-905.

9. Zhou, Weihua et al. "The Calorically Restricted Ketogenic Diet, an Effective Alternative Therapy for Malignant Brain Cancer." Nutrition & Metabolism 4 (2007): 5. PMC. Web. 15 June 2016.

10. Gasior, Maciej, Michael A. Rogawski, and Adam L. Hartman. "Neuroprotective and Disease-Modifying Effects of the Ketogenic Diet." Behavioral pharmacology 17.5-6 (2006): 431–439. Print.

11. Richard D. Feinman, Ph.D.a, , , Wendy K. Pogozelski, Ph.D.b, Arne Astrup, M.D.c, Richard K. Bernstein, M.D.d, Eugene J. Fine, M.S., M.D.e, Eric C. Westman, M.D., M.H.S.f, Anthony Accurso, M.D.g, Lynda Frassetto, M.D.h, Barbara A. Gower, Ph.D.i, Samy I. McFarlane, M.D.j, Jörgen Vesti Nielsen, M.D.k, Thure Krarup, M.D.l, Laura Saslow, Ph.D.m, Karl S. Roth, M.D.n, Mary C. Vernon, M.D.o, Jeff S. Volek, R.D., Ph.D.p, Gilbert B. Wilshire, M.D.q, Annika Dahlqvist, M.D.r, Ralf Sundberg, M.D., Ph.D.s, .Dietary carbohydrate restriction as the first approach in diabetes management: Critical review and evidence base. Nutrition Volume 31, Issue 1, January 2015, Pages 1–13

12. Bhatt, Harikrashna B., and Robert J. Smith. "Fatty Liver Disease in Diabetes Mellitus." Hepatobiliary Surgery and Nutrition 4.2 (2015): 101–108. PMC. Web. 16 June 2016.

13. Roy Taylor, MD, FRC. Type 2 Diabetes Etiology and reversibility. Diabetes Care. 2013 Apr; 36(4): 1047–1055.

14. American Diabetes Association: Diagnosis and classification of diabetes mellitus. Diabetes Care 36 (Suppl.1): S67-S74, 2013a

15. William I. Sivitz, Mark A. Yorek. Mitochondrial Dysfunction in Diabetes: From Molecular Mechanisms to Functional Significance and Therapeutic Opportunities. Antioxidant Redox Signal. 2010 February 15; 12(4): 537–577.

16. International Diabetes Federation - Diabetes Atlas (7th edition)

17. Outi Vaarala,Mark A. Atkinson, and Josef Neu. The "Perfect Storm" for Type 1 Diabetes The Complex Interplay Between Intestinal Microbiota, Gut Permeability, and Mucosal Immunity. Diabetes. 2008 Oct; 57(10): 2555–2562.

Type 2 Diabetes

18. Pihoker C, Lisa K. Gilliam LK, Hampe CS and Lernmark A. Autoantibodies in Diabetes. Diabetes,December 2005, vol. 54, Suppl 2, pages S52-S61

19. Abby G. Ershow. Environmental Influences on Development of Type 2 Diabetes and Obesity: Challenges in Personalising Prevention and Management. J Diabetes Sci Technol. 2009 July; 3(4): 727–734. Published online 2009 July.

20. Frank B. Hu. Globalisation of Diabetes. The role of diet, lifestyle, and genes. From the Departments of Nutrition and Epidemiology, Harvard School of Public Health, Boston, Massachusetts, and the Department of Medicine, Channing Laboratory, Brigham and Women's Hospital and Harvard Medical School, Boston, Massachusetts. Diabetes Care June 2011 vol. 34no. 6 1249-1257

21. Neil J. Snowling, MSC1 and Will G. Hopkins, PHD2.Effects of Different Modes of Exercise Training on Glucose Control and Risk Factors for Complications in Type 2 Diabetic Patients A meta-analysi. Diabetes Care November 2006 vol. 29 no. 11 2518-2527

22. Diabetes Prevention Program. http://www.niddk.nih.gov/about-niddk/research-areas/diabetes/diabetes-prevention-program-dpp/Documents/DPP_508.pdf.

23. Cauza E,Hanusch-Enserer U, Strasser B, Ludvik B, Metz-Schimmerl S, Pacini G, Wagner O, Georg P, Prager R, Kostner K, Dunky A, Haber P: The relative benefits of endurance and strength training on the metabolic factors and muscle function of people with type 2 diabetes mellitus. Arch Phys Med Rehabil2005; 86: 1527– 1533

24. Wycherley TP1, Noakes M, Clifton PM, Cleanthous X, Keogh JB, Brinkworth GD. A high-protein diet with resistance exercise training improves weight loss and body composition in overweight and obese patients with type 2 diabetes. Diabetes Care. 2010 May;33(5):969-76. doi: 10.2337/dc09-1974. Epub 2010 Feb 11.

25. Lori J. Tuttle, corresponding author David R. Sinacore, W. Todd Cade, Michael J. Mueller.Lower Physical Activity Is Associated With Higher Intermuscular Adipose Tissue in People With Type 2 Diabetes and Peripheral Neuropathy. Phys Therapy. 2011 Jun; 91(6): 923–930.

26. Errol B. Marliss1 and Mladen Vranic2.Intense Exercise Has Unique Effects on Both Insulin Release and Its Roles in Glucoregulation Implications for Diabetes. Diabetes February 2002 vol. 51 no. supplement 1 S271-S283

27. Segal KR, Edano A, Abalos A, Albu J, Blando L, Tomas MB, Pi-Sunyer FX: Effect of exercise training on insulin sensitivity and glucose metabolism in lean, obese, and diabetic men. J Appl Physiol 71:2402–2411, 1991

28. Dunstan DW, Daly RM, Owen N, Jolley D, De Courten M, Shaw J, Zimmet P: High-intensity resistance training improves glycemic control in older patients with type 2 diabetes. Diabetes Care25 :1729 –1736,2002.

29. Van der Heijden, Gert-Jan et al. "Strength Exercise Improves Muscle Mass and Hepatic Insulin Sensitivity in Obese Youth." Medicine and science in sports and exercise 42.11 (2010): 1973–1980. PMC. Web. 1 Apr. 2016.

Diabetes - A Global Issue

16. International Diabetes Federation - Diabetes Atlas (7th edition) 2015

30. Bellamy L, Casas J-P, Hingorani AD et al. Type 2 diabetes mellitus after gestational diabetes: a systematic review and meta-analysis. Lancet 2009; 373:1773–1779.

31. Diabetes.Org - Cost of Diabetes - http://www.diabetes.org/advocacy/news-events/cost-of-diabetes.html

32. About Diabetes: Epidemiology of diabetes in Mediterranean Regional overviews A global perspective http://www.mgsd.org/informations-2/about-diabetes/

33. Diabetes.Org - Cost of Diabetes - https://www.diabetes.org.uk/About_us/News/Number-of-people-diagnosed-with-diabetes-reaches-32-million/

Diabetes Diagnostics: Key Measures

34. WHO and International Diabetes Federation (IDF) , 2005, Definition and diagnosis of diabetes mellitus and intermediate hyperglycemia

35. Enzo Bonora, MD, PHD and Jaakko Tuomilehto, MD, MA, PHD2. The Pros and Cons of Diagnosing Diabetes With A1C. Diabetes Care May 2011 vol. 34 no. Supplement 2 S184-S190

36. NICE guidelines [NG17] Type 1 diabetes in adults: diagnosis and management Published date: August 2015 http://www.nice.org.uk/guidance/ng17/chapter/1-Recommendations#blood-glucose-management-2

37. Association of glycaemia with macrovascular and microvascular complications of Type 2 diabetes: prospective observational study. British Medical Journal 2000; 321: 405-412.

38. NICE https://www.nice.org.uk/news/article/new-thresholds-for-diagnosis-of-diabetes-in-pregnancy

Other forms of Insulin resistance

39. Gunnar Stenström, Anders Gottsäter, Ekaterine Bakhtadze, Bo Berger and Göran Sundkvist. Latent Autoimmune Diabetes in Adults Definition, Prevalence, β-Cell Function, and Treatment. Diabetes December 2005 vol. 54 no. suppl 2 S68-S72

40. American Diabetes Association. Gestational Diabetes Mellitus. Diabetes Care January 2003 vol. 26 no. suppl 1 s103-s105

41. Cleary MA, Green A. Developmental delay: when to suspect and how to investigate for an inborn error of metabolism Published: 2005-11-1. Arch Dis Child 2005;90:1128-1132 doi:10.1136/adc.2005.072025

42. Dunaif A, Givens JR, Haseltine F, Merriam GR (eds) 1992 The Polycystic Ovary Syndrome. Blackwell Scientific, Cambridge, MA

43. Franks S 1995 Polycystic ovary syndrome. N Engl J Med 333;853–861

44. "Polycystic Ovary Syndrome (PCOS): Condition Information". http://www.nichd.nih.gov/. 2013-05-23.

45. Insulin Resistance and the Polycystic Ovary Syndrome: Mechanism and Implications for Pathogenesis. Andrea Dunaif. Endocrine Reviews 1997 18:6, 774-800

46. Insulin Resistance and the Polycystic Ovary Syndrome: Mechanism and Implications for Pathogenesis. Andrea Dunaif Endocrine Reviews 1997 18:6, 774-800

CHAPTER 5 - A CLOSER LOOK AT DIABETES MEDICATION

1. Richter B, Neises G. 'Human' insulin versus animal insulin in people with diabetes mellitus. Cochrane Database of Systematic Reviews 2005, Issue 1. Art. No.: CD003816. DOI: 10.1002/14651858.CD003816.pub2

2. Siebenhofer A, Plank J, Berghold A, Jeitler K, Horvath K, Narath M, Gfrerer R, Pieber TR. Short acting insulin analogues versus regular human insulin in patients with diabetes mellitus. Cochrane Database of Systematic Reviews 2006, Issue 2. Art. No.: CD003287. DOI: 10.1002/14651858.CD003287.pub4

3. 18th Expert Committee on the Selection and Use of Essential Medicines (http://www.who.int/selection_medicines/committees/expert/18/applications/Insulin_review.pdf

4. Insulin Administration. American Diabetes Association. Diabetes Care 2002 Jan; 25(suppl 1): s112-s115.

5. Jicheng Yua, Yuqi Zhanga, Yanqi Yea, Rocco DiSantoa, Wujin Suna, Davis Ransona, Frances S. Liglera, John B. Busec, and Zhen Gu, Microneedle-array patches loaded with hypoxia-sensitive vesicles provide fast glucose-responsive insulin delivery. July 7, 2015 vol. 112 no. 27

6. Black C, Cummins E, Royle P, Philip S, Waugh N (2007). "The clinical effectiveness and cost-effectiveness of inhaled insulin in diabetes mellitus: a systematic review and economic evaluation". Health technology assessment (Winchester, England) 11 (33): 1–126.

7. Diabetes Prevention Program Research Group. Long-term safety, tolerability, and weight loss associated with metformin in the Diabetes Prevention Program Outcomes Study. Diabetes Care. 2012;35:731-737

8. Nieuwenhuis-Ruifrok AE, Kuchenbecker WK, Hoek A, Middleton P, Norman RJ. Insulin sensitizing drugs for weight loss in women of reproductive age who are overweight or obese: systematic review and meta-analysis. Hum Reprod Update. 2009;15:57-68.

9. Alan J. Garber, MD, PHD. Long-Acting Glucagon-Like Peptide 1 Receptor Agonists A review of their efficacy and tolerability. Diabetes Care May 2011 vol. 34 no.

10. Amori RE, Lau J, Pittas AGEfficacy and safety of incretin therapy in type 2 diabetes: systematic review and meta-analysis. JAMA 2007;298:194–206.

11. Goldstein BJ, Feinglos MN, Lunceford JK, Johnson J, Williams-Herman DE. Effect of initial combination therapy with sitagliptin, a dipeptidyl peptidase-4 inhibitor, and metformin on glycemic control in patients with type 2 diabetes. Diabetes Care 2007;30:1979–1987

12. Dror Dicker, MD. DPP-4 Inhibitors Impact on glycemic control and cardiovascular risk factors. Diabetes Care May 2011 vol. 34 no. Supplement 2 S276-S278

13. Avandia to Carry Stronger Heart Failure Warning - Forbes.com". Archived from the original on 2007-10-21. Retrieved 2007-08-15.

CHAPTER 6 – NUTRITION

Understanding Food Quantity

1. Manore M. Exercise and the Institute of Medicine recommendations for nutrition. Curr Sports Med Rep. 2005;4(4):193-8.

2. Gibson A, Seimon R, Lee C, Ayre J, Franklin J, Markovic T, et al. Do ketogenic diets really suppress appetite? A systematic review and meta-analysis. Obes Rev. 2015;16(1):64-76.

3. H. J. van Wyk R. E. Davis andJ. S. Davies. A critical review of low-carbohydrate diets in people with Type 2 diabetes. Diabetic Medicine Volume 33, Issue 2, pages 148–157, February 2016

4. Ravussin E, Lillioja S, Anderson TE, Christin L, Bogardus C. Determinants of 24-hour energy expenditure in man. Methods and results using a respiratory chamber. The Journal of Clinical Investigation. 1986;78(6):1568–1578. doi:10.1172/JCI112749.

5. Illner K et al. Metabolically active components of fat free mass and resting energy expenditure in non-obese adults. Am J Physiology Endocrinology Metabolsim. 2000 Feb;278(2):E308-15.

6. Shetty P. Energy requirements of adults. Public Health Nutr. 2005;8(7A):994–1009.

7. Buchholz AC, Schoeller DA. Is a calorie a calorie? American Journal of Clinical Nutrition. 2004;79(5):899S–906S.

8. Levine JA, Schleusner SJ, Jensen MD. Energy expenditure of non-exercise activity. Am J Clin Nutr. 2000;72(6):1451–1454

9. Donahoo WT , Levine JA, Melanson EL. Variability in energy expenditure and its components. Curr Opin Clin Nutr Metab Care. 2004 Nov;7(6):599-605.

Understanding Food Quality

10. Stotland S. Moderation: an alternative to restraint as a mode of weight self-regulation. Eat Behav. 2012 Dec;13(4):406-9.

11. Stewart TM, Williamson DA, White MA. Rigid vs. flexible dieting: association with eating disorder symptoms in non-obese women. Appetite. 2002 Feb;38(1):39-44.

Carbs

12. SACN_Carbohydrates_and_Health.pdf.
https://www.gov.uk/government/uploads/system/uploads/attachment_data/file/4
45503/SACN_Carbohydrates_and_Health.pdf 11.21

13. Nicholas Arpaia, Clarissa Campbell, Xiying Fan, Stanislav Dikiy, Joris van der
Veeken, Paul deRoos, Hui Liu, Justin R. Cross, Klaus Pfeffer, Paul J. Coffer &
Alexander Y. Rudensky. Metabolites produced by commensal bacteria promote
peripheral regulatory T-cell generation. Nature 504, 451–455 (19 December 2013)

14. Aurélien Trompette Eva S Gollwitzer Koshika Yadava Anke K Sichelstiel
Norbert Sprenger Catherine Ngom-Bru Carine Blanchard Tobias Junt Laurent P
Nicod Nicola L Harris Benjamin J Marsland. Gut microbiota metabolism of
dietary fiber influences allergic airway disease and hematopoiesis. Nature
Medicine 20, 159–166 (2014)

15. Cani PD, Neyrinck AM, Fava F, Knauf C, Burcelin RG, Tuohy KM, Gibson GR,
Delzenne NM.. Selective increases of bifidobacteria in gut microflora improve
high-fat-diet-induced diabetes in mice through a mechanism associated with
endotoxaemia. Diabetologia. 2007 Nov;50(11):2374-83. Epub 2007 Sep 6.

16. George A Bray. How bad is fructose?. Am J Clin Nutr October 2007 vol. 86 no.
4 895-896

17. Mei Chung et al. Fructose, high-fructose corn syrup, sucrose, and nonalcoholic
fatty liver disease or indexes of liver health: a systematic review and
meta-analysis. Am J Clin Nutr September 2014 vol. 100 no. 3 833-849

18. Dietary carbohydrate restriction as the first approach in diabetes
management: Critical review and evidence base. Feinman, Richard D. et al..
Nutrition , Volume 31 , Issue 1 , 1 – 13

19. Accurso A, Bernstein RK, Dahlqvist A, Draznin B, Feinman RD, Fine EJ, et al.
Dietary carbohydrate restriction in type 2 diabetes mellitus and metabolic
syndrome: time for a critical appraisal. Nutr Metab (Lond) 2008;5:9.

20. Feinman RD. Fad diets in the treatment of diabetes. Curr Diab Rep
2011;11:128–35.

21. Volek JS, Fernandez ML, Feinman RD, Phinney SD. Dietary carbohydrate
restriction induces a unique metabolic state positively affecting athergenic
dyslipidemia, fatty acid partitioning, and metabolic syndrome. Prog Lipid Res
2008;47:307–18.

22. Westman EC, Yancy WS, Mavropoulos JC, Marquart M, McDuffie JR. The effect
of a low-carbohydrate, ketogenic diet versus a low-glycemic index diet on
glycemic control in type 2-diabetes mellitus. Nutr Metab (Lond) 2008;5:36.

23. American Diabetes Association. Nutrition recommendations and interventions for diabetes–2013. Diabetes Care 2013;36(Suppl 1):S12–32.

24. Atkins RC. Dr. Atkins' new diet revolution. New York: Avon Books; 2002.

25. Gannon MC, Hoover H, Nuttall FQ. Further decrease in glycated hemoglobin following ingestion of a LoBAG30 diet for 10 wk compared with 5 wk in ⬚people with untreated type 2 diabetes. Nutr Metab (Lond) 2010;7:64.

26. Gannon MC, Nuttall FQ. Control of blood glucose in type 2 diabetes without weight loss by modification of diet composition. Nutr Metab (Lond) ⬚2006;3:16. ⬚

27. Nuttall FQ, Schweim K, Hoover H, Gannon MC. Effect of the LoBAG30 diet on blood glucose control in people with type 2 diabetes. Br J Nutr 2008;99:511–9.

28. Al-Khalifa A, Mathew TC, Al-Zaid NS, Mathew E, Dashti H. Low carbohy- ⬚drate ketogenic diet prevents the induction of diabetes using streptozo- ⬚tocin in rats. Exp Toxicol Pathol 2011;63:663–9.

29. Dashti HM, Mathew TC, Khadada M, Al-Mousawi M, Talib H, Asfar SK, et al. Beneficial effects of ketogenic diet in obese diabetic subjects. Mol Cell Biochem 2007;302:249–56. ⬚

30. Nielsen JV, Gando C, Joensson E, Paulsson C. Low carbohydrate diet in type 1 diabetes, long-term improvement and adherence: a clinical audit. Dia- betol Metab Syndr 2012;4:23.

31. Saslow LR, Kim S, Daubenmier JJ, Moskowitz JT, Phinney SD, Goldman V, et al. A randomized pilot trial of a moderate carbohydrate diet compared with a very low carbohydrate diet in overweight or obese individuals with type 2 diabetes mellitus or prediabetes. PLoS One 2014;9:e91027.

32. Pagoto SL, Appelhans BM. A Call for an End to the Diet Debates. JAMA. 2013;310(7):687-688. doi:10.1001/jama.2013.8601.

33. United States Department of Agriculture - http://www.ers.usda.gov/data-products/sugar-and-sweeteners-yearbook-tables.aspx

34. Watt MJ, Krustrup P, Secher NH, Saltin B, Pedersen K, Febbraio MA. Glucose ingestion blunts hormone-sensitive lipase activity in contracting human skeletal muscle. Am J Physiology Endocrinology Metabolism 2004; 286: E144-E150.

35. Jenni S, Oetliker C, Alleman S et al. Fuel metabolism during exercise in euglycaemia and hyperglycaemia in patients with type 1 diabetes mellitus – a prospective single-blinded randomized crossover trial. Diabetologia 2008; 51: 1457-1465.

36. Magnuson BA, Burdock GA, Doull J, Kroes RM, Marsh GM, Pariza MW, Spencer PS, Waddell WJ, Walker R, Williams GM.. Aspartame: a safety evaluation based on current use levels, regulations, and toxicological and epidemiological studies. Crit Rev Toxicol. 2007;37(8):629-727.

37. Blackburn GL, Kanders BS, Lavin PT, Keller SD, Whatley J. The effect of aspartame as part of a multidisciplinary weight-control program on short- and long-term control of body weight. Am J Clin Nutr. 1997 Feb;65(2):409-18.

38. Examine.com http://examine.com/faq/is-diet-soda-bad-for-you/

39. Magnuson BA, Burdock GA, Doull J, Kroes RM, Marsh GM, Pariza MW, Spencer PS, Waddell WJ, Walker R, Williams GM.. Aspartame: a safety evaluation based on current use levels, regulations, and toxicological and epidemiological studies. Crit Rev Toxicol. 2007;37(8):629-727.

40. Kaplowitz GJ. An update on the dangers of soda pop. Dent Assist. 2011 Jul-Aug;80(4):14-6, 18-20, 22-3

Protein

1. Scientific Opinion on Dietary Reference Values for protein. EFSA Panel on Dietetic Products, Nutrition and Allergies (NDA)2. European Food Safety Authority (EFSA), Parma, Italy. EFSA Journal 2012;10(2):2557

2. The National Kidney Foundation: https://www.kidney.org/news/newsroom/factsheets/Diabetes-And-CKD

3. Daniel Landau, Ralph Rabkin, Nutritional Management of Renal Disease (Third Edition) 2013, Pages 197–207 Chapter 13 – Effect of Nutritional Status and Changes in Protein Intake on Renal Function.

4. UNITED STATES RENAL DATA SYSTEM. www.usrds.org

5. Martin, W., Armstrong, L., & Rodriguez, N. (2005). Dietary Protein intake and Renal Function. Nutrition & Metabolism, 2-25.

6. Heaney, R. & Recker, R. (1982). Effects of nitrogen, phosphorus, and caffeine on calcium balance in women. Journal of Laboratory and Clinical Medicine, 99,46-55.

7. Bonjour JP.Dietary protein: an essential nutrient for bone health.Send to: J Am Coll Nutr. 2005 Dec;24(6 Suppl)

8. Churchward-Venne TA, Burd NA, Mitchell CJ, et al. Supplementation of a suboptimal protein dose with leucine or essential amino acids: effects on myofibrillar protein synthesis at rest and following resistance exercise in men.The Journal of Physiology. 2012;590(Pt 11):2751-2765.

9. Scientific Opinion on Dietary Reference Values for protein. EFSA Panel on Dietetic Products, Nutrition and Allergies (NDA)2. European Food Safety Authority (EFSA), Parma, Italy. EFSA Journal 2012;10(2):2557

10. Institute of Medicine Food and Nutrition Board. Dietary Reference Intakes: Energy, Carbohydrates, Fiber, Fat, Fatty Acids, Cholesterol, Protein, and Amino Acids. Washington, DC: National Academies Press; 2002.

11. Forslund AH, El-Khoury AE, Olsson RM, Sjodin AM, Hambraeus L, Young VR: Effect of protein intake and physical activity on 24-h pattern and rate of macronutrient utilization. Am J Physiol. 1999, 276 (5 Pt 1): E964-76.

12. Meredith CN, Zackin MJ, Frontera WR, Evans WJ: Dietary protein requirements and body protein metabolism in endurance-trained men. J Appl Physiol. 1989, 66 (6): 2850-2856.

13. Phillips SM, Atkinson SA, Tarnopolsky MA, MacDougall JD: Gender differences in leucine kinetics and nitrogen balance in endurance athletes. J Appl Physiol. 1993, 75 (5): 2134-2141.

14. Lamont LS, Patel DG, Kalhan SC: Leucine kinetics in endurance-trained humans. J Appl Physiol. 1990, 69 (1): 1-6.

15. Friedman JE, Lemon PW: Effect of chronic endurance exercise on retention of dietary protein. Int J Sports Med. 1989, 10 (2): 118-123.

16. Tarnopolsky MA, Atkinson SA, MacDougall JD, Chesley A, Phillips S, Schwarcz HP: Evaluation of protein requirements for trained strength athletes. J Appl Physiol. 1992, 73 (5): 1986-1995.

17. Lemon PW, Tarnopolsky MA, MacDougall JD, Atkinson SA: Protein requirements and muscle mass/strength changes during intensive training in novice bodybuilders. J Appl Physiol. 1992, 73 (2): 767-775.

18. Westerterp-Plantenga MS: How are normal, high- or low-protein diets defined? Br J Nutr 2007, 97:217-218.

19. Antonio J et al. The effects of consuming a high protein diet (4.4 g/kg/d) on body composition in resistance-trained individuals. Journal of the International Society of Sports Nutrition201411:19 DOI: 10.1186/1550-2783-11-19 https://jissn.biomedcentral.com/articles/10.1186/1550-2783-11-19

20. Jose Antonio, Anya Ellerbroek, Tobin Silver, Steve Orris, Max Scheiner, Adriana Gonzalez and Corey A Peacock.A high protein diet (3.4 g/kg/d) combined with a heavy resistance training program improves body composition in healthy trained men and women – a follow-up investigation. Journal of the International Society of Sports Nutrition201512:39 DOI: 10.1186/s12970-015-0100-0

21. Examine.com – How Much Protein Do I Need Every day? https://examine.com/nutrition/how-much-protein-do-i-need-every-day/

22. International Society of Sports Nutrition position stand: protein and exercise. Journal of the International Society of Sports Nutrition 20074:8

23. Macnaughton et al. Physiological Reports Aug 2016, 4 (15) e12893

Fat

24. Pimpin L et al. Is Butter Back? A Systematic Review and Meta-Analysis of Butter Consumption and Risk of Cardiovascular Disease, Diabetes, and Total Mortality. PLoS One. 2016 Jun 29;11(6):e0158118.

25. Daniel Lieberman. The Story of the Human Body: Evolution, Health, and Disease

26. Mary G. Enig. Know Your Fats: The Complete Primer for Understanding the Nutrition of Fats, Oils and Cholesterol

27. The 2015-2020 Dietary Guidelines for Americans. https://health.gov/dietaryguidelines/2015/guidelines/executive-summary/#footnote-3

28. Steinberg D (2006). "An interpretive history of the cholesterol controversy, part IV: The 1984 coronary primary prevention trial ends it - almost". J Lipid Res 47(1): 1–14. doi:10.1194/jlr.R500014-JLR200.PMID 16227628.

29. Siri-Tarino PW, Sun Q, Hu FB, Krauss RM. Meta-analysis of prospective cohort studies evaluating the association of saturated fat with cardiovascular disease. Am J Clin Nutr 2010;91:535–46

30. Siri-Tarino PW, Sun Q, Hu FB, Krauss RM. Saturated fat, carbohydrate, and cardiovascular disease. American Journal of Clinical Nutrition 2010;91:502–9.

31. Weinberg SL. The diet-heart hypothesis: a critique. J Am Coll Cardiol 2004;43:731–3.

32. Ravnskov U, Rosch PJ, Sutter MC, Houston MC. Should we lower cholesterol as much as possible? Bmj 2006;332:1330–2.

33. Yancy WS Jr, Westman EC, French PA, Califf RM. Diets and clinical coronary events: The truth is out there. Circulation 2003;107:10–6.

34. Jakobsen MU et al. Intake of carbohydrates compared with intake of saturated fatty acids and risk of myocardial infarction: importance of the glycemic index. Am J Clin Nutr2010;91:1764–8.

35. Mozaffarian D, Micha R, Wallace S. Effects on coronary heart disease of increasing polyunsaturated fat in place of saturated fat: a systematic review and meta-analysis of randomized controlled trials. PLoS Med 2010;7:e1000252.

36. Hooper L, et al, Effects of chocolate, cocoa, and flavan-3-ols on cardiovascular health: a systematic review and meta-analysis of randomized trials. Am J Clin Nutr. 2012 Mar;95(3):740-51.

37. Albert, C.M., et al . Dietary a -linolenic acid intake and risk of sudden cardiac death and coronary heart disease. Circulation. 112: 3232-3238, 2005.

38. Brenna JT et al. alpha-Linolenic acid supplementation and conversion to n-3 long-chain polyunsaturated fatty acids in humans. Prostaglandins Leukot Essent Fatty Acids. 2009 Feb-Mar;80(2-3):85-91.

39. Shauna M Downs a, Anne Marie Thow a & Stephen R Leeder. The effectiveness of policies for reducing dietary trans fat: a systematic review of the evidence. Bulletin of the World Health Organization 2013;91:262-269H

40. From burden to "best buys": reducing the economic impact of non-communicable diseases in low- and middle-income countries. Geneva: World Economic Forum & World Health Organization; 2011.

41. Mozaffarian D, Stampfer MJ. Removing industrial trans fat from foods. BMJ2010; 340: c1826

42. Savage DB, Petersen KF, Shulman GI. Disordered lipid metabolism and the pathogenesis of insulin resistance. Physiol Rev 2007;87:507–520pmid:17429039

43. Delahanty LM, Nathan DM, Lachin JM, et al., Diabetes Control and Complications Trial/Epidemiology of Diabetes. Association of diet with glycated hemoglobin during intensive treatment of type 1 diabetes in the Diabetes Control and Complications Trial. Am J Clin Nutr 2009;89:518–524pmid:19106241

44. Ahern JA, Gatcomb PM, Held NA, Petit WA Jr, Tamborlane WV. Exaggerated hyperglycemia after a pizza meal in well-controlled diabetes. Diabetes Care 1993;16:578–580pmid:8462382

45. Howard A. Wolpert, MD, Astrid Atakov-Castillo, BA, Stephanie A. Smith, MPH and Garry M. Steil, PHD. Dietary Fat Acutely Increases Glucose Concentrations and Insulin Requirements in Patients With Type 1 Diabetes. Diabetes Care 2013 Apr; 36(4): 810-816.

Why Most Diet's Fail

46. Pagato SL, Appelhans BM. "A call for an end to the diet debates." JAMA 2013; 310: 687-688.

Supplements

47. Sandoval, W.M. and V.H. Heyward, Food selection patterns of bodybuilders. Int J Sport Nutr, 1991. 1(1): p. 61-8.

48. Sandoval, W.M., V.H. Heyward, and T.M. Lyons, Comparison of body composition, exercise and nutritional profiles of female and male body builders at competition. J Sports Med Phys Fitness, 1989. 29(1): p. 63-70.

49. Walberg-Rankin, J., C.E. Edmonds, and F.C. Gwazdauskas, Diet and weight changes of female bodybuilders before and after competition. Int J Sport Nutr, 1993. 3(1): p. 87-102.

50. Bazzarre, T.L., S.M. Kleiner, and M.D. Litchford, Nutrient intake, body fat, and lipid profiles of competitive male and female bodybuilders. Journal of the American College of Nutrition, 1990. 9(2): p. 136-42.

51. Kleiner, S.M., T.L. Bazzarre, and B.E. Ainsworth, Nutritional status of nationally ranked elite bodybuilders. International Journal of Sport Nutrition, 1994. 4(1): p. 54-69.

52. SACN vitamin D and health report - Gov.uk https://www.gov.uk/government/uploads/system/uploads/attachment_data/file/5 37616/SACN_Vitamin_D_and_Health_report.pdf

53. Urashima M, Segawa T, Okazaki M, Kurihara M, Wada Y, Ida H. Randomized trial of vitamin D supplementation to prevent seasonal influenza A in schoolchildren. Am J Clin Nutr. 2010 May;91(5):1255-60.

54. Mitri J, Dawson-Hughes B, Hu FB, Pittas AG. Effects of vitamin D and calcium supplementation on pancreatic β cell function, insulin sensitivity, and glycemia in adults at high risk of diabetes: the Calcium and Vitamin D for Diabetes Mellitus (CaDDM) randomized controlled trial. Am J Clin Nutr. 2011 Aug;94(2):486-94.

55. Harris SS, Pittas AG, Palermo NJ. A randomized, placebo-controlled trial of vitamin D supplementation to improve glycaemia in overweight and obese African Americans. Diabetes Obes Metab. 2012 Sep;14(9):789-94.

56. Pilz S, Frisch S, Koertke H, Kuhn J, Dreier J, Obermayer-Pietsch B, Wehr E, Zittermann A. Effect of vitamin D supplementation on testosterone levels in men. Horm Metab Res. 2011 Mar;43(3):223-5.

57. Bischoff-Ferrari HA, Dawson-Hughes B, Staehelin HB, Orav JE, Stuck AE, Theiler R, Wong JB, Egli A, Kiel DP, Henschkowski J. Fall prevention with supplemental and active forms of vitamin D: a meta-analysis of randomised controlled trials.BMJ. 2009 Oct 1;339:b3692.

58. Gorham ED, Garland CF, Garland FC, Grant WB, Mohr SB, Lipkin M, Newmark HL, Giovannucci E, Wei M, Holick MF..Optimal vitamin D status for colorectal cancer prevention: a quantitative meta analysis.Am J Prev Med. 2007 Mar;32(3):210-6.

59. Garland CF, Gorham ED, Mohr SB, Grant WB, Giovannucci EL, Lipkin M, Newmark H, Holick MF, Garland FC. Vitamin D and prevention of breast cancer: pooled analysis. J Steroid Biochem Mol Biol. 2007 Mar;103(3-5):708-11.

60. Wang L, Manson JE, Song Y, Sesso HD. Systematic review: Vitamin D and calcium supplementation in prevention of cardiovascular events. Ann Intern Med. 2010 Mar 2;152(5):315-23.

61. Khan H, Kunutsor S, Franco OH, Chowdhury R.. Vitamin D, type 2 diabetes and other metabolic outcomes: a systematic review and meta-analysis of prospective studies.Proc Nutr Soc. 2013 Feb;72(1):89-97.

62. Mohr SB, Garland CF, Gorham ED, Garland FC. The association between ultraviolet B irradiance, vitamin D status and incidence rates of type 1 diabetes in 51 regions worldwide. Diabetologia. 2008 Aug;51(8):1391-8.

63. Khan H, Kunutsor S, Franco OH, Chowdhury R.. Vitamin D, type 2 diabetes and other metabolic outcomes: a systematic review and meta-analysis of prospective studies.Proc Nutr Soc. 2013 Feb;72(1):89-97.

64. Examine.com The Supplement-Goals Reference Guide (Vitamin D)

65. Shiraki M1, Shiraki Y, Aoki C, Miura M. Vitamin K2 (menatetrenone) effectively prevents fractures and sustains lumbar bone mineral density in osteoporosis. J Bone Miner Res. 2000 Mar;15(3):515-21.

66. Ishizuka M, Kubota K, Shimoda M, Kita J, Kato M, Park KH, Shiraki T. Effect of menatetrenone, a vitamin k2 analog, on recurrence of hepatocellular carcinoma after surgical resection: a prospective randomized controlled trial. Anticancer Res. 2012 Dec;32(12):5415-20.

67. Sakamoto N, Nishiike T, Iguchi H, Sakamoto K.. Possible effects of one week vitamin K (menaquinone-4) tablets intake on glucose tolerance in healthy young male volunteers with different descarboxy prothrombin levels.Clin Nutr. 2000 Aug;19(4):259-63.

68. Hyung Jin Choi, MD, Juyoun Yu, BS, Hosanna Choi, BS, Jee Hyun An, MD, Sang Wan Kim, MD, PHD, Kyong Soo Park, MD, PHD, Hak C. Jang, MD, PHD, Seong Yeon Kim, MD, PHD and Chan Soo Shin, MD, PHD. Vitamin K2 Supplementation Improves Insulin Sensitivity via Osteocalcin Metabolism: A Placebo-Controlled Trial. Diabetes Care 2011 Sep; 34(9): e147-e147

69. Examine.com The Supplement-Goals Reference Guide (Vitamin K)

70. Paolisso G, Scheen A, D'Onofrio F, Lefebvre P: Magnesium and glucose homeostasis. Diabetologia 33:511–514, 1990

71. Nadler JL, Buchanan T, Natarajan R, Antonipillai I, Bergman R, Rude R: Magnesium deficiency produces insulin resistance and increased thromboxane synthesis. Hypertension 21:1024–1029, 1993

72. Rosolova H, Mayer O Jr, Reaven GM: Insulin-mediated glucose disposal is decreased in normal subjects with relatively low plasma magnesium concentrations. Metabolism 49:418–420, 2000

73. Resnick LM, Gupta RK, Gruenspan H, Alderman MH, Laragh JH: Hypertension and peripheral insulin resistance: possible mediating role of intracellular free magnesium. Am J Hypertens 3:373–379, 1990

74. Lopez-Ridaura R, Willett WC, Rimm EB, Liu S, Stampfer MJ, Manson JE, Hu FB: Magnesium intake and risk of type 2 diabetes in men and women. Diabetes Care 27:134–140, 2004

75. Kao WH, Folsom AR, Nieto FJ, Mo JP, Watson RL, Brancati FL: Serum and dietary magnesium and the risk for type 2 diabetes mellitus: the Atherosclerosis Risk in Communities Study. Arch Intern Med 159:2151, 1999

76. Held K, Antonijevic IA, Künzel H, Uhr M, Wetter TC, Golly IC, Steiger A, Murck H.Oral Mg(2+) supplementation reverses age-related neuroendocrine and sleep EEG changes in humans. Pharmacopsychiatry. 2002 Jul;35(4):135-43.

77. Kao WH, Folsom AR, Nieto FJ, Mo JP, Watson RL, Brancati FL: Serum and dietary magnesium and the risk for type 2 diabetes mellitus: the Atherosclerosis Risk in Communities Study. Arch Intern Med 159:2151, 1999

78. Yang CY, Chiu HF, Cheng MF, Tsai SS, Hung CF, Tseng YT. Magnesium in drinking water and the risk of death from diabetes mellitus.Magnes Res. 1999 Jun;12(2):131-7

79. The National Academy Press - http://www.nap.edu/read/5776/chapter/8#223

80. Examine Supplement Reference Guide (Magnesium)

81. Flint J et al. The role of the gut microbiota in nutrition and health. Nature Reviews Gastroenterology and Hepatology 9, 577-589 (October 2012)

82. Roberfroid M et al. Prebiotic effects: metabolic and health benefits. Br J Nutr. 2010 Aug;104 Suppl 2:S1-63.

83. Tarantino G. Gut microbiome, obesity-related comorbidities, and low-grade chronic inflammation. J Clin Endocrinol Metab. 2014 Jul;99(7):2343-6.

84. Foster JA. Gut-brain axis: how the microbiome influences anxiety and depression. Trends Neurosci. 2013 May;36(5):305-12.

85. Dinan TG, Cryan JF. Melancholic microbes: a link between gut microbiota and depression? Neurogastroenterol Motil. 2013 Sep;25(9):713-9.

86. Behall et al. Consumption of both resistant starch and beta-glucan improves postprandial plasma glucose and insulin in women. Diabetes Care. 2006 May;29(5):976-81.

87. Johnston K et al. Resistant starch improves insulin sensitivity in metabolic syndrome. Diabet Med. 2010 Apr;27(4):391-7.

88. Resistant starch: the effect on postprandial glycemia, hormonal response, and satiety. Am J Clin Nutr 1994 60: 4 544-51

89. Resistant starch: the effect on postprandial glycemia, hormonal response, and satiety. Am J Clin Nutr 1994 60: 4 544-51

90. Can M, Beşirbellioglu BA, Avci IY, Beker CM, Pahsa A. Prophylactic Saccharomyces boulardii in the prevention of antibiotic-associated diarrhea: a prospective study. Med Sci Monit. 2006 Apr;12(4) PI19-22. PMID: 16572062.

91. SZAJEWSKA. Meta-analysis: non-pathogenic yeast Saccharomyces boulardii in the prevention of antibiotic-associated diarrhoea - - 2005 - Alimentary Pharmacology & Therapeutics

92. Sazawal et al. Efficacy of probiotics in prevention of acute diarrhoea: a meta-analysis of masked, randomised, placebo-controlled trials. The Lancet Infectious Diseases Volume 6, Issue 6, June 2006, Pages 374–382

93. CZERUCKA. Review article: yeast as probiotics –Saccharomyces boulardii - 2007 - Alimentary Pharmacology & Therapeutics

94. Cremonini. Meta-analysis: the effect of probiotic administration on antibiotic-associated diarrhoea - 2002 - Alimentary Pharmacology & Therapeutics

95. Armuzzi - The effect of oral administration of Lactobacillus GG on antibiotic-associated gastrointestinal side-effects during Helicobacter pylori eradication therapy - 2001 - Alimentary Pharmacology & Therapeutics

96. D'Souza Aloysius L, Rajkumar Chakravarthi, CookeJonathan, Bulpitt Christopher J. Probiotics in prevention of antibiotic associated diarrhoea: meta-analysis BMJ 2002; 324 :1361

97. Raúl Ricardo Gamba, Carlos Andrés Caro, Olga Lucía Martínez, Ana Florencia Moretti, Leda Giannuzzi, Graciela Liliana De Antoni, Angela León Peláez, Antifungal effect of kefir fermented milk and shelf life improvement of corn arepas,International Journal of Food Microbiology, 2016, 235, 85

98. Liu JR, Wang SY, Lin YY, Lin CW. Antitumor activity of milk kefir and soy milk kefir in tumor-bearing mice. Nutr Cancer. 2002;44(2):183-7.

99. Hilimire, Matthew R. et al. Fermented foods, neuroticism, and social anxiety: An interaction model. Psychiatry Research , Volume 228 , Issue 2 , 203 – 208

100. Fatemeh Dabaghzadeh, et al. Ginger for prevention of antiretroviral-induced nausea and vomiting: a randomized clinical trial. Volume 13, Issue 7, 2014

101. Raghavendra Haniadka et al. A review of the gastroprotective effects of ginger (Zingiber officinale Roscoe).Food & Function Issue 6, 2013

102. Examine Supplement Reference Guide (berberine)

103. Frid AH et al. Effect of whey on blood glucose and insulin responses to composite breakfast and lunch meals in type 2 diabetic subjects.Am J Clin Nutr. 2005 Jul;82(1):69-75.

104. Examine.com
https://examine.com/nutrition/how-much-protein-do-i-need-every-day/

105. Examine.com
https://examine.com/nutrition/how-much-protein-do-i-need-every-day/

106. Groeneveld GJ, et al Few adverse effects of long-term creatine supplementation in a placebo-controlled trial . Int J Sports Med. (2005)

107. Greenwood M, et al Creatine supplementation during college football training does not increase the incidence of cramping or injury . Mol Cell Biochem. (2003)

108. Lopez RM, et al Does creatine supplementation hinder exercise heat tolerance or hydration status? A systematic review with meta-analyses . J Athl Train. (2009)

109. Greenwood M, et al Cramping and Injury Incidence in Collegiate Football Players Are Reduced by Creatine Supplementation . J Athl Train. (2003)

110. Shao A, Hathcock JN Risk assessment for creatine monohydrate . Regul Toxicol Pharmacol. (2006)

111. Bender A, et al Long-term creatine supplementation is safe in aged patients with Parkinson disease . Nutr Res. (2008)

112. Gualano B, de Salles Painelli V, Roschel H, Lugaresi R, Dorea E, Artioli GG, Lima FR, da Silva ME, Cunha MR, Seguro AC, Shimizu MH, Otaduy MC, Sapienza MT, da Costa Leite C, Bonfá E, Lancha Junior AH. Creatine supplementation does not impair kidney function in type 2 diabetic patients: a randomized, double-blind, placebo-controlled, clinical trial. Eur J Appl Physiol. 2011 May;111(5):749-56.

113. Slowinska-Lisowska M1, Zembron-Lacny A, Rynkiewicz M, Rynkiewicz T, Kopec W. Influence of l-carnosine on pro-antioxidant status in elite kayakers and canoeists. Acta Physiol Hung. 2014 Dec;101(4):461-70. doi: 10.1556/APhysiol.101.2014.008.

114. McFarland GA, Holliday R. Retardation of the senescence of cultured human diploid fibroblasts by carnosine. Exp Cell Res. 1994 Jun;212(2):167-75.

115. Lombardi C, Carubelli V, Lazzarini V, Vizzardi E, Bordonali T, Ciccarese C, Castrini AI, Dei Cas A, Nodari S, Metra M.. Effects of oral administration of orodispersible levo-carnosine on quality of life and exercise performance in patients with chronic heart failure.Nutrition. 2015 Jan;31(1):72-8.

116. Everaert I, Stegen S, Vanheel B, Taes Y, Derave W. Effect of beta-alanine and carnosine supplementation on muscle contractility in mice.Med Sci Sports Exerc. 2013 Jan;45(1):43-51

117. Robertson, D., Frolich, J.C., Carr, R.K., Watson, J.T., Hollifield, J.W., Shand, D.G. and J.A. Oates. 1978. Effects of caffeine on plasma renin activity, catecholamines and blood pressure. New England Journal of Medicine. 298(4):181-6.

118. Keijzers, G.B., De Galan, B.E., Tack, C.J. and Smits, P. 2002. Caffeine can decrease insulin sensitivity in humans. Diabetes Care. 25(2):364-9.

119. Geijlswijk IM, Mol RH, Egberts TC, Smits MG.. Evaluation of sleep, puberty and mental health in children with long-term melatonin treatment for chronic idiopathic childhood sleep onset insomnia.Psychopharmacology (Berl). 2011 Jul;216(1):111-20

120. Luthringer R, Muzet M, Zisapel N, Staner L. The effect of prolonged-release melatonin on sleep measures and psychomotor performance in elderly patients with insomnia.Int Clin Psychopharmacol. 2009 Sep;24(5):239-49

121. Schernhammer ES, Berrino F, Krogh V, Secreto G, Micheli A, Venturelli E, Grioni S, Sempos CT, Cavalleri A, Schünemann HJ, Strano S, Muti P. Urinary 6-Sulphatoxymelatonin levels and risk of breast cancer in premenopausal women: the ORDET cohort.. Cancer Epidemiol Biomarkers Prev. 2010 Mar;19(3):729-37

122. Examine Supplement Reference Guide (Melatonin)

123. Fernández-San-Martín MI, Masa-Font R, Palacios-Soler L, Sancho-Gómez P, Calbó-Caldentey C, Flores-Mateo G. Effectiveness of Valerian on insomnia: a meta-analysis of randomized placebo-controlled trials.Sleep Med. 2010 Jun;11(6):505-11

124. Examine Supplement Reference Guide (Valeriana+officinalis)

125. Jang, H.S., J.Y. Jung, I.S. Jang, K.H. Jang, S.H. Kim, J.H. Ha, K. Suk, and M.G. Lee (2012). L-theanine partially counteracts caffeine-induced sleep disturbances in rats. Pharmacol. Biochem. Behav. 101:217-221.

126. Haskell CF, et al The effects of L-theanine, caffeine and their combination on cognition and mood . Biol Psychol. (2008)

127. Jackson Williams, Jane Kellett, Paul Daniel Roach, Andrew McKune, Duane Mellor, Jackson Thomas and Nenad Naumovski.l-Theanine as a Functional Food Additive: Its Role in Disease Prevention and Health Promotion. Beverages 2016, 2(2),

128. Examine Supplement Reference Guide (Thianine)

129. Yorek MA. The role of oxidative stress in diabetic vascular and neural disease.Free Radic Res. 2003 May; 37(5):471-80

130. Yusuf S et al. Vitamin E supplementation and cardiovascular events in high-risk patients. The Heart Outcomes Prevention Evaluation Study Investigators.N Engl J Med. 2000 Jan 20; 342(3):154-60.

131. Ascorbic acid blunts oxidant stress due to menadione in endothelial cells. May JM, Qu ZC, Li X Arch Biochem Biophys. 2003 Mar 1; 411(1):136-44.

132. Standards of medical care in diabetes--2009. American Diabetes Association.Diabetes Care. 2009 Jan; 32 Suppl 1():S13-61.

133. Merry T et al. Do antioxidant supplements interfere with skeletal muscle adaptation to exercise training? J Physiol. 2015 Dec 7

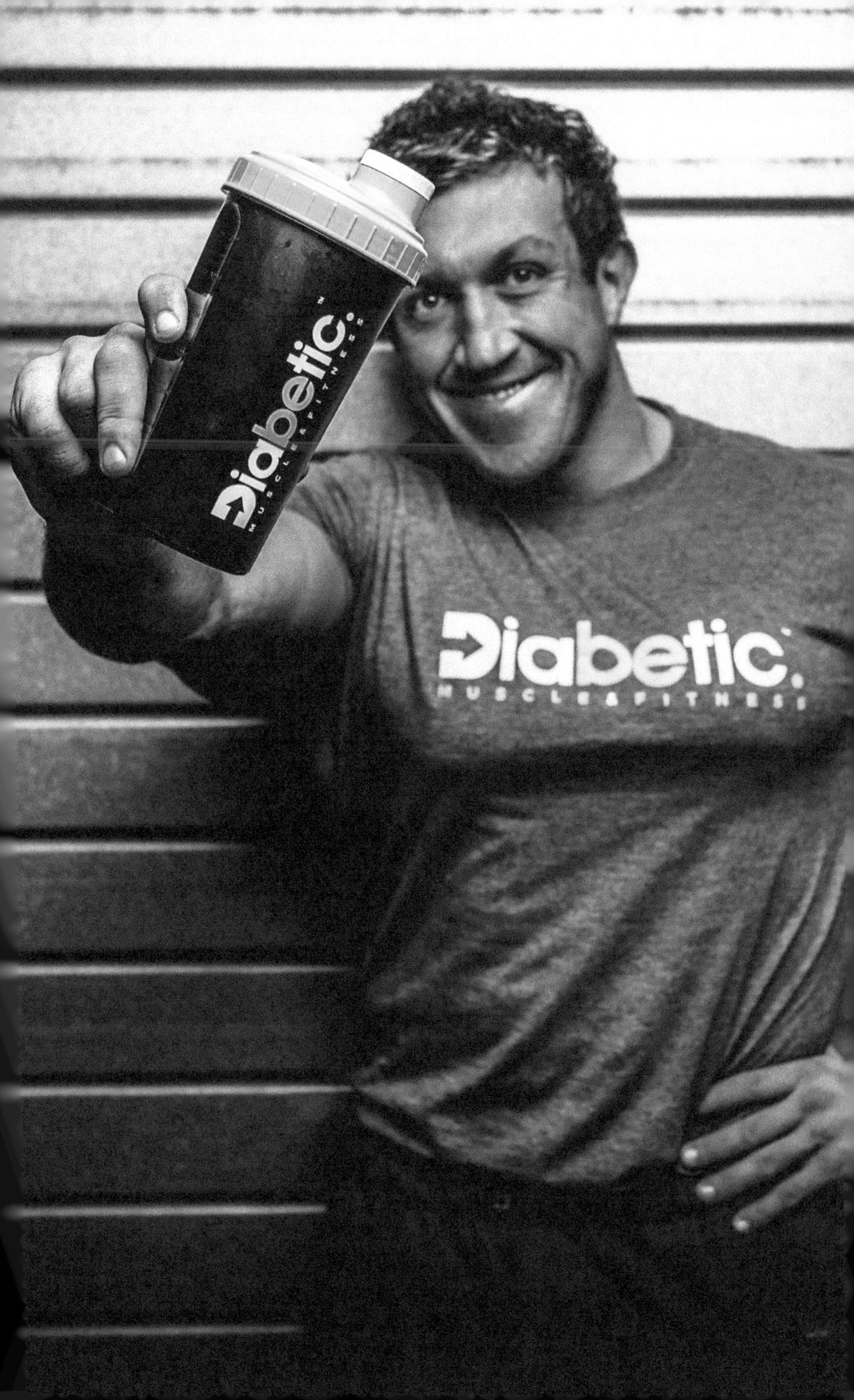
Diabetic
MUSCLE&FITNESS
Diabetic
MUSCLE&FITNESS

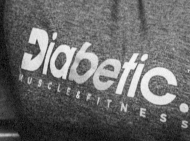

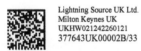

9 780995 762206